Foundations of Therapeutic Recreation

SECOND EDITION

TERRY LONG, PhD
TERRY ROBERTSON, PhD

Editors

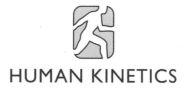

HUMAN KINETICS

Library of Congress Cataloging-in-Publication Data

Names: Long, Terry, 1971- editor. | Robertson, Terry, 1958- editor.
Title: Foundations of therapeutic recreation / Terry Long, PhD, Northwest
  Missouri State University, Terry Robertson, PhD, California State
  University, Long Beach, editors.
Description: Second edition. | Champaign, IL : Human Kinetics, [2020] |
  Revision of: Foundations of therapeutic recreation / Terry Robertson,
  Terry Long (eds.). 2008. | Includes bibliographical references and index.
Identifiers: LCCN 2018032321 (print) | LCCN 2018037853 (ebook) | ISBN
  9781492550440 (epub) | ISBN 9781492543688 (PDF) | ISBN 9781492543671
  (print)
Subjects: LCSH: Recreational therapy. | Recreational therapy--Vocational
  guidance. | People with disabilities--Rehabilitation.
Classification: LCC RM736.7 (ebook) | LCC RM736.7 .F66 2020 (print) | DDC
  615.8/5153--dc23
LC record available at https://lccn.loc.gov/2018032321

ISBN: 978-1-4925-4367-1 (print)

The web addresses cited in this text were current as of November 2018, unless otherwise noted.

Senior Acquisitions Editor: Amy N. Tocco; **Developmental Editor:** Jacqueline Eaton Blakley; **Managing Editor:** Anne E. Mrozek; **Copyeditors:** Erin Cler and Karla Walsh; **Indexer:** Andrea J. Hepner; **Permissions Manager:** Dalene Reeder; **Graphic Designer:** Dawn Sills; **Cover Designer:** Keri Evans; **Cover Design Associate:** Susan Rothermel Allen; **Photograph (cover):** Marc Dufresne/E+/Getty Images; **Photographs (interior):** © Human Kinetics, unless otherwise noted; **Photo Asset Manager:** Laura Fitch; **Photo Production Manager:** Jason Allen; **Senior Art Manager:** Kelly Hendren; **Illustrations:** © Human Kinetics, unless otherwise noted; **Printer:** Sheridan Books

Printed in the United States of America   10 9 8 7 6 5 4 3 2 1

The paper in this book is certified under a sustainable forestry program.

Human Kinetics
P.O. Box 5076
Champaign, IL 61825-5076
Website: www.HumanKinetics.com

In the United States, email info@hkusa.com or call 800-747-4457.
In Canada, email info@hkcanada.com.
In the United Kingdom/Europe, email hk@hkeurope.com.

For information about Human Kinetics' coverage in other areas of the world,
please visit our website: **www.HumanKinetics.com**   E6934

Contents

PART II Potential Areas of Practice   83

Preface

The purpose of this book is to introduce you to the profession of therapeutic recreation. Exploring therapeutic recreation from both a personal and a professional perspective is critical for students considering a career in therapeutic recreation. This text was designed to facilitate that exploration. You are encouraged to examine what therapeutic recreation is all about, but it is equally important that you consider what therapeutic recreation can provide to you and will require of you. Within this broad profession, there are many career-related possibilities to consider. Figuring out where you best fit as a person and a professional is a process you can start right now.

Therapeutic recreation is a relatively new occupation, but its roots are as old as civilization. These roots have grown into a diverse array of applications and an equally broad range of potential benefits. To adequately reflect this diversity, this book draws from the combined wisdom, experience, and technical expertise of 22 contributing authors and leaders within the therapeutic recreation profession. Numerous stories, case examples, professional profiles, and other learning tools will help you enjoy and personalize the exploration of this exciting and rewarding human services profession.

This introductory therapeutic recreation textbook has been written to meet the needs of those who are seeking fundamental knowledge and practice; therefore, emphasis is placed on foundational information that is essential to acquiring a general understanding of this profession. This information is a building block to developing the knowledge required of a competent professional and will be useful as you prepare to obtain your certification or licensure. In addition, we have attempted to challenge the status quo in a way that pushes some of the long-established boundaries of therapeutic recreation and encourages innovative programs and services. Through this process, the material will also challenge the expectations of many experienced therapeutic recreation professionals and educators. At the same time, we advocate for a consistent application of research-based information that will help to further establish evidence-based practices within therapeutic recreation.

We also assert that these purposeful therapeutic recreation interventions are built on theories of play, leisure, and recreation; therefore, associated interventions should be designed, engineered, and delivered to be enjoyable, beneficial, and rewarding. This perspective also supports the notion that positive functional outcomes can be successfully built and delivered from numerous strength-based approaches to intervention, particularly when evidence-based practice is implemented.

The book includes a clear expectation that you will work to develop the appropriate knowledge, skills, discernment, and disposition to be a successful professional. We challenge those entering the profession to think about their personal, civic, and related professional responsibilities; their ethics; and their level of professional commitment. Times and circumstances change at an increasingly faster pace, and if we continue to share our knowledge and experiences openly and without fear or territorial barriers, our profession will grow to meet these changes.

The second edition of this text does include some changes that are specifically designed to achieve the objectives just described. Past readers have helped us identify the most useful aspects of the first edition, and these elements have been preserved in this edition. However, the need to emphasize more contemporary models and philosophies for practice to develop awareness of evidence-based practice and present a more global perspective on therapeutic recreation is a theme that we have attempted to infuse into this edition. Of course, there are updates related to the many specific details that have changed in the past 10 years. For example, there are updates to information pertaining to diagnostic categories, appropriate terminology, innovative philosophies and modalities being used in the profession, legislative changes, and a variety of other details pertaining to the profession (e.g., professional associations, credentialing guidelines, standards of practice). Last, we have continued our effort to develop a reader-friendly text that can be easily digested by students who are just beginning their journey into the profession. Our desire has been to create an inviting text that provides accessible answers to the curious student.

The second edition is divided into two parts. Part I, Introduction to Therapeutic Recreation, has maintained its core content and includes updates relevant to the current state of the profession. Chapter 1, Considering Therapeutic Recreation as Your Profession, explores the process of choosing a profession that is right for you and presents basic information on what therapeutic recreation entails. Chapter 2, History of Therapeutic Recreation, has been streamlined and includes more contemporary content related to professional associations, credentialing trends, and other external issues affecting the profession at the national and global levels. Chapter 3, Professional Opportunities in Therapeutic Recreation, explores professional preparation and includes new material on the importance of becoming a culturally competent professional as well as a more detailed discussion on professional standards. As before, chapter 4, Person-First Philosophy in Therapeutic Recreation, reviews person-first philosophy but has been expanded to introduce the idea of focusing on strengths. Chapter 5, Models and Modalities of Practice, represents a significant improvement, with a more comprehensive presentation of practice models, including strengths-based models. A more comprehensive discussion of treatment modalities is presented in this chapter in an effort to capture more contemporary and culturally diverse perspectives on therapeutic recreation.

Part II, Potential Areas of Practice, begins with a comprehensive overview of the APIE (assessment, planning, implementation, and evaluation) process in chapter 6, The Therapeutic Recreation Process. Then, a series of chapters begins on specific areas of practice, including mental health (chapter 7), developmental disabilities (chapter 8), physical rehabilitation (chapter 9), youth development (chapter 10), and senior populations (chapter 11). Each of these chapters explores common needs and opportunities within the designated area, common modalities associated with achieving goals, and suggestions for ensuring best practices within the designated area.

Part II wraps up with two chapters that provide a global examination of the therapeutic recreation profession. Chapter 12, A Global Perspective of Therapeutic Recreation, attempts to present a truly global profile of how recreation and leisure are being purposefully used to achieve therapeutic outcomes. And finally, chapter 13, Envisioning the Future: Therapeutic Recreation as a Profession, explores the implications regarding public policy, technology innovations, service demand trends, social crisis and disaster relief, and the increasing importance of multicultural and multiethnic training and service delivery, all from a global perspective.

It should also be noted that significant improvements have been made to the supplemental resources available to instructors. For instructors, the slide presentations for each chapter have been significantly improved, and the test bank has been updated and expanded. The second edition instructor guide includes resources for each chapter, including an overview; an outline; updated learning objectives; sample classroom activities and assignments; and web links.

Stay involved, and keep sharing and caring! This profession is not for everyone, but it may be right for you. The challenge to you is to examine your own interests and motivations for a career in therapeutic recreation and then examine the expectations for practicing professionals working in recreation therapy. In the end, this information will help you decide for yourself whether this occupation—this profession—is right for you. The challenge for the educator is to continue discovering the opportunities and benefits of our profession and to share them with others. Enjoy!

Acknowledgments

It is with great pleasure and sincere hearts that we are allowed to publicly acknowledge and thank many of those who have encouraged, supported, and helped us in the creation of this book. First and foremost, we would like to thank our spouses (Shelly and Anne). Thank you for your patience, encouragement, and understanding during this process. We could not have done this without you and your support. We also hope that our time away on this project will be far surpassed by the time spent with you and our families in the near future.

We also want to recognize the efforts of past and current Human Kinetics team members. Thank you to Gayle Kassing, PhD, for her willingness to support us through the initial ideas and up to the completion of this text; to Jacqueline Blakley and Amy Tocco, for their patience and support on this second edition; and to numerous other HK personnel who helped in other ways. We are grateful for their professional commitment to this project.

Next, we would like to thank all the authors who have contributed their time, thought, and dedication to our profession. Each of the contributing authors is a recognized expert within the area that he or she wrote in, and we appreciate each one's willingness to be part of this project. We would also like to thank those who submitted personal and professional data to create Exemplary Professionals sidebars within each chapter. The included individuals represent only a small number of the many professionals willing to share, so we would also like to thank everyone who expressed interest and supplied support information, including pictures and case information.

We would be of poor character if we did not also acknowledge our colleagues at Northwest Missouri State University and California State University, Long Beach, who have supported our effort in one way or another. Similarly, we want to thank the thousands of students and professionals who have encouraged us over the years to write a book that was more "reader and faculty friendly" and yet maintained high expectations for those who will eventually go into practice. Specifically, we would like to thank the following folks for their professional support, teaching, mentoring, and leadership: Dr. David L. Holmes, Dr. Gerald O' Morrow, Dr. Marcia Carter, Dr. David Compton, Dr. Gary Ellis, Mrs. Sandy Negley, Dr. Norma Stumbo, Dr. David Austin, Dr. Jean Keller, Dr. Syd Post, and Dr. Steven Bell.

We also owe a great deal of appreciation to a number of professional associations and their elected officials and staffs: American Therapeutic Recreation Association; Missouri Association for Health, Physical Education, Recreation and Dance; Missouri Park and Recreation Association; National Recreation and Park Association; Nevada Recreation & Park Society; Nevada State Association for Health, Physical Education, Recreation and Dance; Utah Recreation & Parks Association; Utah Recreation Therapy Association; and National Council for Therapeutic Recreation Certification. Finally, a very special thank you to Dr. Gerald Hitzhusen for supporting our careers in countless ways, most notably as leader of the Midwest Therapeutic Recreation Symposium and as a mentor and friend.

Introduction to Therapeutic Recreation

Considering Therapeutic Recreation as Your Profession

Terry Robertson | Terry Long

Welcome to the challenging and rewarding profession known as therapeutic recreation. You have chosen an area of study that, for the right person, is full of opportunities. That's right—therapeutic recreation is not for everyone. But for those who find themselves drawn to helping others in a dynamic and engaging environment, this may be the perfect career. A lifetime of discovery, creativity, and problem solving awaits the future professional.

The editors and authors of this text believe that it can be useful to all students regardless of major. If you have not committed to an academic major, this book can provide you with information about a potential career choice. If you have committed to a major other than therapeutic recreation, developing a better understanding of disability-related issues can help you later in your career to better serve all members of society. Finally, if you are a therapeutic recreation major, this text can provide you with a core understanding of your chosen profession. We hope that by reading this book, you will develop confidence in and commitment to your choice of a therapeutic recreation major.

What Is Therapeutic Recreation?

Agreeing on a definition of therapeutic recreation has always been a challenge. As the profession has evolved, many perspectives on the nature of therapeutic recreation have been presented. The development of diverse perspectives and alternative viewpoints is similar to that seen in other professions. For example, psychologists have a common name, but their views on therapy and the mechanisms by which it functions are diverse. Likewise, the effectiveness of these therapy mechanisms varies depending on client needs, and no single form of therapy is the best approach for everyone. Fortunately, psychologists have managed to embrace what they have in common and still recognize the value of different approaches.

With this perspective in mind, an applied definition is presented here that focuses on basic, commonly accepted elements of therapeutic recreation. The purpose of the presented definition is not to replace formal definitional statements put forth by professional organizations such as the Canadian Therapeutic Recreation Association (CTRA), the American Therapeutic Recreation Association (ATRA), or Diversional & Recreation Therapy Australia (DRTA). Instead, the purpose is to provide students and other interested individuals with a practical explanation of the core ingredients of therapeutic recreation.

Therapeutic recreation (TR) is the purposeful use and enhancement of leisure as a way to maximize a person's overall health, well-being, or quality of life. To understand this definition, carefully consider the chosen terminology.

The first key word in this definition is *purposeful*. Therapeutic recreation specialists should always think about the purpose of whatever elements or strategies they include in their programs. What to include is important, of course, but so is how to include it. How a challenge, problem, concept, or skill is presented to a client will affect the outcomes of the experience. Purposeful planning should be used to determine the content of every therapeutic recreation session. The purpose is typically described through formally written goals and targeted **outcomes**. In therapeutic recreation, all clients or participants have goals that they are expected to achieve through their participation. If the therapeutic recreation specialist fails to intentionally plan and implement his or her work with clients, any observed benefits will depend largely on luck. Such an approach is irresponsible and unethical. In contrast, outcome-driven interventions allow the therapeutic recreation specialist to maximize client benefits.

The next two key words in the definition are *use* and *enhancement*. Specifically, this portion of the definition refers to using and enhancing one's leisure. Using leisure involves actively engaging leisure interests, choices, abilities, and behaviors to maintain or improve ability levels in leisure and other areas of functioning. Simply put, recreation is used as a therapy tool. For example, using leisure in therapeutic recreation could involve regular participation in memory and object recognition games to improve or maintain cognitive abilities.

Enhancement of leisure refers to the fact that therapeutic recreation specialists should always consider potential leisure-related needs and wants of the client, and services should ultimately lead to improvement in leisure functioning. Client goals often focus on rebuilding lost leisure skills, identifying new interests, learning new skills, or finding alternative ways to perform skills. Examples of leisure enhancement might include working with a person struggling with substance abuse to develop a drug-free leisure lifestyle or teaching a person with a spinal cord injury how to snow ski. Keep in mind that the use and the enhancement of leisure are interrelated; each element contributes

Therapeutic recreation professionals work under many job titles. Therapeutic recreation specialist, recreation therapist, recreational therapist, activity therapist, leisure therapist, diversional therapist, life enrichment coordinator, and inclusion specialist are some of the many common job titles that can appear on job advertisements or on your business card. The use of so many titles results from several factors, such as the role of the professional, the nation in which one is employed, government-mandated laws and regulations, or the philosophy and preferences of the agency. For the job seeker, this mix of names can sometimes be confusing, but keep in mind that each title reflects a potential employment opportunity for an aspiring therapeutic recreation professional.

Because there are so many title variations in therapeutic recreation, *therapeutic recreation specialist* is used across all chapters of this book unless the nature of the discussion requires otherwise. Therapeutic recreation specialist was chosen because the title is not tied to any particular setting or situation and it reflects a certain skill set that characterizes what it means to be part of the profession. Mastering and applying this skill set is what characterizes a therapeutic recreation professional regardless of title.

---

to the other at some level. Read the Client Portrait: Terrance for an example of this interrelatedness.

The most important word of all in this definition is *leisure*. It differentiates therapeutic recreation from other therapies and involves physical, cognitive, social, or emotional activity that is freely chosen and intrinsically motivated. Structured leisure activities are often referred to as recreation, but therapeutic recreation interventions can include any aspect of leisure. Organized sports, creative arts, meditation, outdoor activities, traveling, and bird-watching could all be part of a therapeutic recreation program. Even work activities may reflect leisure, depending on the perspective and experiences of the participant. Ultimately, developing such leisure abilities allows one to choose and participate in activities that are enjoyable and personally rewarding. Individuals who lack such leisure abilities will find it more difficult to live a healthy, happy life.

The use and enhancement of leisure can greatly improve health and well-being, which is the ultimate goal of therapeutic recreation. The extent to which the client achieves this goal depends largely on the care and thoughtfulness applied by the therapeutic recreation specialist in planning and implementing interventions that focus on the targeted outcomes (client and program goals).

Two criteria can be used to identify whether an intervention or activity can be considered therapeutic recreation. The first criterion is ensuring that outcomes are grounded in a leisure context. In many cases, the leisure context is inherent but not necessarily immediate because of the current therapy needs of the patient. For example, playing card games can be a useful therapeutic tool when working with stroke patients. Enhancing number recognition or the ability to grasp objects may be primary therapy goals when working with such patients, whereas learning to play the game would seem somewhat trivial until those basic skills improve. Still, leisure is embedded in the intervention and separates it from other forms of therapy. Even if playing games is not an immediate concern of the client, the leisure context of this activity may be of use when the client begins to focus on returning home and living a satisfying life. In addition, time spent playing games can provide much needed relief from the physical and psychological strains of therapy. At other times, the therapeutic recreation professional may be more direct in communicating the leisure context of therapy to the client. Later sessions with the same stroke patient might involve direct efforts to develop activity skills or discussion of opportunities for recreation participation through adapted sports organizations.

The second defining characteristic of therapeutic recreation is purposeful intervention. As already mentioned, the therapist must make a deliberate effort to bring about targeted therapy outcomes. Goals are established through use of client assessment, and therapeutic recreation interventions are built around achieving these goals. Progress is then monitored through periodic evaluation of the client.

Note that using outcome-driven interventions alone is not therapeutic recreation. All legitimate therapies establish and track the achievement of goals, and therapeutic recreation is just one of those therapies. Likewise, all leisure activities that have the potential for enhancing health or well-

Terrance is a 62-year-old man who had a left-brain stroke. As a result, he cannot lift his arm above his shoulder and can hold his arm at shoulder level for only a few seconds. He also has difficulty grasping objects, especially small items such as shirt buttons or shoestrings. A few weeks after his stroke, Terrance is still working to regain the skills required to do the basic things necessary to get by in life (activities of daily living).

Terrance works with a certified therapeutic recreation specialist (CTRS), a professional credential often required by employers of therapeutic recreation professionals (this credential is explained further in chapter 3). The CTRS meets with Terrance for about an hour each day to work on improving grasp, range of motion, and activity tolerance. The CTRS knows what activities to do with Terrance based on an intake assessment that the two completed when Terrance was admitted to the rehabilitation center. The CTRS then works with Terrance to develop goals for treatment. To address these goals, Terrance selects from a variety of activities suggested by the CTRS, all of which involve exercising the targeted functional skills. The activities could include choices such as checkers (grasping skills) or model construction (requiring more endurance) or challenges such as stacking blocks (requiring a progressively higher reach). Early on, simple leisure activities are chosen to accommodate Terrance's level of functioning, but as he masters each activity, more complex forms of leisure are both implemented as therapy and integrated into Terrance's daily life activities. As a result, both his immediate functional skills and long-term

potential for satisfying leisure are enhanced through well-planned, leisure-based intervention.

Leisure Context

The leisure context of Terrance's program can be seen in the nature of the activities that the CTRS provides. By encouraging the client to use these existing leisure interests and abilities, he is able to improve functional limitations associated with the stroke. Also important is the fact that the client is empowered to choose activities that are of interest to him. A core element in providing therapeutic recreation programs is that clients be given as much freedom and control as possible, which ultimately helps ensure that the program is grounded in leisure.

Purposeful Intervention

Because the CTRS identified client needs through an assessment, established goals related to assessment results, and developed activity choices in line with these goals, Terrance's therapeutic recreation program can be considered purposeful. A common error in this area is to choose activities based solely on the interest of the client or, even worse, on the interest of the CTRS. Although choice is important, all program elements should be in line with treatment goals. Remember that therapeutic recreation goals for Terrance may also include enhancing his leisure, even while he stays at the rehab center. As such, some of his program may be oriented around having fun, relaxing, and escaping the worries associated with his condition.

---

being are not necessarily therapeutic recreation. Many leisure activities are beneficial to a person but are not purposefully developed and delivered therapeutic interventions. Therapeutic recreation intervention exists only when leisure context and purposeful intervention are paired together.

A Diverse Profession

Therapeutic recreation has emerged from a dynamic and ever-evolving mix of perspectives, converging schools of thought, borrowed and original theories, and unique interventions and services. This diverse background offers potential for a large variety of service applications. Some have referred to therapeutic recreation as being eclectic in nature. Others have referred to it as

a **strengths-based approach**. Some suggest that therapeutic recreation is unique in that it involves use of recreation or leisure. Others say that it is a mix of philosophy, psychology, the arts, and physical therapy and occupational therapy techniques—all used by a trained professional to bring about functional change within another person or group of people.

Regardless of the perspective chosen, therapeutic recreation is a profession that has tremendous potential for growth and evolution. The diverse philosophical positions or perspectives within the profession provide numerous opportunities for flexible application and professional growth. This diversity tends to produce a well-rounded college graduate who is capable of working within, on the fringes of, or outside of therapeutic recreation. Likewise, therapeutic recreation training programs have traditionally been ideal for those seeking a bachelor's degree before moving into a graduate degree program. A therapeutic recreation degree has also helped professionals enter community-based recreation and administrative positions within a variety of fields. If you are searching for a degree that could prepare you for a wide variety of occupations or you are looking for a specific career, then therapeutic recreation may be right for you. Are you still interested?

Choosing a Profession

As a bright person capable of choosing from among many occupations, you should think about why you are interested in therapeutic recreation. Are you interested in helping others? Are you interested in physical activity or psychological processes? Do you or any members of your family have a disability? Are you deciding between this major and some other therapy-oriented degree such as occupational therapy, physical therapy, or nursing? Maybe you are interested in broader topics such as social justice, aging, or health and wellness, or maybe you simply know someone in this major or profession. You are the only one who can answer the why questions. If you have not done so, try to answer the question for yourself right now—why choose this profession?

Your interest and motivation in this course and profession will have an effect on what you study, how you study, and whether you will succeed in your academic performance. Your motives can also influence who you might study or work with as well as where you might eventually work and ultimately live. So do you know where or with whom you might want to work? Do you know how this course could benefit you regardless of your major? If you answered no or have other questions, ask the course instructor and your advisor for some individual attention.

If the answer to either question is yes, then we would simply ask that you keep yourself open to more possibilities as you go through this text and course. If you are unsure about how all of this information is relevant to you, then we would ask that you try to focus a bit and select a temporary answer to these questions to help you reflect on and understand concepts as you move through the book and explore this profession. Whether you answered yes or no, before you try to finalize your decisions, you should learn the basic **therapeutic recreation process**, understand some of the

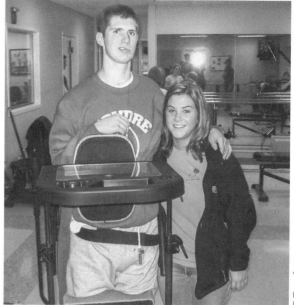

You may have already witnessed the positive influence of therapeutic recreation through the experiences of a family member.

basic techniques utilized during this process, and become familiar with what therapeutic recreation services have to offer clients who participate in this process (what benefits might come to clients from provision of this service). Later chapters will explore these topics in detail.

Finding a Personal Fit

Success in the therapeutic recreation profession requires commitment, forethought, and a willingness to engage others. The working professional generally has the ability to organize experiences, motivate others, be flexible, and work on several tasks simultaneously. The ability to communicate to diverse audiences (e.g., individuals, groups, and other professionals) in a variety of ways (e.g., oral, written, in person, electronically) and to be both understanding and assertive are also important characteristics. In plain words, therapeutic recreation is a people profession; a major job skill for a therapeutic recreation professional is to relate to people in an understanding and accepting way. Because creating effective interactions and experiences requires use of a systematic method, the successful professional must be competent at planning, organizing, solving problems, and managing several tasks and programs at once. To succeed in this profession, a person must be responsible, knowledgeable, and genuinely compassionate.

Employment Options

Therapeutic recreation specialists work in a variety of settings, and often those settings include a mix of clientele. Breaking down the profession based on client population reveals that about 37 percent work in mental health, 29 percent work in geriatrics, 20 percent work in physical medicine, and 14 percent work with individuals with developmental disabilities (National Council for Therapeutic Recreation Certification [NCTRC], 2015). The nature of therapeutic recreation services for each of these populations is addressed further in chapters 7 to 11, but this diversity is mentioned here to illustrate the options that are available to professionals. In addition, these categories are very general, and you will find that there are many specializations within each area.

Work-setting options for therapeutic recreation professionals are equally diverse and include hospitals, psychiatric facilities, long-term-care facilities, and community-based settings. It is also true that the boundaries between these settings are difficult if not impossible to define. The categories presented here can help you sort through what your future might entail, but keep in mind that more specialized settings exist both within these categories and in other areas.

Hospitals

Hospitals employ about 38 percent of the therapeutic recreation specialists who hold national certification (NCTRC, 2015), and the services provided within these hospitals include both psychiatric care and physical medicine. There are well over 5,000 hospitals in the United States, about 2,000 of which are located in rural settings (American Hospital Association [AHA], 2017). As you would guess, each hospital is unique, but there are some general types to consider here. Acute care hospitals provide short-term care to individuals with conditions that are more severe and require immediate care. The average stay in such a facility is 4.8 days, which limits the time the therapeutic recreation professional has to work with a client (National Center for Health Statistics, 2010). Services can include both mental and physical health programs. Therapeutic recreation staff may work across both units, or they may be assigned to either one or the other.

For physical medicine, acute care is often followed by either rehabilitation services or outpatient care. **Rehabilitation hospitals** can sometimes exist within an acute care facility, but they can also be freestanding hospitals in another location. The purpose of a rehabilitation hospital is to provide any necessary long-term treatment to the patient once the initial health threat has stabilized. Outpatient care provides services that require the client to stay at home and come to the hospital for periodic therapy or treatment sessions. For example, chemotherapy or physical therapy services are often provided in an outpatient manner, where the client comes to the hospital for periodic treatments. In therapeutic recreation, outpatient care is less common but can exist in different forms. For instance, clients may return to participate in adapted sports clinics or for an outpatient fitness and wellness program.

A large portion of hospital-based therapeutic recreation services are focused on psychiatric care. As with physical rehabilitation, psychiatric care can be provided through both inpatient and outpatient services. Acute care facilities often house mental health services, but there are approximately 400 nonfederal freestanding psychiatric hospitals in the United States as well (AHA, 2017).

In addition, there are 152 Veterans Administration Medical Centers in the United States, which provide military veterans with mental and physical health care services, including therapeutic recreation (U.S. Department of Veterans Affairs, 2016). Specialized hospitals for children are another niche that often are locations for therapeutic recreation services, such as the 22 Shriners Hospitals for Children located in the United States, Canada, and Mexico.

Geriatric Care

There is no doubt that the world's population is aging. Americans generally think of the baby boomer generation and all of its associated challenges as a problem for the United States, but aging is really a global issue. The total number of people who are 60 or older will double by 2050, and the number who reach 80 by 2050 will triple (United Nations, 2015). Worldwide, the senior population is taxing the health care system, and the need for quality and efficient services increases daily. The need for therapeutic recreation professionals within this realm is equally significant. The *Occupational Outlook Handbook*, published by the U.S. Department of Labor, indicates that therapeutic recreation professionals "who specialize in working with the elderly or who earn certification in geriatric therapy may have the best job prospects" within the field (Bureau of Labor Statistics, 2015).

In light of this projected growth, it is important to examine some of the settings where this growth may occur. It is useful to consider such settings on a continuum that varies based on the level of care provided. Any of the following settings can be a potential delivery point for therapeutic recreation services:

- **In-home services.** In-home services can vary widely but generally involve a health care professional coming to one's home to provide some type of assistive or medical service. Services can be divided into two categories: in-home care and home health care. The former typically involves assistance with activities of daily living, such as housekeeping, food preparation, and other nonmedical needs. Home health care involves assistance with personal care and medical needs, such as bathing, medication, and nursing care.

- **Adult day facilities.** Adult day facilities provide care during daytime hours. Such services allow for a loved one to be cared for while primary caregivers go to work or take respite. Those who attend these facilities may have physical limitations, need social support, or have cognitive impairments (e.g., dementia).

EXEMPLARY PROFESSIONAL

TRACEY CRAWFORD, CTRS, CPRP

Education: BS in Therapeutic Recreation, University of Iowa
Position: Executive Director
Organization: Northwest Special Recreation Association, Chicago, Illinois
Special Awards
- Presidential Award, National Therapeutic Recreation Society (2001)
- Meritorious Service Award, National Therapeutic Recreation Society (2004)
- Member of the Year Award, National Therapeutic Recreation Society (2004)
- IPRA Chairman's Award, Illinois Park and Recreation Association (2005, 2014)
- Rolling Meadows Chamber of Commerce 2017 Community Leader of the Year

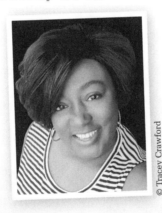
© Tracey Crawford

My Career

I was appointed executive director at Northwest Special Recreation Association (NWSRA) in late 2011. NWSRA partners closely with 17 park districts in the northwest suburbs of Chicago to provide and facilitate year-round recreation programs for children and adults at all levels of ability. Services include weekly recreation programs, clubs, leisure education, special events, day camps, trips, collaborative programming—including the PURSUIT adult day programs, the STAR Academy after-school programs, and the Snoezelen sensory room, where we provide sensory therapy.

My pathway to this position included a variety of opportunities, beginning with nine years as the inclusion coordinator/therapeutic recreation specialist and assistant director at Fox Valley Special Recreation Association (FVSRA) in Aurora, Illinois. I also spent two and a half years as the manager of inclusion services, nine years as the superintendent of recreation, and one and a half years as the superintendent of development and interim director at Northern Suburban Special Recreation Association (NSSRA).

Throughout my career, I have taken part in a variety of professional service roles. I have served on the board of directors for the National Therapeutic Recreation Society and the American Therapeutic Recreation Society. I have also served local and state organizations such as the Special Leisure Services Foundation and the Illinois Park and Recreation Association. These service opportunities have been a critical part of my professional development and networking.

My Advice To You

I feel that the field of therapeutic recreation is one of the most rewarding professions. It is a career and not a job. I encourage those new to the field to experience different avenues and gain maximum exposure. This exposure is what will help students make those future career choices. I also encourage students to seek mentors.

- *Assisted living facilities.* Assisted living is residential care that provides meal services, assistance with medication, and minimal assistance with self-care skills that enables a person to still live as independently as possible. One common requirement for living in such a facility is the ability to perform activities of daily living with assistance from no more than one person. Once clients require two helpers to transfer, shower, or use the restroom, they may need to move to a long-term-care facility.
- *Nursing home facilities.* Nursing home facilities are licensed by the state to provide nursing care, room and board, and convalescent care for seniors on a 24-hour basis. Residents often have physical, emotional, or cognitive impairments and require a significant level of care that exceeds what may be available in assisted living.
- *Dementia care facilities.* Dementia care facilities are designed to provide residential care and support for individuals who are experiencing the challenges that come with memory loss and disorientation. Dementia care can be housed within assisted living or nursing home facilities but may also be a stand-alone facility.

Community-Based Services

Community-based therapeutic recreation programs are a major aspect of our profession. Not only are there programs that are solely housed within community settings, such as park and recreation agencies or schools, but there are also programs that extend from hospitals or residential settings into the community. In fact the clinical versus community distinction is one that is misleading and potentially counterproductive. Acknowledging this limitation, it is useful to consider community-based therapeutic recreation programs when exploring career options. Again, there are many therapeutic recreation programs that exist within municipal park and recreation programs. What distinguishes these programs from standard recreation participation programs is the key factor mentioned earlier: purposeful intervention.

Therapeutic recreation specialists are well equipped to address the needs of general recreation program participants who just happen to have disabilities, and they often discover that careers focused on helping these individuals can

be very rewarding; however, such programs are not therapeutic recreation unless they include purposeful intervention. Community-based therapeutic recreation programs will always involve some form of client assessment that guides program planning in a way that targets desired outcomes. This plan can come in the form of an individualized education program in the schools, an inclusion plan at summer camp or a neighborhood recreation center, or even a substance abuse treatment plan that is delivered through the local homeless shelter. In fact, nonprofit agencies are a significant part of the therapeutic recreation world, including organizations such as the National Ability Center in Park City, Utah (www.discovernac.org); the National Sports Center for the Disabled in Denver, Colorado (www.nscd.org); and Community Living Opportunities Midnight Farm in Lawrence, Kansas (www.midnight-farm.org). Take a look at these websites and explore what the programs entail.

Because "community" is a less-than-ideal descriptor for clearly defining a place of employment, it is difficult to quantify how many people work in this realm. However, a recent survey of nationally certified therapeutic recreation specialists (i.e., CTRSs) found that 7.3 percent of respondents reported their primary service setting as an adaptive recreation program, 4.3 percent as a parks and recreation organization, 3.5 percent as a day care, 2.2 percent as a disability support organization, and 1.8 percent as a school (NCTRC, 2015). When asked to report "primary level of service," 15.5 percent reported "community." Certainly, there are many professional opportunities that involve working outside of residential or hospital settings. Be sure to take the time to explore the many types of agencies that provide therapeutic recreation services and keep an open mind when it comes to possibilities.

Occupational Profiles

You will likely find it helpful to look at some examples of where professionals work and what they do as a part of their professional duties. Here are a few brief descriptions to further clarify what possibilities are available in the profession.

- Isabelle works at the Veterans Administration (VA) in central California with veterans who have disabilities and are homeless. She works with clients to solve or resolve issues such as homelessness, poverty, starvation, substance abuse, violence, stress management, and depression.

- Jerome works for a large municipality in the Midwest that provides programs for school-aged youth with spinal cord injuries who are interested in participating in sport-related activities. Jerome develops and implements recreation-based programs designed to achieve goals related to access to space, adequate coaching, and establishing friendships with nondisabled peers.

- Bernita works in upstate New York at a residential camp that provides temporary or respite services to elderly men and women who are recovering from either stroke or heart-related problems. Bernita's programs are designed to work on regaining strength, range of motion, and coordination as well as establishing a sense of dignity and respect.

- Hiro works in a small private hospital in the Pacific Northwest that specializes in working with people who have issues with substance abuse. Clients who participate in Hiro's program typically work toward regaining old friendships, healthy leisure activities,

and family relationships. Hiro is currently working with several clients on identifying triggers that create stress and lead to further drug use. In his "expressions" group, Hiro provides clients with space, material, and metaphors to express their feelings through music, poetry, art, or creative movement.

- Steve works in a small community center in a suburb of Houston, Texas, that specializes in providing services exclusively for people with disabilities. His work focuses on advocacy through his assistance to community members in developing skills and strategies for exercising their right to both physical access and social inclusion. The challenges they tackle include housing discrimination, inadequate access to voting equipment, and being denied adequate access to facilities such as local libraries, golf courses, parks, pools, and movie theaters.

- Greta works in a maximum-security prison. The unit she works in houses inmates with mental illness. Greta is working to help the inmates identify and acquire new leisure interests and activity skills, stress man-

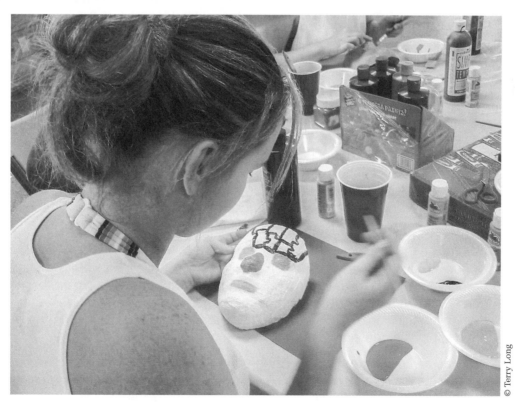

© Terry Long

Therapeutic recreation specialists often use creative and expressive activities as alternative outlets for communication and self-expression.

agement techniques, and alternative decision-making strategies.

- Charlie works in a Canadian residential care facility designed for elderly people who have significant disabilities. Major goals for his clients include resolving issues of boredom, apathy, depression, and anger as well as fulfilling opportunities to pursue both lifelong and recently developed leisure interests.
- Arlene works at the Olympics training camp with elite-level soccer athletes who use prosthetic devices to ambulate (walk and run). Arlene's programs focus on improving strength and conditioning as well as sport-specific skill development.

These examples are only a portion of the potential work opportunities available to therapeutic recreation specialists. Your future work could ultimately include any age or population, as all people are impacted by leisure-related determinants of quality of life.

Summary

Therapeutic recreation is a relatively young profession that has evolved from a long and rich history of people helping other people and their communities and sharing their knowledge, skills, and insight with others. It is a profession made up of thousands of people around the world who seek to improve the quality and longevity of life.

Just as people and their perspectives change over time, so do professions and their practices and techniques. At present, the broad profession of therapeutic recreation is unified by many concepts, theories, and practices. At the same time, various professional groups or organizations represent differing perspectives. In all cases, we have tried to remain neutral while also providing various perspectives for consideration.

We hope that you have developed an understanding of how the contents of this text and the accompanying course will benefit you. You should also have an idea of typical settings in which therapeutic recreation professionals might work, the clientele whom they might serve, and the type of skills that are necessary for exemplary practice. In particular, you should have a basic understanding of what differentiates therapeutic recreation from other therapy or leisure realms.

As you work through the first section of the book, these concepts will become more complex, enabling a deeper understanding of the overall profession. Open discussion related to the presented topics is critical in mastering these concepts, so take the time to read and talk about the following discussion questions with classmates and the instructor. Doing so will help clarify your opinions and understanding of issues that someday you will be required to address.

DISCUSSION QUESTIONS

1. There are several definitions of therapeutic recreation. Search for one or two definitions that differ from the one presented in this text, and compare them to what you have read in this chapter. Discuss similarities and differences with classmates and your course instructor. Ask your instructor for his or her perspective, and inquire about influences that led to that viewpoint.

2. What do you think the most important characteristics of a therapeutic recreation professional would be? Do you think that those who work in helping professions are "born with it" or rather, that people can learn such skills? Make a list of what you think are the most critical skills for working in a helping profession, and apply this question to each skill.

3. Discuss with a partner or in small groups what your understanding of therapeutic recreation was before you read this chapter. Have your views changed? If so, how? What professional opportunities have you learned about that you were previously unaware of?

4. Review the career examples presented in the Occupational Profiles section. Are any of these scenarios of interest to you? Do you have another example that you could share? Is there some combination of the examples that interests you? Are there examples that you would have no interest in? Why or why not? Discuss with your instructor whether he or she believes that all the examples represent something that a therapeutic recreation specialist might do.

5. Review the definition of therapeutic recreation provided in the What Is Therapeutic Recreation? section, and consider the following scenario. Is the intervention leisure-based? Is it purposeful? Would you consider the program to be utilizing leisure, enhancing leisure, or both?

Jason is a 10-year-old boy who is impulsive in social situations, often struggling to wait his turn in cooperative play activities or interrupting others in conversations. When adults tell him what to do, he becomes argumentative, frequently throws tantrums, and refuses to comply. Jason also occasionally pushes and shoves other kids when he feels threatened or embarrassed. He is especially sensitive to social play situations, particularly when he struggles to perform a skill or "loses" in the presence of others. Because of these behaviors, his peers have rejected him. When he does play, he rarely finishes an activity without incident.

After several behavior-related incidents at the local recreation center, Jason was suspended from participation. When his mother revealed Jason's disability to the recreation center, staff referred the family to Steve, who was the therapeutic recreation specialist responsible for developing inclusion plans for kids with disabilities. Steve met with Jason and his mother to assess Jason's leisure interests and abilities as well as his current behavior difficulties. Steve worked with the boy to develop ways to remember to take his turn and listen to others. Steve also advised other staff members about strategies to use when communicating with Jason, such as making eye contact before making a request, allowing adequate time for a response, and giving choices whenever possible. Steve also worked with recreation staff to create opportunities for Jason to develop activity skills and experience success in his play, such as by providing appropriate difficulty levels in sports drills. Finally, Steve worked with Jason and his mother to develop a behavior management plan intended to establish not only behavior supports but also behavioral expectations and consequences of inappropriate behavior. Jason's return to the center was contingent on his being able to maintain safe and reasonably appropriate behavior. Over the next 4 weeks, Steve tracked Jason's behavior and his ability to play successfully with others in a fun and rewarding way. Over time, Jason's improved behavior led to his having more friends and being a happier child.

2

History of Therapeutic Recreation

Rodney Dieser

LEARNING OUTCOMES

At the end of this chapter, students will be able to

- articulate why therapeutic recreation students should have a good understanding of the history of the profession,
- demonstrate how medical authority was used to justify leisure experiences,
- identify how the profession developed from both community and medical environments,
- identify how various sociological events affected the development of therapeutic recreation,
- reveal how past (and current) philosophical battles affected the profession, and
- articulate the difference between the leisure orientation and therapy orientation of therapeutic recreation.

In the novel *Frankenstein* (Shelley, 1818/2003), the fictional Swiss scientist, Victor Frankenstein, truly wanted to help people. He was attempting to understand the secrets of heaven and earth so he could prevent death and the physical and emotional pain associated with it (in the Hollywood movies, Frankenstein is the monster; in the novel, Frankenstein is the scientist). Unfortunately, his ambitions became framed in dangerous extremes and absolutes, resulting in the destruction of his life and any meaningful relationships (Campbell, 1997). In many ways, the *Frankenstein* story is relevant to the history of therapeutic recreation. Like Victor Frankenstein, therapeutic recreation leaders (both educators and practitioners) at times cause destructive consequences from genuine intentions. For over 50 years, prominent therapeutic recreation leaders have debated whether therapeutic recreation should have a therapy orientation or a leisure orientation, often using arguments that are extreme, binary, and based on absolutism. These philosophical battles are damaging the professional standing of therapeutic recreation. The aim of this chapter is to explain the development of therapeutic recreation from the late 1700s to the present and underscore the continuing internal struggles regarding the nature and essence of therapeutic recreation.

Importance of History

Students of therapeutic recreation should understand the history of their professional field for three paramount reasons. First, understanding past successes and failures helps professionals avoid repeating past mistakes, learn from past successes, and predict the consequences of individual and organizational actions.

Second, understanding the history of a professional field provides a source of professional identity. According to Sylvester (1989), "A field without history, though, is like a person without a memory. . . . [W]ithout sources of identity drawn from a meaningful past, purposeful direction is unlikely" (p. 19). What makes therapeutic recreation a distinct profession in human services? What are the differences between therapeutic recreation and occupational therapy? How are social work and therapeutic recreation similar? Should therapeutic recreation professionals implement programs that increase self-esteem or well-being? These questions and many more can be answered when a professional identity is in place.

Third, and related to professional identity, historical research creates perceptions of reality in the present (Hutcheon, 1989). That is to say, the present can be affected by how the past is interpreted. A historical accounting that interprets the history of therapeutic recreation as being closely aligned to a clinical past (e.g., **hospital recreation**) constructs a contemporary therapeutic recreation identity that makes clinical therapeutic recreation dominant and renders community therapeutic recreation marginal and inferior. Historical research must go beyond chronicling past activities and engage in critical thinking that explores past professional choices and the alternative thoughts that were bypassed and are sometimes forgotten (Hemingway, 2016). This chapter is based on historical analysis and will discuss not just the good aspects of therapeutic recreation but also a holistic view of the history of therapeutic recreation, even if it underscores certain unsightly and ugly events.

Origins of the Profession (Late 1700s to Mid-1900s)

Most books that examine the history of therapeutic recreation begin by highlighting how the efforts of various medical experts represent the early history of therapeutic recreation (e.g., Carter & Van Andel, 2011). The "play ladies" of community-oriented settlement houses (e.g., Hull-House), who are viewed as the first therapeutic recreation specialists, are simply missing in most therapeutic recreation books that examine history (see Bedini [1995] to learn more about the play ladies of early therapeutic recreation). The origins of therapeutic recreation developed in both community and clinical arenas. The following section will explain antecedents in medicine and community programs that eventually developed the profession of therapeutic recreation.

European and American Medicine

European medical practices and programs during the later 1700s to early 1900s were antecedents to the eventual development of therapeutic recreation in the United States. This section considers several examples about how medical efforts during this time were embedded in the values of recreation and leisure experiences.

Philippe Pinel and William Tuke

Philippe Pinel (1745-1826) of France and William Tuke (1732-1822) of England are often cited as two of the most influential pioneers of the **humanitarian treatment movement**. Humanitarian treatment, which emerged in the 18th century and became pervasive in Western Europe in the 19th century, was an approach to helping people who were suffering by focusing on humane psychosocial care and moral discipline. Pinel was appointed director of the Bicêtre insane asylum in 1793, which was the largest hospital for people with insanity in Paris. Following his appointment, Pinel removed patients from dungeons and chains, allowed patients to reside in sunny rooms, and encouraged patients to exercise and move freely on the hospital grounds. Tuke, an English merchant and philanthropist, founded the York Retreat (opened in 1796), a pleasant country home where people with mental illness worked in a kindly Quaker environment. Although Tuke was not trained as a medical expert, he used a medical and scientific approach to human services work. These two human services pioneers seemed to have no connection; they worked independently of each other, but their ideas and programs were the same. Both reformers influenced medical experts of the time, such as Samuel Hitch, a prominent English medical psychologist, and Benjamin Rush, founder of American psychiatry. Beyond planting the seeds of humane psychological intervention, Pinel and Tuke are also credited with planting the seeds of therapeutic recreation; Pinel believed people with mental illnesses were capable and deserved compassionate treatment. This approach included the use of purposeful recreational activities and work experiences to restore mental and physical health (Carter & Van Andel, 2011).

By the close of the 1800s, the use of humane approaches to treatment, which often incorporated leisure and recreation programs, was widespread in Europe and the United States (Mobily & MacNeil, 2002). Although it is accurate to say that Pinel and Tuke changed the course of human services and used recreation and leisure in a therapeutic manner, moral treatment interventions had a dark side. As an example, there are historians who believe that the humanitarian treatment movement was a stigmatizing response to a myth of a dreaded disease that spread from the houses of confinement (Foucault, 1965). That is, the countryside retreat that Tuke developed as a quiet country estate where individuals were encouraged to garden, talk with attendants, and take walks in the countryside was a method to remove people with mental illness from mainstream society.

In this regard, early therapeutic recreation and leisure services may have been used as a method to manipulate people into accepting the values of the dominant culture, thus using recreation and leisure in both a beneficial and a controlling manner (Dieser, 2002a).

Medical Spas and Thermal Baths of Europe

The development of medical spas and thermal baths throughout Europe, and in particular France, from the early 1800s through the mid-1900s eventually led to an understanding of the therapeutic consequences of leisure (Mackaman, 1998). Although medical doctors prescribed different types of spa baths (e.g., cold and hot showers, vapor box bathing, circular showering, and hosing and rubbing treatments), the essence of spa and thermal medicine was to experience leisure and freedom during a time in which leisure was not justified (1800s to mid-1900s). That is to say, European medical recreation in the form of spas and thermal baths was rooted in the leisure experience but needed medical authority to justify it so it did not appear as waste, idleness, or sloth (Mackaman, 1998).

Hence, the purpose of the European spas and thermal baths appeared to be recreation therapy or purposeful activity, but the true essence of medical spas was simply to justify leisure experiences. For that reason, medical spas and thermal facilities offered diverse leisure programs and services, such as grand hotels, casinos, musical performances and concert halls, tennis courts, lakes for boating, dance halls, theater houses, libraries, ballrooms, games and billiard rooms, and many other leisure facilities and services (Mackaman, 1998). These medical facilities were resorts full of leisure experiences and opportunities.

With medical authority to justify leisure, rest cures became popular psychiatric practices throughout the United States in the middle 1800s and early 1900s (Shorter, 1997). Silas Weir Mitchell, a nationally respected American psychiatrist who trained in France, created **rest cures**, based on rest and recreation to help restore mental health. For example, to treat a client known as Mrs. G for deep exhaustion, Dr. Mitchell's medical recommendation was enjoyment-based exercise and a massage and rub (see Shorter, 1997, pp. 131-132).

By 1900, rest cures had become a dominant treatment intervention for neurasthenia throughout the United States, "but it soon became apparent to many doctors that the essence of the Weir

Mitchell cure was the physician's authority, and not the specific physical components of the cure itself" (Shorter, 1997, p. 133). Just as in European medical spas, the essences of rest cures were simply to justify leisure experiences. The medical spas and thermal baths of Europe and rest cures of America clearly underscored that medical recreation was embedded in the leisure experience.

Leisure for Enjoyment at the Mayo Clinic

In the United States, William Worrall Mayo (1819-1911), William James Mayo (1861-1939), and Charles Horace Mayo (1865-1939)—the medical doctors and pioneers who started the world-renowned Mayo Clinic—were actively involved in a surplus of leisure and parks programs to help patients experience enjoyment and hope at the Mayo Clinic. That is to say, leisure for freedom and enjoyment has always had a place at the Mayo Clinic (see Mayo Foundation for Medical Education and Research, 2014; Nelson, 1990).

The essential purpose of art, for example, at the Mayo Clinic was to "enhance the environment of Mayo for patients, relatives, and staff, and to enrich the experience of patients and visitors at Mayo through cultural, recreational, and educational opportunities" (Roesler, 1987, pp. 16-17). Nelson's (1990) historical writings outline that these three Mayo doctors were early supporters of music, art, and parks and recreation at the Mayo Clinic and in the city of Rochester, Minnesota. To that end, when William Worrall Mayo was elected mayor in 1882, his pet project was to develop parks around the Mayo Clinic, and in the process, he had to wage a battle with the city council and the people of Rochester (Clapesattle, 1969). Following their father's example, in 1907 and 1909 the Mayo brothers (Charles and William James) advocated for and contributed to the development of Mayo Park (30 acres), which was only a few blocks away from the Mayo Clinic. In 1908, they purchased four and one-half acres of land and donated it to the city so that St. Mary's Park could be right next to St. Mary's Hospital on the Mayo campus. In 1910, the Mayo brothers presented nine and one-half acres of land northeast of the Mayo Park to create the Mayo Fields, where patients attended semipro baseball games (Edginton, Lankford, Dieser, & Kowalski, 2017). These three Mayo doctors wanted the original Mayo Clinic to be surrounded by parks so that patients and their families could experience leisure enjoyment at and around the Mayo Clinic. In speaking to the editor of *Better Homes and Gardens* about healthy living from a preventive perspective, in 1934 Charles Mayo stated,

> Business men should take more time for recreation—walking, horse-back riding, golf. . . . Too many men work until they drop, and never get to enjoy life. Every man should have an avocation. It might be geology or gardening or painting or astronomy or toolcraft or literature—anything to get the mind away from the humdrum things, freshen it, and occupy spare time. (cited in Peterson, 1934, p. 64)

The sidebar titled "A Legacy of Leisure at the Mayo Clinic" provides a broad overview of how leisure enjoyment has continued at Mayo Clinic today. Close to 30 years after Charles Horace and William James Mayo had died (both in 1939) and having never met or referred to how the Mayo doctors thought about the role of leisure in medicine, Paul Haun (1965), a kindred spirit in his thinking about recreation and leisure in medical institutions, continued the Mayo philosophy by arguing that "the unique value of providing recreation services to patients lies in their not being clinical" (p. 54). He believed that such services

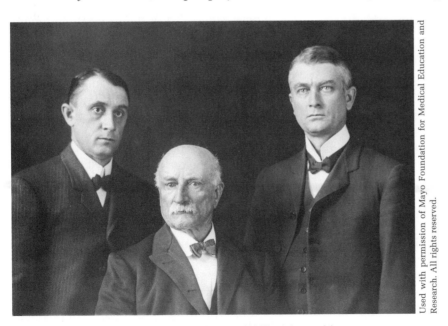

Charles Horace Mayo, William Worrall Mayo, and William James Mayo.

Year after year, the *U.S. News and World Report*, along with other publications, ranks the Mayo Clinic as one of the best hospitals in the United States (see Eisenman, 2014). The Mayo Clinic employs 4,100 physicians/scientists and 53,600 practitioners in **allied health professions** and sees more than 1 million patients each year (Olsen & Dacy, 2014).

Leisure for enjoyment has a long history at the Mayo Clinic, dating back to 1914 (Mayo Foundation for Medical Education and Research, 2014). "Man and Recreation," the large sculpture on the south façade of the Mayo building, represents the importance of rest, play, joyful moments, physical activities, rejuvenation, introspection, and enjoyment of nature (Mayo Clinic, 1984). Through a cafeteria and quality-of-life programming approach, the Mayo Clinic provides a plethora of diverse leisure activities through many organizational units. For example, the Peregrine Falcon Program at the Rochester campus allows patients to view and interact with Peregrine falcons that nest on the top of the 20-story Mayo and Gonda buildings (see http://history.mayoclinic.org/tours-events/mayo-clinic-peregrine-falcon-program.php).

The art collection at the Rochester campus presents thousands of art pieces from the media of glass, textiles, paintings, prints, ancient/ethnographic/folk art, sculptures, photography, and ceramics. Internationally known artists, such as Barbara Hepworth and Ivan Meštrović, are represented. Each year, the Art and Ability exhibit at the Rochester campus celebrates artworks from people with disabilities.

The Center for Humanities in Medicine at the Mayo Clinic Jacksonville (Florida) campus has professional musicians perform daily concerts in hospital lounges and local artists work one on one at the bedside with patients and families, exploring creative expression (see www.mayoclinic.org/patient-visitor-guide/humanities-in-medicine/florida-schedule). A 56-bell carillon on top of the Plummer building on the Rochester campus is rung regularly throughout the week (Mayo Clinic, 2006); patients can sit in the many outdoor courtyards and atriums or in the Feith Family Statuary Park in the center of campus to hear this musical performance. In keeping with a strengths-based approach, sometimes called the "Mayo way . . . to look at the strengths of individuals rather than at the deficiencies" (p. 150), grand pianos are placed at certain locations on the Rochester campus so that patients can perform impromptu concerts with crowds of other patients and staff singing or listening (Berry & Seltman, 2008; see also Mayo Clinic, 2001).

The Florida campus has a large park with lakes and a bridge to Louchery Island, where patients can contemplate and reflect (Mayo Clinic, 2011). The Scottsdale/Phoenix (Arizona) campus has a one-third-mile trail that includes more than 40 species of cacti and plants, where patients sometimes encounter roadrunners, quail, or horned owls (Mayo Clinic, 2011).

The St. Mary's Hospital Patient Library, on the Rochester campus—a community-based patient library—provides DVDs, music CDs, books/audiobooks, magazines and newspapers, desktop and laptop computers with Internet access, board games, video consoles and games, and crafts for patients and their families as well as a daily morning coffee social activity (St. Mary's Patient Library, 2016).

These examples illustrate how leisure remains an inherent part of the Mayo philosophy and culture. This philosophy, linked to a community parks and recreation approach, has allowed therapeutic recreation to exist not only as a formal service within the Mayo system, but also as a fundamental element of care and the overall patient experience.

---

should be focused on changing the medical environment (ecological thinking) so that patients can forget about their pain and misery through recreation programming. Haun advocated following a parks and recreation programming model for recreation delivery in hospital settings in which recreation provides fun and pleasure. He considered clinical-based recreation in healthcare settings (what is known today as "recreation therapy") to be a type of counterfeit psychology or imitation of occupational therapy. This sentiment is clear as Haun (cited in Phillips, 1957) elaborates about the value of recreation in the hospital setting:

> In such a setting the unique value of providing recreation services to patients lies in their not being clinical . . . Contemporary medicine is coming to think less about the disease and more about people with disease. The strength of the recreation movement is that it thinks about people, and in so doing goes beyond the limitations of medicine . . . While not curative in itself, it helps create the milieu for successful treatment . . . Recreational pursuits

attack the patient's loneliness by making it easy and attractive to be with other people . . . recreation as potential environmental normalizer, making the hospital a friendlier and more familiar place to the patient, easier to come to, easier to accept, easier to leave" (p. 54-57)

Haun felt that while recreation programming was not curative in itself, it helps create the milieu for successful treatment in healthcare settings. His book *Recreation: A Medical Viewpoint* (1965) is considered a classic text that should be read by every therapeutic recreation student. Most recently, Dieser, Edginton, and Ziemer (2017) demonstrated how Dr. Haun's ideology of recreation programming is at the core of the Mayo Clinic treatment of care.

Florence Nightingale

Florence Nightingale is often cited as an early medical expert (**nurse**) who highlighted the therapeutic effects of recreation while working in British hospitals during the Crimean War (1854-1856; Avedon, 1974; Carter et al., 2003; James, 1998). Nightingale observed that after surgery, patients were left to lie in their cots in dreary hospital environments with little custodial care.

Nightingale also observed that many soldiers were going to bars and using alcohol and other drugs as an unhealthy coping method to deal with the horrors of war. To remedy these issues, Nightingale advocated for and provided recreation programs in hospital environments, such as opportunities to listen to and perform music and theater, do needlework, play games (e.g., football and chess), write, and care for pets. In September 1855, Nightingale established the **Inkerman Cafe**, a small wooden hut located at the center of the hospital complex. The cafe had a large recreation room and a coffeehouse (James, 1998). A safe place where soldiers could escape their problems and find friendship, the Inkerman Cafe gave competition to local bars that profited on the dreadfulness of war. As Nightingale remarked, "Give them books and games, and amusements and they will leave off drinking" (cited in Woodham-Smith, 1951, p. 166).

The Two World Wars

Nightingale's ideas that recreation had therapeutic consequences led to the further development of therapeutic recreation programs in the United States during both World War I and World War II. The American Red Cross built recreation huts on military bases, homelike structures that provided convalescing soldiers with libraries, movies, entertainment, tables, games, and pianos. Each hut served 2,000 beds, which were staffed by four or five women (Bedini, 1995).

When the United States became involved in World War II, the Red Cross hired a great number of women with college degrees in any area of study and provided them 7 weeks of educational training (4 weeks in recreation leadership and a 3-week internship in military hospitals) for hospital recreation (James, 1998). During the period of both world wars, there was a consistent pattern of hiring hospital recreation staff during the war and eliminating recreation staff and programs after the war. For example, after the end of World War I, the Red Cross staffed only 26 of the original 52 hospitals with recreation leaders. At the conclusion of World War II, the first proposed graduate program curriculum conference for therapeutic recreation, which was requested by the Red Cross in 1945, lost its revenue base and was deleted (James, 1998).

Settlement Houses and Community Therapeutic Recreation

The play ladies involved in settlement houses and community schools during the 1800s were some of the first therapeutic recreation professionals in the United States (Bedini, 1995). A **settlement house** was an established human services agency developed purposely in city slums where human services workers provided human services (e.g., education, citizenship classes, community development, immigration protection, and recreation) and engaged in social action on behalf of the poor living nearby (Schram & Mandell, 2012). The settlement house movement was at its zenith in the late 19th and early 20th centuries. The primary mission of the settlement workers was to develop a holistic understanding of the conditions and causes of poverty by living with and learning from poor neighborhood residents (Stivers, 2000). By becoming neighbors of the poor, settlement workers developed friendships with them. Friendships and shared experiences would eventually lead to a holistic understanding of poverty, which would then make possible holistic problem solving and community programs to mediate the struggles of poverty. This section will highlight how community social programs in the United States, like the practices in European medicine, represent some of the early efforts to elicit the therapeutic outcomes of recreation and leisure experiences.

Jane Addams and the Women of the Hull-House Settlement

In September 1889, Jane Addams, Ellen Gates Starr, and Mary Keyser opened **Hull-House**, a settlement house in a poor district of Chicago. Hull-House, like most settlement houses of that era, established agencies in city slums where residents provided human services and engaged in social action on behalf of people with special needs (Schram & Mandell, 2012). Although Addams provided pioneering work in public recreation, she was also a pioneer in therapeutic recreation through her use of recreation and leisure to help improve the health and well-being of people with special needs, such as people with substance dependency or people living in poverty (Dieser, 2004a). Like Florence Nightingale, Addams established a coffee shop (in 1893) and provided an assortment of recreation programs and facilities (e.g., gymnasium, music and theatrical groups, art, needlework, creative writing, and games) at the center of a poverty-stricken community to promote an alternative meeting place to saloons (Bryan & Davis, 1990). The coffeehouse, which served nonalcoholic beverages, had a men's club, billiards, card tables, baths, food services, and the latest newspapers and magazines so that working immigrants could experience recreation, develop

friendships, and be informed about community and national events (Bryan & Davis, 1990). Like Nightingale's Inkerman Cafe, Addams' coffee shop was a safe place where immigrants could escape their problems, find friendship, and become educated citizens. Table 2.1 presents the similarities between Nightingale and Addams, (the only real difference was that Nightingale worked in a clinical setting and Addams worked in a community setting). Drawing on the historical research of Dieser (2004a), the following sections underscore how Addams and numerous women of Hull-House (e.g., Ellen Gates Starr, Julia Lathrop, and Alice Hamilton) used the recreation programs of expressive arts, bibliotherapy, and leisure education in a therapeutic manner in the later 1800s and early 1900s.

Expressive arts are the employment of visual arts, music, dance, or drama techniques with the intent to produce and achieve a final product (Devine & Dattilo, 2000; Silver, 1989). Numerous Hull-House programs provided expressive arts to people with special needs. For example, Hull-House developed a circulating art program of pictures and paintings as a method for developing freedom and resilience among tenement residents of Chicago. Regarding this program, Addams (1895/1990) commented,

> Another good mother [using the circulating painting and picture program] . . . who is battling with life against the odds too often found in a tenement-

Table 2.1 Therapeutic Recreation Similarities Between Florence Nightingale and Jane Addams

Florence Nightingale	Jane Addams
Highlighted how the dreariness of hospitals was counterproductive.	Highlighted how the dreariness of poverty-stricken communities was counterproductive.
Explained that the monotony endured by patients affected their recovery and motivation.	Explained that the monotony endured by poor immigrants affected their motivation.
Wrote of the benefits of caring for pets, listening to and performing music, doing needlework, and writing.	Wrote of the benefits of listening to and performing music, doing needlework, and writing.
Established Inkerman Cafe, a recreation room and coffeehouse.	Established the coffee shop—a recreation room and coffeehouse.
Established theatrical groups and social activities (e.g., dances and singing).	Established theatrical groups and social activities (e.g., dances and singing).
Recreation centers competed against bars that surrounded the hospital and military installations.	Recreation centers competed against bars, which saturated the community.
Provided multiple leisure experiences.	Provided multiple leisure experiences.

Reprinted by permission from R.B. Dieser, *Jane Addams and Hull-House Programs: Forgotten Pioneers in Therapeutic Recreation*, paper presented at the American Therapeutic Recreation Association Research Institute, (Kansas City, MO. 2004).

house, of a drinking husband and ever increasing poverty takes the pictures from the collection . . . [as a method] which will enable her to realize for her children some of the things she dreamed out of them. The oldest one of her eight children saw the light in a pretty suburban house. . . . this mother borrowed Mrs. Jameson's "Sacred and Legendary Art" and read the story of St. Genevieve to her children while they had Puvis de Chavanne's St. Genevieve pictures, and she took the Fra Angelico "Paradise" a second time because she thought it gave the children a pleasant idea of Heaven." (pp. 41-42)

This mother used the art program to develop freedom, resiliency, hope, and self-determination in her children. Likewise, Addams (1909/1972) used theater as a medium by which youthful imagination could roam free, in sharp contrast to the otherwise grim lives of most immigrant families (e.g., joining gangs or the sex and drug trade). Addams observed young people leaving theaters "with the magic of the play still thick upon them" (p. 75).

Hull-House also used other expressive arts—dances and social events—within the framework of contact theory to bridge cross-cultural differences (Dieser, 2005c). Hilda Satt, a Polish immigrant who worked at Hull-House, highlighted how dances and social gatherings at Hull-House built bridges of cross-cultural understanding and developed freedom (Polacheck, 1989).

Beyond art, theater, and dance, other expressive art activities such as therapeutic writing and drama were used to help people with special needs experience the beneficial outcomes of enjoyment, meaning, accomplishment, freedom, and self-determination (Elshtain, 2002; Hackett, 1925/1990; Starr, 1896; Weil, 1913/1990).

Bibliotherapy utilizes reading materials, such as novels, plays, short stories, booklets, and pamphlets, to help clients become aware that other people share similar problems, gain new insights, and structure their lives (Austin, 2004). Jane Addams and Hull-House programs used readings to help people with special needs realize that they were not alone and to gain personal insights. For example, to help Italian immigrants deal with poverty and loneliness, a George Eliot reading group formed in which the first novel selected was *Romola*, read in Italian (Elshtain, 2002). To help immigrant children deal with poverty and discrimination, Addams held Abraham Lincoln's birthday social celebrations at Hull-House and gave copies of the book *Appreciation of Abraham Lincoln* to immigrant boys who were members of the Hull-House boys club (Addams,

1910/1981). By showing these boys that Abraham Lincoln celebrated cultural diversity by reading books, Addams aimed to help them understand that they should not be ashamed of their cultural backgrounds and, instead, they should celebrate them (Addams, 1910/1981).

Furthermore, the reading of poetry and short stories was often used to help Hull-House participants structure their lives (Addams, 1905/1990; Monroe, 1912/1990). For example, Carmella Gustaferre (1914/1990), a young Italian immigrant girl, wrote a short story called "What Type of Home I Would Like," in which she explained her life ambition was to have a nice house, garden, piano, backyard with a swing, beautiful trees to provide shade to read under, and a parlor full of flowers. This short story provided structure, motivation, and insights to this young immigrant girl.

Leisure education is a developmental process through which a person or group of people increase their understanding of leisure and the relationship among leisure, lifestyle, and society (Mundy, 1998). Jane Addams and Hull-House programs provided leisure-oriented community education to help people with special needs. Community leisure education was offered in literature, the arts, physical activity, and cooking, just to name a few (see Bryan & Davis, 1990; Fischer, 2004). However, the **Labor Museum** exemplifies how community leisure education was a developmental process in which groups of people increased their understanding of leisure and the relationship among leisure, lifestyle, culture, and society.

The Labor Museum developed from Addams' twofold concern for the disdainful attitudes that immigrant children had toward their parents' old-world traditions and culture and the contemptuous attitudes that Americans had toward poverty-stricken immigrants who were living in Chicago (Addams, 1910/1981). Addams wanted to bridge the gap between immigrant parents and children by highlighting how old-world spinning and weaving were a cultural tradition that showcased the leisure skills of immigrant adults and parents (Addams, 1910/1981). By allowing immigrants to display their creative skills through a community leisure education program, the Labor Museum provided people freedom and enjoyment from their depressing lives and educated the masses about the talents of immigrant people. For example, Washburne (1904/1990) reported that an Irish immigrant woman who had experienced physical abuse from a husband and had had two children with disabilities commented: "Oh, I can smile and laugh with the best when I am at work here [spindling at the Labor Museum]" (p. 80).

Other Community Antecedents to Therapeutic Recreation

Other social settlement houses and community settings besides Hull-House also showcased the therapeutic value of play, recreation, and leisure experiences (regarding the role and value of recreation in social settlement houses throughout the United States, see Woods & Kennedy, 1970). For example, in 1919 Ada Sophia McKinley, a retired schoolteacher and a leader in the African American Southside Settlement House in Chicago, volunteered as the head recreational host of the War Camp Club. The club used recreational and civic activities to help returning soldiers and their families make a transition into American society (e.g., dealing with posttraumatic stress syndrome or finding employment and housing; see www .adasmckinley.org).

Philosophical Battles in Therapeutic Recreation (1945-1965)

After the end of World War II, both medical and community programs and settings began to take a more direct approach to observing and documenting the therapeutic value of leisure and recreation. For example, clinical and medical staff at the nationally known Menninger Clinic in Topeka, Kansas, were explicit in explaining the therapeutic value of providing play, recreation, and leisure experiences to clients who were struggling with psychological disabilities (Carter et al., 2003). Menninger and McColl (1937) advocated that patients go out for dinner or go shopping to create a sense of freedom and renewal.

In essence, Menninger and McColl argued that a distinguishing feature of therapeutic recreation was its clear and direct association to recreation and leisure. The leisure experience was what made therapeutic recreation distinct from occupational therapy and educational therapy. The view that leisure in hospital settings should be focused on freedom and enjoyment and not on therapy was supported by other hospital workers and medical staff. In addition, various authors at this time outlined that providing leisure for curative or therapy purposes was based on the principles of occupational therapy and that providing leisure for enjoyment and freedom was the quintessential aspect of therapeutic recreation, making therapeutic recreation different from occupational therapy (see Romney, 1945) or mental health counseling (see Nice, 1948).

In fact, the **leisure orientation to therapeutic recreation**—the idea that the distinctness of therapeutic recreation is its clear association with programming recreation and leisure services—was the underlying philosophy when hospital recreation became a special-interest option or branch of the American Recreation Society (ARS) in 1949 (James, 1998). One of the most powerful founding members, Harold D. Meyer, was able to develop a hospital recreation curriculum that was aligned to recreation and physical education programs (instead of medicine or applied health programs), and he pioneered the phrase "I am a rec-re-a-tor *first*!" (James, 1998).

As the hospital recreation section of ARS was developing, a group of therapeutic recreation professionals who followed the **therapy orientation of therapeutic recreation** began to design a rival organization that stressed the curative aspects of hospital recreation. This group believed that the essence of therapeutic recreation was to use or prescribe recreation and leisure for medical purposes. In 1952 B.E. Phillips (1952b) and a group of like-minded Veterans Administration professionals eventually formed the Recreational Therapy Section within the Recreation Division of the American Association for Health, Physical Education and Recreation (AAHPER) with "its primary purpose . . . to assist physicians in their treatment of patients" (p. 2). Phillips (1952a) further commented that "[recreational therapy is a] means toward patient recovery rather than an end in itself. This concept dictates the selection of activities primarily on the basis of needs and capabilities, and secondary on the basis of interests" (p. 29). In 1953, Charles Cottle, who shared Phillips' perspective, formed the **National Association of Recreation Therapists (NART)** to dissociate the therapy orientation from the recreation and physical education curriculum of AAHPER and to respond to the lack of attention by ARS to clinical outcomes and the role of recreation in bringing functional improvements to clients (Mobily & Ostiguy, 2004).

Therapeutic recreation was poised to become a respected profession after the end of World War II. Instead it became a fragmented and disjointed profession that had no fewer than three organizations

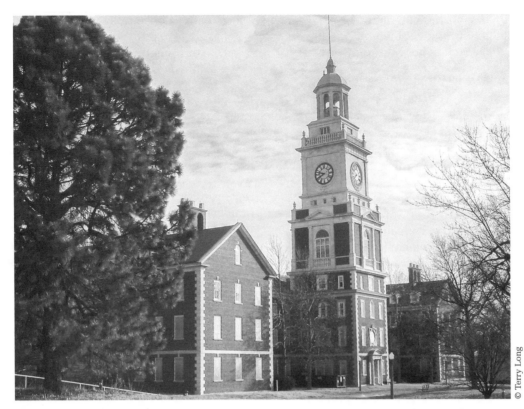

Prior to its relocation to Houston, Texas, in 2003, the world-renowned Menninger Clinic had been based out of this Topeka, Kansas, facility. C.F. Menninger started the clinic with his two sons, Karl and Will, in 1925, and they went on to become pioneers in the development of psychiatry.

claiming to be the voice of therapeutic recreation (According to van der Smissen [personal communication, June 16, 2005], a fourth voice was the National Association of Recreation Services for the Handicapped, which began in 1953).

Binary and absolute thinking, the kind of thinking used by Victor Frankenstein, was used to conceptualize therapeutic recreation. In one corner were professionals who followed the philosophy of recreation as therapy, emphasizing the use of recreation and leisure as therapy tools. In the other corner were professionals who believed quality leisure to be the primary goal of therapeutic recreation, recognizing recreation and enjoyment as basic human needs that can be enhanced to allow people with special needs (e.g., people with spinal cord injuries) the opportunity to experience freedom, choice, pleasure, and meaningfulness. In this case, therapy is a byproduct of the leisure experience. These differing philosophies and the professional organizations associated with them followed separate developmental paths up until the 1960s. As the boundaries of practice between the two camps began to fade and the political, professional, and social benefits of unity grew

stronger, a historical reorganization of the profession was just over the horizon.

The Utopian Years of Therapeutic Recreation (1966-1984)

Following the philosophical battles that occurred from 1945 to 1965, a social movement began in the early 1960s to unite all leisure-oriented professionals together into one loosely structured organization (James, 1998; van der Smissen, 2005). In 1965, five organizations began to align to form the **National Recreation and Park Association (NRPA)**, which officially began on January 1, 1966 (van der Smissen, 2005):

- National Recreation Association (NRA), founded in 1906
- American Institute of Park Executives (AIPE), founded in 1898
- National Confederation on State Parks (NCSP), founded in 1921

- American Association of Zoological Parks and Aquariums (AZA), founded in 1924
- American Recreation Society (ARS), with its six sections, including therapeutic recreation–hospital recreation, founded in 1938

The **National Therapeutic Recreation Society (NTRS)**, a branch of NRPA, was also born when NRPA was created. Regarding therapeutic recreation, James (1998) noted,

> The underlying principles supporting such an alliance were so attractive to members of NART and of the Hospital Section of ARS that they put aside their philosophical differences, voted to merge, agreed to a charter and bylaws and elected officials, all within a year. On Sunday, October 9, 1966, the Board of Trustees of NRPA approved the Charter of the National Therapeutic Recreation Society. (p. 25)

In a reflective narrative, Compton (1997) referred to this era as the **utopian years of therapeutic recreation** because the merger brought together various factions of the leisure field and developed a strong lobbying voice in Washington, DC. Besides developing a pool of federal dollars that was used to establish therapeutic recreation curricula and professionalism across the nation, the development of both NRPA and NTRS brought into focus the social and moral issues of rights for people with disabilities.

Austin's (2002) historical observations confirmed the existence of a utopian era, when therapeutic recreation was a unified profession. Austin also described the benefits of having a unified therapeutic recreation profession:

> For almost 20 years, the National Therapeutic Recreation Society (NTRS) singly advocated for the professionalization of therapeutic recreation in the United States. During these years a number of advances were made by NTRS. The *Therapeutic Recreation Journal* began publication in 1966. Guidelines were published for community-based programs for special populations in 1978, as well as for clinical standards in 1979. . . . University curricula in therapeutic recreation expanded, and accreditation standards were established. . . . Finally, in 1981, the National Council on Therapeutic Recreation Certification was instituted. (pp. 279-280)

Simply stated, the period from the mid-1960s to the mid-1980s was a wonderful time for therapeutic recreation, namely because members of the profession came together, worked in collaboration, and were unified.

As alluded to earlier, this era witnessed a strong focus in community therapeutic recreation programs. In particular, the principle of normalization, which is a conceptual cornerstone in providing therapeutic recreation services delivery (Bullock & Mahon, 2000; Howe-Murphy & Charboneau, 1987; Pedlar & Gilbert, 1997; Searle, Mahon, Iso-Ahola, Sdrolias, & van Dyck, 1995; Searle et al., 1998; Sylvester, Voelkl, & Ellis, 2001), developed in this era under the framework of recreation inclusion. The heightened focus on the rights of people with disabilities developed a theoretical framework for helping people with disabilities become included in mainstream society. In particular, the **normalization principle** makes "available to persons with intellectual and other impairments or disabilities patterns of life and conditions of everyday living which are as close as possible or indeed the same as the regular circumstances and ways of life of their communities" (Nirje, 1992, p. 16).

Building on the normalization principle and significant acts of legislation that were enacted for people with disabilities in the 1960s and 1970s, this era witnessed community-based therapeutic recreation approaches oriented toward **inclusive recreation**, which created recreation opportunities so that people with disabilities could experience leisure in mainstream society. Therapeutic recreation programs developed in various community and human services organizations, such as public recreation and parks programs, nonprofit organizations, outpatient programs in hospitals and rehabilitation centers, group homes and transitional living facilities, youth services, community councils, and consortiums of public agencies that represented community needs. From a therapeutic recreation perspective, inclusive recreation can be provided in three ways:

- Community reintegration programs (e.g., providing therapeutic recreation services to recently discharged rehabilitation patients during the period of transition from hospital to home or community)
- Community integration programs (e.g., helping people with disabilities develop leisure skills so they can experience interdependent or independent leisure participation)
- Community development approach (e.g., building accessible and inclusive community recreation facilities and services; Sylvester et al., 2001)

To this end, community development inclusive recreation occurred during the early 1970s with

MEAD B. JACKSON, CTRS, CPRP, RECREATION THERAPY CERTIFIED (CALIFORNIA CERTIFICATION)

Education: BS in Social Science, Southern University

Postgraduate Program in Physical Medicine, Valley Forge Army Medical Center

Position: Director of Psychiatric Rehabilitation Therapy Services

Organization: Los Angeles County–University of Southern California Medical Center, Los Angeles, California

Special Awards

- Outstanding Therapist of the Year, California Park and Recreation Society, 1974

- Pacific Southwest Professional of the Year, National Recreation and Park Association, 1984

- Distinguished Service Award, National Therapeutic Recreation Society, 1989

- Lifetime Achievement Award, California Park and Recreation Society, 1998

- Special Award, "In Recognition of Outstanding Contributions as a Pioneer in the Origin and Development of the National Therapeutic Recreation Society," National Therapeutic Recreation Society National Congress, 2006

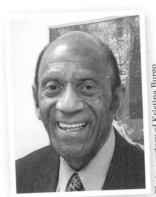

Photo courtesy of Kristina Burgo

My Career

My first professional job was junior high school teacher, in 1959. At the end of my first year as a teacher, I was drafted into the army. I was fortunate to be one of the eight military personnel with a college degree selected for the physical medicine training program at Valley Forge Medical Center. Upon completing the academic phase of the program, I completed an internship in the psychiatric unit at Valley Forge General Hospital. After completing the internship, I was assigned to the physical medicine department of Brooke Army Medical Center at Fort Sam Huston, Texas. I completed my military tour of duties in the activity therapy department of Brooke General Psychiatric Hospital, where I served from 1961 to 1963. After my discharge from the Army, I moved to California and was hired in 1963 by the physical medicine department at Los Angeles County–University of Southern California Medical Center (LAC+USC), which is one of the largest public hospitals in the country. LAC+USC provides a full spectrum of emergency, inpatient, and outpatient services. These include trauma and surgical emergency, obstetrical, gynecological, and pediatric services, as well as psychiatric services for adults, adolescents, and children.

I worked my way up from a level I recreation therapist to an appointment as the recreation therapy director in 1975. When the occupational therapy and recreation therapy departments were administratively consolidated in 1995 to create the Division of Psychiatric Rehabilitation Services, I was appointed director of the division. As director, I am responsible for planning, organizing, directing, controlling, and coordinating rehabilitation therapy services for a patient population with severe mental, social, or physical disabilities. I am responsible for administering intensive treatment programs of occupational and recreational therapy designed to restore or maintain the patients' physical, social, and mental functioning abilities. In this position, I also administer the rehabilitation therapy education programs.

What I like about the job is that it provides me with the opportunity to make major contributions to the health care delivery system and the professional organizations. I have the privilege of interacting with a group of dedicated medical and allied health personnel on a daily basis. I also have the opportunity to travel around the country to serve on committees and boards at the local, state, regional, and national levels and to network with known experts on matters affecting the rehabilitation therapy delivery system. Based on my numerous contributions to the therapeutic recreation profession at the local, state, and national levels, I am highly respected as a leader in the profession. This is verified by the numerous prestigious awards I have received over the years.

My Advice To You

My advice to undergraduate students is to get practical experience in all areas of therapeutic recreation before selecting an agency to complete your internship. Select the agency that meets your needs and interests. Be prepared to work hard and go above and beyond the minimum requirements for the internship experience to improve your knowledge and skills. Do not be afraid of making a mistake, but learn from your mistake and move forward—this is how you will become a good leader and therapist.

the creation of numerous special recreation programs, such as the Special Olympics, and special recreation associations throughout the United States, which provided recreation programs and services specifically for adults and children with disabilities (Bullock & Mahon, 2000). For example, the Northern Suburban Special Recreation Association (NSSRA) of Chicago, which formed in 1970 and was the first special recreation association in Illinois and among the first of its kind in the United States, was and still is an intergovernmental partnership of 10 park districts, one city, and one village. NSSRA provides year-round recreation programs and services for over 5,000 people with various disabilities per year (see www.nssra.org).

Furthermore, the utopian years of therapeutic recreation also witnessed the development of the **National Council for Therapeutic Recreation Certification (NCTRC)** in 1981. NCTRC is an independent credentialing agency that oversees the national certification program in therapeutic recreation (see www.nctrc.org). NCTRC has identified through years of research minimal competency skills that a certified (or competent) therapeutic recreation specialist should possess. NCTRC was able to trademark the title *certified therapeutic recreation specialist* (CTRS) in 1993 in the United States.

The Fragmentation Years of Therapeutic Recreation (1985-2000)

During the utopian years (1966-1984), therapeutic recreation was a promising and emerging profession under a unified banner, but tension still existed between the recreation therapy approach and the leisure orientation approach. For example, in the early 1980s, Meyer (1980) argued that there were two subspecializations to therapeutic recreation—the therapist and the special recreator. As such, Meyer suggested that the two subspecializations functioned in different worlds, with different purposes, work settings, and accountability structures. Meyer predicted that it would only be a matter of time before one of these specializations would seek its independence from the other.

Compton's (1997) personal reflections provide additional understanding of the tension that was occurring during this era. He described the growing unrest between NTRS and NRPA during the early 1980s, notably the doubts that many NTRS leaders had about the commitment that NRPA made to NTRS. Furthermore, Compton explained how nasty allegations were thrown back and forth between NRPA and NTRS, and he can still "vividly remember sitting in the office of NRPA refereeing a shouting match between the president of NTRS and the executive director of NRPA over the relationship of NTRS and NRPA and some other rather seminal issues. It was not a pretty sight and affected the relationship of the 'parent' and 'child' for years to come" (p. 43).

In an attempt to develop a philosophical statement and mission for therapeutic recreation, Meyer (1980) articulated four possible positions (see table 2.2). Positions 1 and 2 represented a resurfacing of the historical conflicts between ARS and NART. Positions 3 and 4 were attempts to maintain unity while acknowledging a broader purpose or set of purposes.

After spirited and ugly debate, the NTRS membership turned toward a democratic method and allowed its therapeutic recreation membership to vote on the four positions. The results were decisive: 62.9 percent voted for the leisure ability approach; 22.9 percent, for the therapy approach; 10.6 percent, for the umbrella, or combined, approach; and 3.7 percent, for the recreation service approach (NTRS, 1982, cited in James, 1998). In May 1982, NTRS adopted the leisure ability approach as its official philosophical position (for more information on the leisure ability approach, see the Leisure Ability Model section in chapter 5).

But this decision did not end the tension within NTRS. Although 77.2 percent of the NTRS membership voted against a strict therapy-oriented approach to therapeutic recreation and believed that the leisure ability approach maintained unity while acknowledging a broader purpose or set of purposes (both therapy and leisure), members who followed the therapy orientation continued to believe that NRPA was too controlling, and they eventually developed a **separatist mentality**. James (1998), one of the leaders of the separatist movement, explained that in the late 1970s and early 1980s NRPA did not focus on health care issues that were relevant to therapeutic recreation, such as home health care legislation, and was too focused on issues not relevant to therapeutic recreation, such as developing positive relationships with the Bureau of Outdoor Recreation.

After NTRS made a motion that NRPA become less centralized and study alternative

Table 2.2 Four Positions of Therapeutic Recreation

Approach	Definition
Recreation services approach	The primary purpose of therapeutic recreation was to provide recreation services to people with special needs. The role of a therapeutic recreation specialist was to help or enable people with disabilities to experience leisure and its benefits.
Therapy approach	The primary purpose of therapeutic recreation was to treat and ameliorate the effects of illness and disabilities. Therapeutic recreation was a means to a curative end.
Umbrella, or combined, approach	The primary purpose of therapeutic recreation involved two roles. Therapeutic recreation could be shifted to provide recreation services to people with special needs and to ameliorate the effects of illness. Hunnicutt (1980) posited that "therapeutic recreation is unique because it rests on recreation's subjective quality (the individual's own state of mind, his fun) at the same time it provides tangible evidence that real medical and health goals are served through recreation" (p. 132). That is, therapeutic recreation may be used simultaneously as a medium for therapeutic change and as an enjoyable outcome that is pursued for its own sake.
Leisure ability approach	According to the academic work of Gunn and Peterson (1978) and Peterson and Gunn (1984), the primary purpose of therapeutic recreation was to integrate three phases—therapy or treatment, leisure education, and recreation participation—along a continuum, and the ultimate goal was to help people with disabilities establish an independent leisure lifestyle. A therapeutic recreation specialist would choose which phases to work within based on the context and needs of the client.

organizational structures and NRPA officials defeated that motion, many like-minded therapeutic recreation specialists who believed in the therapy approach began a separatist mentality (James, 1998). During the 1983 NRPA Convention in Kansas City, the separatist group met in the hotel room of David Park, a former executive secretary and past president of NTRS, and made a formal commitment to start an independent therapeutic recreation organization focused on the therapy approach and clinical practice.

On June 12, 1984, followers of this movement formed the **American Therapeutic Recreation Association (ATRA)**. As was the case with NART, the early ATRA leaders felt that therapeutic recreation should emphasize that therapeutic recreation is a treatment for therapeutic change and should separate from its historical roots with parks and recreation and its distinct association with leisure (Austin, 2002). Within a year, the membership of ATRA had grown to 300 (James, 1998), and by 1999, ATRA had over 4,000 members (Crawford, 2001). But many therapeutic recreation leaders had concerns about the possible short- and long-term negative consequences of ATRA, suggesting it would divide and eventually weaken the profession of therapeutic recreation (see Nesbitt, 1984).

Although ATRA membership was growing, internal conflicts and problems plagued the organization. In particular, early ATRA leaders had difficulty agreeing on a statement of purpose before they eventually created one, which underscored that therapeutic recreation had "two functions: treatment services and recreation services. Denoting them both as therapeutic recreation, however, reverted the [purpose] statement to the umbrella dilemma" (James, 1998, p. 31). In short, the original statement of purpose that ATRA drafted did not align with a therapy focus; rather, it aligned with an umbrella, or combined, focus, similar to the leisure ability model.

NTRS clearly suffered when ATRA was formed, with membership falling slightly below 2,000 in 1999 (Crawford, 2001). Despite this change, NTRS maintained its goals to (1) unite therapeutic recreation personnel, (2) encourage the professional development of therapeutic recreation personnel, (3) be an advocate for the leisure rights of individuals with disabilities, (4) encourage research to improve the quality of therapeutic recreation practice, and (5) promote the relationship between therapeutic recreation and other professions concerned with the health and well-being of people with disabilities (Mobily & Ostiguy, 2004). To bolster its commitment to health and rehabilitation, in 1992 NTRS became an associate member of the Commission on Accreditation of Rehabilitation Facilities (CARF) and joined the Joint Commission on Accreditation of Healthcare Organizations (JCAHO) Coalition of Rehabilitation Therapy Organizations (see the NTRS website at www.nrpa.org).

In 2000, NTRS, following its parent organization NRPA, developed the "Therapeutic Recreation—The Benefits Are Endless" training program, which is a communication medium to stakeholders regarding the beneficial outcomes of therapeutic recreation, recreation, and leisure (see the NTRS website at www.nrpa.org). This training program and resource guide enabled therapeutic recreation specialists to (1) promote therapeutic recreation programs in terms of benefits and outcomes produced, (2) develop and justify programs based on documented benefits and outcomes, and (3) manage programs in a manner that highlights efficacy (see Broida, 2000). However, a problematic aspect to this training framework is its suggestion that therapeutic recreation always produces benefits and never produces harmful outcomes. Therapeutic recreation, like all human services programs, can unknowingly harm participants and clients. Examples of such potential dangers are explored in the chapter 3 discussion on ethics in practice.

Although this era was fragmented, there were some positive developments in the profession of therapeutic recreation. For example, ATRA and NTRS worked in partnership on special events such as the Joint Task Force on Credentialing to assist agencies in becoming recognized health care providers in their home states (James, 1998), and in 1998, the organizations mutually developed a resolution and a letter of agreement acknowledging that two national organizations represent therapeutic recreation professionals (Wenzel, 1998). In 1998, ATRA and NTRS created the **Alliance for Therapeutic Recreation**, an entity that brings together board members of both organizations to communicate and work in partnership on certain issues (Carter et al., 2003).

One of the most positive events during the fragmentation years was the production of solid qualitative and quantitative research that showed that therapeutic recreation programs affect the health and well-being of people. During the late 1980s and early 1990s, one of the most complete and wide-ranging attempts to consolidate research findings took place—the National Conference on the Benefits of Therapeutic Recreation, sponsored by the therapeutic recreation program at Temple University and National Institute on Disability and Rehabilitation Research (NIDRR) of the United States Department of Education (Malkin, Coyle, & Carruthers, 1998). The result of this conference was the development of an extensive and precise typology of therapeutic recreation benefits (Shank, Kinney, & Coyle, 1993), which appeared in the lengthy publication *Benefits of Therapeutic Recreation: A Consensus View* (Coyle, Kinney, Riley, & Shank, 1991). The typology of therapeutic recreation benefits highlighted that therapeutic recreation influenced health care outcomes in

- physical health and health maintenance,
- cognitive functioning,
- psychosocial health,
- growth and personal development,
- personal and life satisfaction, and
- societal and health care system outcomes.

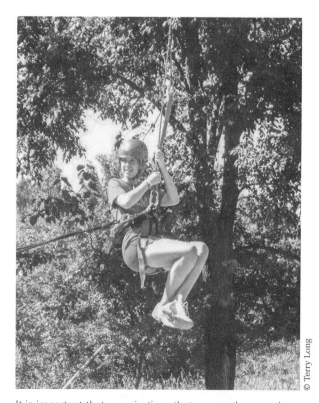

It is important that organizations that govern therapeutic recreation continually come together to monitor treatment practices and standards so that patients can experience the greatest benefits—including a sense of accomplishment and fun.

Therapeutic Recreation in the 21st Century

Perhaps one of the most salient developments in therapeutic recreation in the 21st century was the dissolution of NTRS as a branch of NRPA in 2010 (Carter & Van Andel, 2011) and the development of the NRPA online Inclusion and Accessibility Network. At its core, this network created an online forum for discussion related to providing leisure services to people with special needs or health conditions. Unfortunately, the network was in no way designed to directly support professional needs of therapeutic recreation specialists as NTRS had once done.

In the United States, ATRA is now the sole professional association of therapeutic recreation/recreation therapy and continues to develop its therapy orientation. In 2010, ATRA was accepted as a sponsoring member by the Commission on Accreditation of Allied Health Education Programs (CAAHEP), and the Committee on Accreditation of Recreational Therapy Education (CARTE) was accepted by CAAHEP (see Carter & Van Andel, 2011). Today, therapeutic recreation/recreation therapy academic programs are accredited by two accreditation agencies: the Council on Accreditation of Parks, Recreation, Tourism and Related Professions (COAPRT) and CARTE. The accreditation process and the nature of these accrediting bodies are presented in more detail in Chapter 3.

Therapeutic recreation gained more worldwide attention in the 21st century from journals dedicating special issues on the global perspective of therapeutic recreation. One significant conclusion drawn by multiple scholars has been that successfully delivering therapeutic recreation services in other countries and cultures is possible only if cultural norms are acknowledged and integrated into the delivery approach. For example, researchers who have studied therapeutic/fukushi recreation in Japan have asserted that the American principles and competencies of therapeutic recreation need to assimilate toward Japanese culture rather than Japanese culture assimilating to American values. Research suggests that American therapeutic recreation benefits do not demonstrate positive outcomes in the Japanese culture (Nishino, Chino, Yoshioka, & Gabriella, 2007). In 2015, the *World Leisure Journal* also had a special issue on global therapeutic recreation. Others have noted that the American model of therapeutic recreation, and in particular the NCTRC credentialing framework,

is not compatible with Quebec/French Canadian realities and culture (Carbonneau et al., 2015; Hebblethwaite, 2015) and has caused significant problems in the province of Alberta (Dieser, 2012; Dieser, 2014). Another suggestion related to therapeutic recreation spreading in South Africa is to draw on but not replicate ATRA and NCTRC frameworks that are appropriate to South African culture. In summary, globalization of therapeutic recreation will require a level of cultural sensitivity and relevance that is likely to challenge the traditional medical model that has dominated American therapeutic recreation (Mobily, 2015).

Perhaps one of the most paramount changes in thinking regarding therapeutic recreation in the 21st century was the development of a strengths-based paradigm (see Anderson & Heyne, 2012a; Anderson & Heyne, 2012b; Heyne & Anderson, 2012). In particular, a strengths-based approach can help people reach their goals by emphasizing their strengths or capabilities rather than focusing on their deficits. The approach is in contrast to the deficit approach, which is associated with the medical model that emphasizes what is wrong or abnormal about a person and where a professional is viewed as an expert who can "fix" a person with disabilities. A strengths-based model sees individuals with disabilities (and their families) as their own expert and is dedicated to human flourishing and driven by an ecological approach that focuses on changing environments. In short, this approach empowers participants to take the lead in the therapeutic process rather than depend on the all-powerful therapist to repair their deficits and abnormalities. Furthermore, a strengths-based approach will help people with disabilities experience flow (enjoyment). To this end, the recent leisure education toward happiness model, which is based on a strengths-based and positive psychology framework, examines how a person can use his or her own signature strengths as a serious leisure endeavor to experience enjoyment/flow and an optimal leisure lifestyle (see Dieser, 2013).

Summary

The purpose of this chapter was to explain the development of therapeutic recreation from the late 1700s to the present and describe the continuing internal struggles about the nature and essence of therapeutic recreation. In this last section, I would like to make some summary remarks based on historical observation and return to where I began the chapter—the story of Victor Frankenstein.

When Victor Frankenstein created his monster, his intentions were good; he wanted to help society by overcoming death. But the result was tragic—both Victor Frankenstein and the monster became binary thinkers who followed the doctrines of absolutism and constantly battled each other. Both died a cold death (Shelley, 1818/2003). Frankenstein's "quest for a grand achievement . . . [became] his own undoing" (Kelly, 2000, p. 80).

This absolutism has limited our ability to thrive as a profession by creating confusion in external stakeholders regarding the profession (Skalko, 1997). More important, absolutism limits our ability to serve the many people who might benefit from therapeutic recreation services. In short, the quest for grand achievement has become our own undoing. Although other important economic, social, and political factors have hurt the profession of therapeutic recreation, collectivistic actions of conflict related to accreditation have marred the profession from its very beginning and continues into the 21st century. Likewise, economic, social, and political forces helped therapeutic recreation flourish during the utopian years (1966-1984), but therapeutic recreation flourished because of the unified efforts of leaders who were able to demonstrate high collectivistic ego development by having a solid understanding of the needs of others, welcoming and thinking in diverse ways, and acting for the common good. However, part of the reason therapeutic recreation has less effect on health care legislation and the health insurance industry is because of a divided profession that has a history of conflict (Mobily & Ostiguy, 2004). That is, therapeutic recreation is a wonderful and important profession with a solid body of research regarding its beneficial outcomes in both community and clinical services, but internal conflicts have challenged its legitimacy and credibility.

At the end of the *Frankenstein* novel (Shelley, 1818/2003), Victor Frankenstein is close to death somewhere in the cold Arctic when another ambitious scientist and explorer, Robert Walton, attempts to save him. Walton is a kindred spirit who is also driven by a quest for grand and glorious achievement. But Walton is in grave danger because his boat is stuck in ice and his rebellious men want to turn back to England. Even so, Walton wants to continue pursuing his extreme and absolute professional and scientific mission. Frankenstein shares his story with Walton and urges him to "learn of my miseries and do not seek to increase your own" (p. 200). On his deathbed, Frankenstein urges Walton to "seek happiness in tranquility and avoid ambition, even if it be only the apparently innocent one of distinguishing yourself in science and discoveries" (p. 208).

In writing this chapter, my desire was that young therapeutic recreation students and professionals (and all readers) would come to know their professional history and learn from past mistakes and successes. My suggestion is to follow the advice of the fictional Victor Frankenstein and seek professional development in tranquility by avoiding ambition focused in absolutism. Do not destroy something good. As future leaders in therapeutic recreation, you can help manage or resolve the damaging conflict that has harmed the credibility of this wonderful profession.

DISCUSSION QUESTIONS

1. Explain why students of therapeutic recreation should understand the history of their profession.

2. Regarding medical spas, thermal baths, and rest cures, explain why medical authority was needed to justify a leisure experience. Likewise, explain why the world-renowned Mayo Clinic, historically and in the contemporary era, provides a plethora of leisure experiences. To this end, do you agree or disagree with the following statement: a distinct feature of therapeutic recreation is its clear and direct association to recreation and leisure. Support your answer.

3. Regarding the history of therapeutic recreation, how are Jane Addams and Florence Nightingale similar? How are they different?

4. How did both world wars (as sociological events) affect the development of therapeutic recreation?

5. How did the development of Hull-House and other settlement houses affect community-based therapeutic recreation?

6. What conclusions can you draw about the philosophical battles in therapeutic recreation from 1945 through 1966? Do these past philosophical battles exist in the profession of therapeutic recreation today?

7. Explain why the utopian years of therapeutic recreation occurred from 1966 through 1984.

8. In your opinion, after the NTRS membership turned to a democratic method to identify its philosophical position, was it ethical for therapy-oriented therapeutic recreation specialists to break off and develop ATRA? Further, has the creation of ATRA helped or harmed the profession of therapeutic recreation?

9. In your interpretation of the history of therapeutic recreation, who is Victor Frankenstein and who is the monster? To this end, do you agree or disagree that the quest for grand achievement in therapeutic recreation has become the undoing of the profession?

10. Explain the difference between a strengths-based and deficits-based approach to therapeutic recreation practice.

11. Do you believe therapeutic recreation can become a global profession and find homes in other countries, such as Canada and South Africa or European countries? Explain your answer.

3

Professional Opportunities in Therapeutic Recreation

Michal Anne Lord | Ramon B. Zabriskie

LEARNING OUTCOMES

At the end of this chapter, students will be able to

- accurately explain terminology associated with careers and professionalism,
- accurately describe the characteristics of a profession,
- communicate the importance of and mechanisms for professional development,
- accurately describe primary mechanisms of professional credentialing,
- identify, explain, and use ethical concepts and decision-making models,
- differentiate between professional and nonprofessional occupations,
- accurately describe mechanisms of accreditation, and
- identify professional organizations relevant to the therapeutic recreation profession.

Therapeutic recreation is a profession. Certainly, if you ask those who have made a career of delivering therapeutic recreation services and programs, most of them will respond that therapeutic recreation is indeed a profession. But what is it that makes the practice of therapeutic recreation a profession as opposed to just a job? How does therapeutic recreation go beyond being an occupation? A **job** is a regular remunerative position; a person is paid for the completion of assigned tasks. A person with a **profession** directs his or her efforts toward service rather than only financial remuneration. A person's profession is a personal choice and reflects his or her personality, creativity, interests, and goals.

Characteristics of a Profession

A profession is a calling that requires specialized knowledge and often long academic preparation. A profession can also refer to the collective body of people engaged in a "calling." All professions include several common elements: a systematic body of knowledge, professional development, professional authority, professional credentialing, standards of practice, and a code of ethics.

Body of Knowledge

A primary prerequisite of a profession is that it must have a distinct set, or systematic body, of knowledge. Edginton, Hudson, and Scholl (2005) noted that the unique body of knowledge in the field of recreation and leisure is considered professional knowledge and consists of information drawn from three sources. These three sources, which apply to therapeutic recreation as well, are the following:

- *Scientific disciplines.* Areas of study that provide the theoretical notion of man, the environment, and how the two relate (e.g., sociology, psychology, biology, and botany)
- *Values that we profess and subscribe to.* Belief among therapeutic recreation professionals that all people have the right to recreation and leisure experiences or that recreation is the medium used to bring about physical, cognitive, emotional, or social behavioral changes in the individual
- *Applied and engineered skills.* Skills required by the professional to perform the job, such as leading an activity to assess client functionality or writing goals and objectives

Professional Development

Professional development is the exchange and transmission of professional knowledge through professional associations' conferences, workshops, and publications. A critical responsibility of being a therapeutic recreation professional is to maintain one's skills and knowledge base within the field of therapeutic recreation. A therapeutic recreation professional should be committed to professional development. Moreover, employers generally expect their employees to engage in professional development. Professional development includes continuing education, professional and civic contributions, research, and evaluation.

The therapeutic recreation professional should take advantage of continuing education opportunities available through conferences, workshops, and publications sponsored by professional associations. A responsible and committed professional attends conferences and workshops, reads professional journals and books on related topics, and advocates for in-service training opportunities

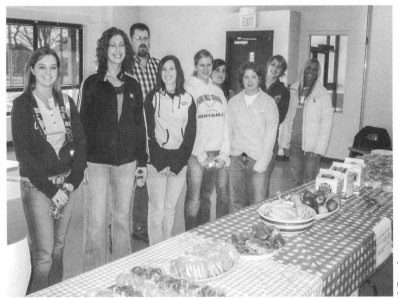

Service is a key aspect of the individual's professional development and personal growth.

© Terry Long

within his or her agency and willingly participates in them.

Involvement in professional and civic organizations provides leadership development opportunities. Opportunities may include serving on committees or boards of professional associations and organizations. Community involvement with civic organizations demonstrates professional behavior, which moves the professional beyond just doing the job. Service is a key aspect of professional development and often is an avenue to career advancement.

Responsible professionals use research related to therapeutic recreation and recreation. Therapeutic recreation professionals regularly read research in the *Therapeutic Recreation Journal*, *Annual in Therapeutic Recreation*, *American Journal of Recreation Therapy*, or other related professional journals or magazines. When appropriate, they conduct or participate in research projects. They cooperate on applied research programs within their agencies or programs. Although a faculty member or graduate student from a university or college may approach a therapeutic recreation professional to participate in research, the therapeutic recreation professional should not hesitate to initiate a research idea with university personnel. Likewise, the therapeutic recreation professional should consistently carry out evaluative research on his or her own programs and services. Evaluations and research findings can provide greater credibility of therapeutic recreation services, refine and develop standards of practice in the profession, and document the value of programs and their effect on consumers.

Career Resilience

Career resilience is an emerging aspect of professional development. The therapeutic recreation specialist should take control of his or her future by seeking out appropriate training, at his or her own expense if necessary, to be in the best position

CLIENT PORTRAIT: KIERA'S JOURNEY IN THERAPEUTIC RECREATION

One of the biggest challenges for therapeutic recreation specialists is helping clients deal with behavior management problems. Kiera, a 42-year-old woman with intellectual impairment, was one such client. Kiera lived in a group home; worked in a sheltered workshop; and regularly went with her home mates to organized recreation events, such as Special Olympics and movie night. A number of people worked with Kiera, including several certified therapeutic recreation specialists (CTRSs) who were on staff at the group home.

Current Challenge

A problem developed when Kiera started stealing things on a daily basis. Typically, the items were small things. She would steal her roommate's lunch at work, another person's soda at home, or small items from the mall. Frustrated by the disturbances that her behavior was causing at work, the group home administrator threatened to terminate Kiera's employment unless the behavior changed. Other residents at the group home started to act out toward Kiera because of her continued disregard for other people's personal property. Although Kiera had always had a history of helping herself to things that were not hers, the stealing had escalated to the point that her living situation and employment were threatened. Reprimands from the staff were becoming ineffective, and Kiera was at risk of losing her job.

Changes

When Kiera's CTRS attended a conference, she was able to speak with other specialists who were helping clients with similar problems. In fact, she found that problems like Kiera's were commonly discussed at conferences. At one presentation, she learned that negative behaviors are typically inappropriate ways of achieving some type of goal. She also learned that providing an alternative goal, or reward, is an effective way of discouraging negative behavior. Finally, she learned that a token economy can be used to delay final reward and sustain behavior over time. After talking with the presenter at the evening social, she took some ideas back to the group home staff. The staff decided to try a token economy system. For every day that Kiera refrained from stealing, she received a coupon signed by the minister at her church. Because Kiera was religious, she viewed the coupon as an especially valuable reward. After Kiera earned 10 coupons, she was rewarded with dinner at a restaurant of her choice (food was also a major motivator for her stealing). After implementation of this system, Kiera's stealing became almost nonexistent, with only one incident over the following 2 months.

for a desired career track. A person's willingness to take planned risks and guide his or her future rather than react to it will potentially provide a win–win outcome. Career resilience as outlined by Joseph A. Bucolo (2003) is the ability to

- initiate or respond to changes in the workplace,
- initiate new learning,
- reinvent oneself,
- take past successes and experiences and leverage them into future successes that will help the organization meet its anticipated goals, and
- determine one's value-added ingredient.

Building Career Resilience in Therapeutic Recreation

People can create added value and career resilience for themselves by assessing their value, just as a therapeutic recreation specialist would assess a client's needs, by asking themselves, "What is it that I do better than others in the organization? What are my specific talents or areas for future development?" As individual professionals assess their value, they should consider not only their perspective but also that of their employers or prospective employers. For example, if an agency or organization needs the therapeutic recreation specialist to do more with less, what can the therapeutic recreation specialist offer or do that will not only satisfy the immediate business needs of the employer but also advance his or her personal career objectives? Career resilience is the result of being able to deal with change positively, to use it as an opportunity for skill development and knowledge transference that can enhance the person's capabilities and future career prospects.

For example, a therapeutic recreation specialist in a Chicago rehabilitation facility recognized that the administration was cutting staff in all departments because of financial challenges (reduced income). Noting that the chief administrator had stated that all unnecessary, nonrevenue-generating services would be cut first, the therapeutic recreation specialist began to consider how he could create value as a therapeutic recreation specialist for the agency. During a subsequent staff meeting, the administrator noted that the facility had received a donation of a car with adapted driving controls from a local car dealer who hoped that the facility would start a driving program as part of its rehabilitation services. But the administrator noted that although a driving program could generate some income for the facility, the budget included no money to hire an instructor. The therapeutic recreation specialist realized that if he volunteered to do the driving program in addition to performing his therapeutic recreation services responsibilities, he would be creating value by generating income while enabling the rehabilitation facility to carry out the wishes of a donor. Additionally, the therapeutic recreation specialist would be adding to the menu of therapeutic recreation services as well as to his own résumé and skill set. Because of the therapeutic recreation specialist's initiative, the driving program was implemented, a critical need of consumers was met, a donor's wish was recognized, the value of therapeutic recreation services was enhanced, and the therapeutic recreation specialist kept his job despite the downsizing of the rehabilitation facility.

Professional Authority

Professional authority is the ability of a profession to hold its members accountable. Professional authority generally starts with a dialogue on professional values and acceptable tenets of practice, which ultimately translates into professional standards of practice. Professional authority is how a professional responds in light of shared socialization (the norms of accepted practice) and internalized expertise (knowledge and personal expertise—individual skill and judgment). Professional authority depends on a person's technical skills rather than position or office. Edginton, Compton, and Hanson (1989) said that professional authority "is created and exists when an occupation is, generally speaking, free from the consequences of its actions and has monopolized services" (p. 55).

Therapeutic recreation specialists tend to be the sole providers of therapeutic recreation services (monopolized services). In a few settings, other health care providers may endeavor to offer activities, but they usually lack the philosophical or theoretical background necessary to provide effective services. In contrast, therapeutic recreation as a profession has had professional standards of practice for the past 30 or more years and more recently has added standards of practice for paraprofessionals and guidelines for internships.

Professional Credentialing

Professional credentialing serves to document the fact that society accepts the authority of a profession; the profession thus has the sanction of the community. A profession (through professional organizations or associations) defines who it is or what it does, and credentialing bodies establish the minimum standards required to perform the professional duties and responsibilities. The basic purpose of a professional association is to improve the level of practice within the profession. Promoting professional competence is extremely important.

The purpose of credentialing is multifaceted. Credentialing provides evidence that a professional has acquired a body of knowledge and competencies that includes theory, philosophy, and practice within a given field. It also provides insurance that an individual has met specific standards or criteria regarding education, experience, and continuing professional development. Finally, credentialing is a strategy of risk management in that services provided by a credentialed professional offer reasonable protection for the consumer, safeguarding the public from incompetent, unauthorized people claiming to be within the profession. Thus, credentialing enables the public, government, or third-party payers to distinguish between those who have attained some qualifying level of competency from those who have not. Credentialing enhances the credibility of the individual and the profession. Another benefit of credentialing is that, in the case of licensure, it establishes a legal definition and requirement for professional practice within state law.

Professional credentialing can occur at the state or national level. The nationally recognized certifying body for therapeutic recreation professionals is the National Council for Therapeutic Recreation Certification (NCTRC), which oversees the national certification program for CTRSs. Some states have therapeutic recreation credentialing bodies and processes as well. As of 2018, Utah, North Carolina, Oklahoma, New Hampshire, and the District of Columbia (Washington, DC) had state licensure requirements for practicing therapeutic recreation professionals. Additionally, a therapeutic recreation professional may seek to become a certified parks and recreation professional (CPRP), which is governed by the National Certification Board (NCB) and affiliated with the National Recreation and Park Association (NRPA), through either the direct national program or the certification program of the state association.

The three main types of professional credentialing are registration, certification, and licensure. **Registration** and **certification** are forms of voluntary credentialing, whereas **licensure** is a legal requirement that must be met by anyone who wishes to practice the profession in a particular state. Professional credentials are generally in effect for a specified period (2 to 5 years) and are maintained or renewed by completing a required number of continuing education units (CEUs), submitting verification of CEUs or other professional contributions (professional presentations or publications or leadership service), and paying a fee. Some credentials, such as the CTRS, require the certified professional to pay an annual maintenance fee. Table 3.1 shows the similarities and differences among the types of credentialing.

Professionals can take two professional credentialing paths, academic or equivalency, to document their ability to meet minimum knowledge, skill, and experience standards. Eligibility requirements for the CTRS may be met through the academic path or one of two equivalency paths (see table 3.2). The academic pathway is more useful for college students seeking a degree in recreation or therapeutic recreation, whereas the equivalency paths are often useful for individuals who have discovered the profession after having received a degree in another area. Note that these pathways are regularly updated by NCTRC, and individuals seeking certification should verify current eligibility requirements with the council. For example, all three paths will require a sixth course in therapeutic recreation (TR) after January 1, 2022.

Code of Ethics

A **code of ethics** represents the official moral ideology of the professional group. In the helping professions, a code of ethics is a basic requirement for recognition as a professional body. An ethical code governing professional behavior is a characteristic shared by the majority of human services occupations and symbolizes autonomy of the professional body.

Ethics deals with the duties and obligations of professionals to their consumers (service recipients), the profession, and the wider public. Professional ethics considers **moral conduct**, or how one should act; **moral character**, or what sort of person one ought to be; and **moral community**, or how society should be constructed to enable ethical people to act ethically. Moral conduct, character, and community make ethical behavior possible and sustain moral acts. Ignorance, or lack of knowledge, of professional ethics may well be the primary cause of misguided, inappropriate professional behavior.

Table 3.1 Types of Professional Credentialing

Aspects	Registration	Certification	Licensure
Purpose	Provides a record in official directory	Authorizes adequate training, ensures minimum competencies	Gives permission to practice
Responsibility	Created and monitored by professional organization	Monitored by state, national, or autonomous credentialing board	State board created by law
Effects	The person—voluntary	The person—voluntary	The practice—required by state law
Process	Application and fee, optional exam	Application and fee, required exam	Application and fee, required exam
Criteria	Minimum standards met through application, tend to be flexible and reflect constantly changing criteria	Minimum standards set regarding education and experience, specified criteria for changes through policies and procedures or bylaws	Specific standards set regarding minimum competencies, specified criteria for changes through legislative amendments
Outcome	Directory or list of professionals registered	Professional certificate	License to practice
Renewal	May be contingent on professional development (CEUs)	Contingent on professional development (CEUs)	Contingent on professional development (CEUs)

Ethical principles (norms) prescribe responsibilities for the individual. They allow for professional discretion and judgment. They do not necessarily determine what ought to be done in a given situation. Instead, they serve as a guide for decision making, which may require a person to weigh and balance multiple principles, one against another.

The ethical principles found in the American Therapeutic Recreation Association (ATRA) Code of Ethics are the standards for ethical behavior in the therapeutic recreation profession. Below is an outline of the 10 principles in the ATRA Code of Ethics:

- *Principle of beneficence.* The duty to promote good to further a person's health and welfare by actively making efforts to provide for his or her well-being; maximizing possible benefits; and relieving, lessening, or minimizing possible harm. In other words, a therapeutic recreation professional ought to do good to others.
- *Principle of nonmalfeasance.* Relates to beneficence and means that one has a duty not to injure or harm another person. A

professional has the obligation to use his or her knowledge, skills, abilities, and judgment to help persons while respecting their decisions and protecting them from harm. Above all do no harm.

- *Principle of autonomy.* The duty to preserve and protect the right of each individual to make his or her own choices. Each individual is to be given the opportunity to determine his or her own course of action in accordance with a plan freely chosen. In the case of individuals who are unable to exercise autonomy with regard to their care, professionals have the duty to respect the decisions of their qualified legal representative.
- *Principle of justice.* Includes the responsibility of ensuring that individuals are served fairly and that there is equity in the distribution of services. Individuals should receive services without regard to race, color, creed, gender, sexual orientation, age, disability/disease, or social and financial status.
- *Principle of fidelity.* Includes the obligation, first and foremost, to be loyal and faithful

Table 3.2 CTRS Eligibility Paths

	Academic path	Equivalency path A	Equivalency path B
Education: baccalaureate degree or higher	Major in TR or recreation with TR emphasis Minimum of 18 hours in TR or recreation with a minimum of 15 hr specifically in TR 18 hr of support course work to include anatomy or physiology (3), abnormal psychology (3), human growth and development throughout the life span (3), and the remaining hours from social sciences and humanities	Degree (area of degree is not specified by NCTRC) Minimum of 18 hr in TR or recreation with a minimum of 15 hr specifically in TR 24 hr of support course work from social sciences and humanities	Degree (area of degree is not specified by NCTRC) Minimum of 18 hr in TR or recreation with a minimum of 15 hr specifically in TR 18 hr of support course work to include anatomy or physiology (3), abnormal psychology (3), human growth and development throughout the life span (3), and the remaining hours from social sciences and humanities
Experience: work or internship	Internship under an on-site CTRS to include 560 hr over 14 consecutive weeks	Minimum of 5 years of full-time paid experience (minimum of 32 hr per week in direct TR services)	1 year of full-time paid experience (minimum of 1,500 hr or 52 weeks) under supervision of a CTRS and no more than 5 years before applying

Note: All hours above reflect semester hours. Refer to NCTRC regarding quarter hour requirements. Refer to NCTRC.org for the most current certification standards. All three tracks will require a 6th course in therapeutic recreation (TR) after January 1, 2022.

and meet commitments made to persons receiving services. In addition, professionals have a secondary obligation to colleagues, agencies, and the profession.

- *Principle of veracity.* The duty to be truthful and honest. Deception, by being dishonest or omitting what is true, should always be avoided.
- *Principle of informed consent.* Is related to providing services characterized by mutual respect and shared decision making. Professionals are responsible for providing each individual receiving service with information regarding the services; benefits; outcomes; length of treatment; expected activities; risks; and limitations, including the professional's training and credentials. Informed consent is obtained when information needed to make a reasoned decision is provided by the professional to competent persons seeking services who then decide whether to accept the treatment.
- *Principle of confidentiality and privacy.* Includes the duty to disclose all relevant information to persons seeking services; professionals also have a corresponding duty not to disclose private information to third

parties. If a situation arises that requires disclosure of confidential information about an individual (i.e., to protect the individual's welfare or the interest of others), the professional has the responsibility to inform the individual served of the circumstances.

- *Principle of competence.* Includes the responsibility to maintain and improve one's knowledge related to the profession and demonstrate current, competent practice to persons served. In addition, professionals have an obligation to maintain their credentials (licensure, certification, and/or registration).
- *Principle of laws and regulations.* Includes the responsibility to comply with local, state, and federal laws and regulations and ATRA policies governing the profession of recreational therapy.

The therapeutic recreation professional and agencies or institutions who employ them have a responsibility to demonstrate that the community can trust the profession and the behaviors of its workers will not injure consumers. A profession's code of ethics provides guidance to professionals for maintaining high standards of ethical behavior in the workplace.

Ethical Decision Making

One of the more challenging aspects of any profession is identifying and addressing ethical dilemmas. At first, this task seems to simply be a matter of doing the right thing and following the formal codes written by ATRA or the service-providing agency. In truth, making real decisions is rarely this simple. For example, accepting valuable gifts from a long-standing client in a mental health facility would typically not be seen as ethical. Essentially, a client–therapeutic recreation specialist relationship is different from a friendship because the balance of power is not equal. This

fact opens the door for the professional to manipulate and take advantage of the client. At the same time, accepting a token of appreciation, such as a framed photo of the client and therapist on an outing together, may be acceptable if the meaning of the gift is clear. The challenge in this example is determining when a gift becomes an ethical compromise. Does this judgment rest on the value of the gift, the context in which it is given, or both?

In addressing such dilemmas, structured codes of ethics as well as guidelines for decision making can be helpful. Figure 3.1 illustrates an example of an ethical decision-making model (Long, 2000). Note that the model focuses on identifying all

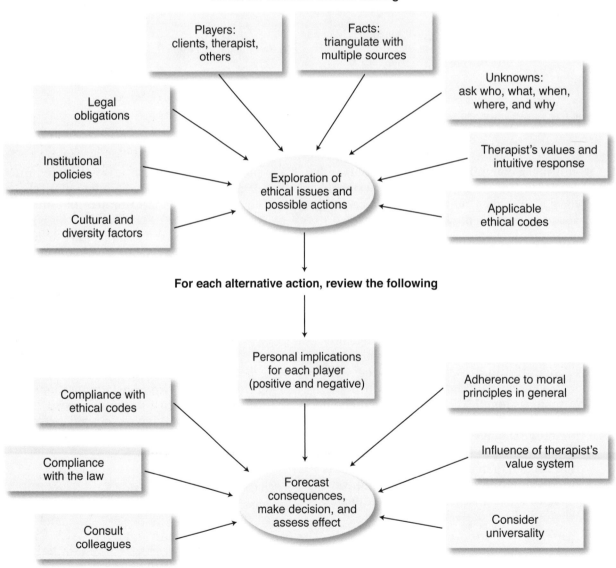

Figure 3.1 Problem-solving model for ethical decision making.

available information and repeatedly reviewing the consequences of any potential action to be taken. The model assumes that the most ethical decision is to be determined by weighing the amount of positive or negative consequences resulting from each possible action. Even with a structured guide for gathering and analyzing information, determining what is best requires honest, objective consideration of difficult scenarios. Thus, a competent professional becomes familiar with available sources of information, including the advice of other professionals.

Consider the ethical scenarios that follow. Is enough information provided to make a decision? What additional information would you seek before making a decision or judgment? Which of the 10 ethical principles listed earlier apply to each scenario? The first scenario is a hypothetical situation, whereas the last three scenarios are real-life situations that have been reported in the past.

- A CTRS has been working with a client who is recovering from an automobile accident that caused a severe injury to both of his legs. After 4 months of intense rehabilitation, the client and CTRS began attending adapted sports clinics and events together as part of an outpatient leisure education program. They also spent several scheduled sessions in the community participating in leisure activities to identify and address physical and environmental barriers related to the client's injuries. On their last outing, the client invited the CTRS to attend a jazz concert at a local nightclub. When the therapist replied that she didn't work on that particular night, the client stated, "I know, that's why I'm asking."

- A CTRS working in a substance abuse program was asked on occasion by the substance abuse counselor to fill in as the lead therapist during group therapy sessions. Because the CTRS demonstrated that she could adequately run the group, the counselor asked the CTRS to cover one particular group on a full-time basis. When the substance abuse counselors all received pay adjustments, the CTRS filed a complaint with the administrators that she had not received the same adjustment despite her work with the program.

- A mental health patient complained to hospital administrators that one of her

therapists has been using "lap hugs" as an intervention during self-esteem groups. The client reported that the therapist periodically instructs patients to sit on his lap or the lap of a fellow client for hugs of encouragement during sessions. When approached about the issue, the therapist replied that the technique is legitimate and that he told the clients that the activity is voluntary.

- A professional working with a depressed 22-year-old homosexual male suggested to his client that most of his problems stem from his homosexuality and that his family is likely to continue to reject him unless he "changes." The professional also told the client that unless he finds God and gives up his sexual lifestyle, his family will never accept him. Two weeks after breaking up with his boyfriend, the client was admitted to a residential therapy program for depression.

Enforcement of Ethical Codes

The current code of ethics for therapeutic recreation professionals is the ATRA Code of Ethics. The principles in this code are accepted by the profession, and violation of the code can result in reprimands from credentialing organizations, such as state licensure boards or the NCTRC. Possible reprimands could be as severe as loss of license or certification but sometimes involve probationary periods and requirements for additional participation in various continuing education efforts. As an example, in reference to the last case study, if the therapeutic recreation professional did not lose his license or certification, he may be asked to take part in professional training regarding best practices for working with gay/lesbian clients. In addition, service-providing agencies may develop internal codes of ethics and enforce additional reprimands, such as probation, training, and termination. Finally, ethical code violations that violate laws or harm others may leave the therapeutic recreation professional open to criminal or civil legal action.

Standards of Practice

Wouldn't it be great, particularly for a new therapeutic recreation specialist entering the profession, to have a clear and comprehensive set of guidelines and expectations (what to do and how to do it) outlining how to provide the very best, consistent, and effective therapeutic recreation services possible? That is exactly what **professional standards of practice** are. Professional standards of practice are a set of guidelines for providing quality and effective services that are continually updated and refined by experienced professionals. The professionals understand the necessary competencies, regulatory and reimbursement protocols, and best practices and services that lead to consistent effective therapeutic outcomes. Such standards for our profession can be found in *Standards for the Practice of Recreational Therapy* (ATRA, 2013). "These standards and criteria and the self-assessment guide are designed to assist the recreational therapy professional to assure the systematic provision of safe, effective, and quality recreational therapy treatment and care that results in outcomes that are achieved on a consistent and predictable basis valued by stakeholders" (ATRA, 2013, p. 9). The current standards of practice are listed here with a brief description of each standard.

1. *Assessment.* The recreational therapist conducts an individual assessment to collect the systematic, comprehensive, and accurate data necessary to determine a course of action and subsequent individualized treatment plan.

2. *Treatment planning.* The recreational therapist plans and develops an individualized treatment plan that identifies goals and evidence-based treatment intervention strategies.

3. *Plan implementation.* The recreational therapist implements an individualized treatment plan, using evidence-based practice, to restore, remediate, or rehabilitate functional abilities in order to improve and maintain independence and quality of life as well as to reduce or eliminate activity limitations and restrictions to participation in life situations caused by an illness or disabling condition.

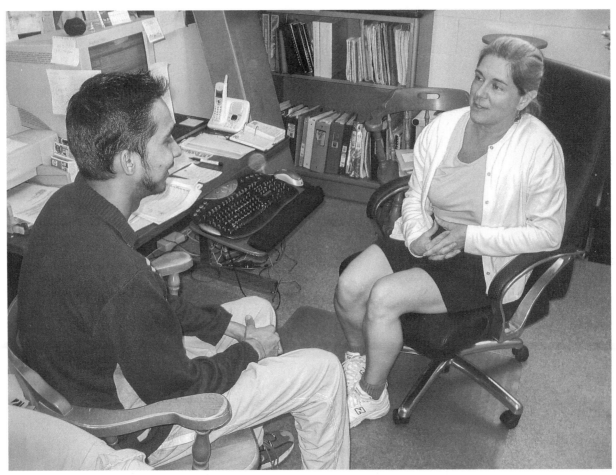

Professional standards of practice outline expectations for providing the best therapeutic recreation services.

4. *Reassessment and evaluation.* The recreational therapist systematically reassesses, evaluates, and compares the patient's/client's progress relative to the individualized treatment plan.

5. *Discharge and transition planning.* The recreational therapist develops a discharge plan in collaboration with the patient/client, family, significant others, and the treatment team members in order to discharge the patient/client or to continue treatment and aftercare, as needed.

6. *Prevention, safety planning, and risk management.* The recreational therapist systematically plans to improve patient/client and staff safety by planning for prevention and reduction of risks in order to prevent injury and reduce potential or actual harm.

7. *Ethical conduct.* The recreational therapist adheres to the *ATRA Code of Ethics* in providing patient/client treatment and care that are humane and professional.

8. *Written plan of operation.* Recreational therapy treatment and care are governed by a written plan of operation that is based upon the *ATRA Standards for the Practice of Recreational Therapy*, state and federal laws and regulations, requirements of regulatory and accrediting agencies, and payers and employer's policies and procedures as appropriate.

9. *Staff qualification and competency assessment.* Recreational therapy staff meet the defined qualifications, demonstrate competency, maintain appropriate credentials, and have opportunities for competency development.

10. *Quality improvement.* There exist objective and systematic processes for continuously improving patient/client safety and for identifying opportunities to improve recreational therapy treatment and care and patient/client outcomes.

11. *Resource management.* Recreational therapy treatment and care are provided in an effective and efficient manner that reflects the reasonable and appropriate use of resources.

12. *Program evaluation.* Recreational therapy staff engages in routine, systematic program evaluation and research for the purpose of determining the appropriateness and effectiveness of recreational therapy treatment and care provided.

Adapted by permission from American Therapeutic Recreation Association, *Standards for the Practice of Recreational Therapy* (Reston, VA: ATR, 2013), 9.

Standards of practice in any profession not only provide guidelines and expectations for quality effective services, but they also help standardize practice and curriculum in professional preparation. Another interesting thing about standards of practice is that a professional in the field is not "required" to use them. They are simply voluntary guidelines developed by the best therapeutic recreation professionals and educators, including decades of cumulative knowledge, experience, and expertise for the overall practice and provision of therapeutic recreation. It certainly seems that the knowledge and use of these standards of practice would be absolutely essential and invaluable for any therapeutic recreation professional.

Professional Culture

A **professional culture** is made up of the customary beliefs, norms, or traits of the profession. Professional associations often define the professional culture. The typical professional culture of a therapeutic recreation specialist is consumer focused. Serving as an advocate on behalf of the person with disabilities is an important responsibility of a therapeutic recreation specialist, whatever the setting or delivery system. Therapeutic recreation professionals believe that leisure and recreation are basic human rights and critical to the health and well-being of people and to their quality of life and life satisfaction. Therefore, therapeutic recreation professionals are committed to providing services that are beneficial, dignified, and empowering. Therapeutic recreation specialists are committed to making a difference in the lives of those whom they serve through a continuum of care. Therapeutic recreation professionals believe that only professionals with training, education, and credentials in therapeutic recreation should provide therapeutic recreation services.

Professional Preparation in Therapeutic Recreation

Those who want to work at the professional level in therapeutic recreation must complete a program of study at an accredited college or university. Those seeking certification may also choose to attend a college or university that offers an accredited curriculum in therapeutic recreation or an accredited curriculum in recreation with a therapeutic recreation emphasis. (Ask your instructor or adviser about which type of program your school offers.) Professional preparation programs generally require students to complete an internship under qualified supervision (a certified therapeutic recreation specialist). Ultimately, those who complete a professional preparation path will receive a bachelor's degree or, for teaching or administrative positions in therapeutic recreation, a master's or doctoral degree.

Accreditation

Accreditation is the credentialing of an academic institution. In other words, it is the process of evaluation for an academic institution involving the institution and a third party (an external accreditation body) in order to be held accountable to certain standards in the provision of higher education. The purpose of accreditation is and always has been to protect the consumer and assure quality of the educational experience (Schray, 2006). There are basically two kinds of accreditation in higher education today, institutional accreditation and specialized, or programmatic, accreditation. Institutional accreditation is the process that evaluates the quality of postsecondary institutions as a whole and confirms "that an institution fulfills its mission and goals and is equal in quality to other comparable intuitions" (Zabriskie & McCormick, 2000, p. 32). This kind of accreditation is provided by regional accrediting bodies, such as the North Central Association of Colleges and Schools, and there are more than 7,800 accredited institutions across the United States today (Council for Higher Education Accreditation [CHEA], 2012).

Specialized, or programmatic, accreditation focuses on a specific school, department, or professional preparation curriculum that prepares students to enter a given profession. This kind of accreditation process is conducted by external accrediting bodies related to a specific profession and assures that knowledge, skills, and abilities considered important or essential by standards of practice, professional competencies, and professionals in the profession are being transmitted effectively to students in the higher education process. There are well over 22,600 accredited programs in health-related professions alone in the United States and Canada today (CHEA, 2012).

In the profession of therapeutic recreation, there are currently two programmatic accrediting bodies that accredit undergraduate therapeutic recreation programs. The Council on Accreditation of Parks, Recreation, Tourism and Related Professions (COAPRT) has published *Guidelines for Learning Outcomes for Therapeutic Recreation Education* (COAPRT, 2012). COAPRT allows an undergraduate therapeutic recreation program the option to become accredited as either a stand-alone program in therapeutic recreation or one program among others in a department seeking COAPRT accreditation. To see those standards and guidelines, visit the COAPRT Standards web page (www.nrpa.org/certification/accreditation/coaprt/coaprt-standards/). The Commission on Accreditation of Allied Health Education Programs (CAAHEP) through the Committee on Accreditation of Recreational Therapy Education (CARTE) also provides programmatic accreditation for undergraduate programs (Skalko, 2013). Their standards and guidelines can be found by viewing the Standards and Guidelines for the Accreditation of Educational Programs in Recreational Therapy document (www.caahep.org/documents/file/For-Program-Directors/CARTEStandardsand-Guidelines.pdf). Both of these accrediting bodies and their programmatic accreditation processes are recognized by CHEA. Most therapeutic recreation academic programs in the United States and Canada are accredited by one or sometimes both of these accrediting bodies. If you don't already know, you should certainly talk to one of your faculty members to see whether your program is currently accredited. This kind of accreditation doesn't only provide verification that a college's or university's academic program meets minimum standards in professional preparation and student learning outcomes; "the process also serves to reduce variation in academic preparation in a given profession and therefore ensures some level of consistency in professional practice among graduates" (Skalko, 2013, p. 246). Overall, accreditation is the mechanism that continually improves the quality of academic preparation within a profession and helps students identify acceptable universities to acquire the competencies necessary to enter professional practice.

Gaining Experience in Therapeutic Recreation

Professional preparation is more than just academic course work. Experience is a valuable teacher. Students and new professionals should seek volunteer opportunities to gain knowledge

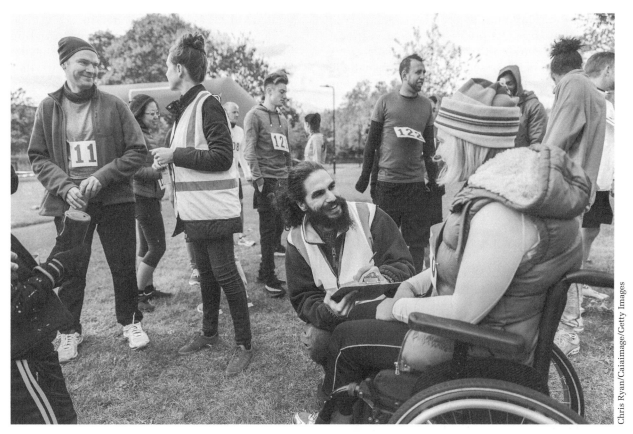

Volunteering gives aspiring professionals valuable experience with the variety of individuals they might one day expect to serve as clients.

and experience as well as build their résumés. Volunteer experience is often as marketable as work experience. Volunteer experience can help students or new professionals gain experience with other special population groups and complement their work experience. The goal is to gain experience with a variety of disability groups, ages, and delivery systems. If a person works or interns in a clinical setting, he or she should seek volunteer opportunities in the community. If a person serves an adult clientele during work or an internship, he or she should consider volunteer experience with children. For example, perhaps the therapeutic recreation professional or student's first job or internship is with a physical rehabilitation facility that serves primarily patients who have experienced a stroke. The person could seek volunteer opportunities with Special Olympics (for those with intellectual disabilities) or Easterseals (youth with disabilities), coach a beep baseball team (for those who are visually impaired), or assist with a community wheelchair basketball or tennis program.

Certainly, a depth of experience with one disability group or age group is valuable when seeking a job in that particular area, but having volunteer experience with other disability groups, ages, and delivery systems will help prepare the student for other available therapeutic recreation positions. Additionally, a person can glean program activity ideas, instructional techniques, and behavioral management strategies from volunteer experiences that could have application in future internship positions or work settings.

Professional Organizations

Professional organizations exist to support professionals within a chosen field. Their purpose is to articulate the practice and benefits of the profession, to promote and foster the advancement and growth of the profession, and to improve the services of those who practice it. People in therapeutic recreation, in both clinical and community settings, are supported by and can become involved in national and state professional organizations. Many state parks and recreation associations also have branches or sections with a specialized focus, such as therapeutic recreation. In some locales, state or national organizations have local or regional units. For example, state associations may have geographic regions or districts that serve the function of sharing information and networking, providing professional development, advocating for public policy, or enhancing public awareness at a grassroots level.

Benefits of professional association membership may vary to some degree, but associations generally offer benefits in five areas:

- *Sponsoring informative meetings and educational programs.* Training and educational development are central to fulfilling the mission of the professional organization.
- *Publishing literature that reflects the body of knowledge of the profession and could contribute to improving practice within the profession.* Professional organizations may commission research projects that will contribute to the body of knowledge, but more often, they distribute findings and other relevant information through their publications, conferences, and meetings.
- *Providing for credentialing or maintenance of professional credentials.* Organizations promote and support credentialing through CEUs to maintain licensure or certification.
- *Defining professional behavior.* Professional organizations develop and promote such things as professional codes of ethics and standards of practice. Professional behavior, also known as **professionalism**, occurs when professionals perform competently and demonstrate high moral character in fulfilling obligations to their constituents.
- *Recognizing change factors that could influence the profession of therapeutic recreation and the careers of those within the field.* Professional organizations strive to keep the profession current and relevant.

American Therapeutic Recreation Association

The current national membership organization in the United States is the American Therapeutic Recreation Association (ATRA). ATRA was incorporated in 1984 as a nonprofit grassroots organization and is the national membership organization representing the interests and needs of therapeutic recreation professionals today. It currently has over 2,200 professional members, including many from several other countries. The association is directed by an elected board of directors and has over 35 volunteer committees and task forces focused on issue-vital professional areas, such as public policy, coverage and reimbursement, diagnostic specialty groups, higher education, and evidence-based practice. To find out more about ATRA and become a member, you can visit their website (www.atra-online.com/).

Canadian Therapeutic Recreation Association

The Canadian Therapeutic Recreation Association (CTRA) is the national association of practitioners in the field of therapeutic recreation in Canada and was formally incorporated in 1996. Its mission is to advocate for the therapeutic recreation profession and its membership. The primary focus of the organization is to unite therapeutic recreation specialists across Canada by providing opportunities for members to be informed of trends and opportunities to further enhance practice and advocacy efforts. CTRA strives to work in partnership with members by cohosting its annual general meeting and conference with a provincial association. In 2009, the CTRA membership voted in favor of endorsing the NCTRC's CTRS credential as the national credential in Canada. There has been a 400 percent increase in the number of certified professionals in the past 12 years. Currently, CTRA has 930 members. To find out more about CTRA and to become a member, you can visit their website (http://canadian-tr.org/).

Diversional & Recreation Therapy Australia

Although there are several small professional therapeutic recreation–based networks operating within the various state and territory health systems in the Australia setting (e.g., Queensland Leisure Therapy Network), Diversional & Recreation Therapy Australia (DRTA) has emerged in recent years as the principal voice of the therapeutic recreation movement in Australia. The association and its state affiliates, with a membership in excess of 2,000 nationwide, are committed to promoting, fostering, and advancing

THOMAS "ANDY" FERNANDEZ, CTRS, CPRP

Education: BA in Psychology (Minor in Special Ed/Rehab), University of Arizona
MA in Recreation, University of Northern Colorado
Position: Adaptive Recreation and Older Adult/Senior Services Manager
Organization: City of Eugene Adaptive Recreation Services, Eugene, Oregon
Special Awards

* LILAC Award, Lane Independent Living Alliance (2011)

* Staff Recognition Award, International Human Rights, Eugene City (2007)

* Organizational Citation, National Therapeutic Recreation Society (2006)

* Presidential Citation, National Therapeutic Recreation Society (2000, 2002)

* New Professional of the Year Award, National Therapeutic Recreation Society (1999)

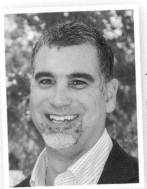

Courtesy of T. Andy Fernandez.

My Career

I specifically chose positions with premier agencies that would give me the opportunity to gain valuable experience in community-based therapeutic recreation. I have worked with the University of Arizona adaptive athletics program, the Breckenridge Outdoor Education Center, the City of Boulder EXPAND program, and the City of Las Vegas adaptive recreation program, and I was the creator and supervisor of the City of Reno inclusion services program. I currently manage the older adult services in the adaptive recreation services division of the City of Eugene. My responsibilities include managing a team of 10 full-time employees, four facilities, over 60 community partnerships, and a $1.5 million budget. I supervised the restructure of two recreation service areas into one service section and am currently managing a $5 million renovation to our senior center. I have also facilitated community needs assessments for both older adults and adaptive recreation ser-

vices. I believe our ability to provide meaningful community-based health and wellness programs to our aging population is key to improving quality of life while reducing the costs for people of all abilities.

The adaptive recreation services division is the primary public provider of community recreation services for people with disabilities in Eugene, Oregon. Direct services include recreation programs adapted to serve people with disabilities, individualized and group skills training, assistance to make activities accessible, adapted equipment, and referral or information assistance. Our staff provides training, consultation, and adapted equipment to city departments and community groups to facilitate the inclusion of people with disabilities in their programs, including compliance with the Americans with Disabilities Act. The division also provides students and volunteers with crucial hands-on experience and training while working with a variety of disabilities and populations.

At this point in my career, I recognize the huge impact a community-based program can have on the people we serve. It can sometimes be a grind, but systematic changes in policies and procedures, funding, accessibility, and barrier removal can do as much as or more than clinical programs to enhance quality of life and change perceptions of disability.

My Advice to You

Always apply for a position you are interested in, even if it's just to test whether you qualify or not. Get involved professionally on projects, committees, and programs. Volunteer for whatever project you can get involved in. Say *yes* to everything and get the experience. Experience is the top résumé builder and is what separates the job candidates from the job applicants.

the development of the profession of diversional therapy in Australia and internationally. Its stated mission is to ensure that the practice of diversional therapy continues to be viable and relevant and contributes to the well-being of clients and the community while encouraging educational,

professional, and personal development in its members. Diversional therapy is considered to be a client-centered practice and recognizes that leisure and recreational experiences are the right of all individuals. Professionals design and facilitate interventions intended to support, challenge, and enhance the psychological, spiritual, social, emotional, and physical well-being of individuals. To find out more about DRTA and become a member, you can visit their website (http://diversionaltherapy.org.au/).

Professional Networking

Networking, an important tool for advancement, leadership, power, and influence, is related to organizational variables such as socialization, motivation, commitment, and innovation. Networking, as an individual skill, is the ability to create and maintain an effective and diverse system of resources, made possible by using relevant information, having good working relations, and maintaining and communicating a good track record. The professional should know the players within a network and their responsibilities, perspectives, personalities, and sources of power. The professional should be able to identify and articulate the goals of each group and person involved in the network as well as his or her willingness to act on goals.

As a critical strategy in the field of therapeutic recreation, networking serves several useful purposes:

- To develop skills and accomplish activities
- To bridge the gaps between or within functions of a job or an organization
- To foster communication, both formal and informal
- To gather and manage information
- To facilitate exchange or interchange of resources

Professionals working within the field of therapeutic recreation and recreation are often masters of networking because collaboration with others is a prerequisite to getting projects, programs, and events accomplished. Collaboration is particularly important for the one- or two-person therapeutic recreation work unit within an agency or institution. Networking is a process of sharing information, resources, or technical assistance for the purpose of achieving common goals. Information sharing eliminates the need to reinvent the wheel and often strengthens a person's resolve to pursue a cause or innovative idea; knowing that others share similar thoughts can foster increased confidence within a professional entity. Through

the sharing of information and resources by professionals or agencies, a professional association can voice concerns and identify issues to policy makers or regulatory bodies, demonstrate the effect and value of service delivery, or heighten public awareness. Through networking, organizations or groups can demonstrate that many people are involved and the scope of involvement—geographic, professional preparation, financial, political, and social—is broad.

Organizational networking is either **intraorganizational**, that is, operating within an organization to reach a shared goal and ultimately advance the organization, or **interorganizational**, that is, operating among organizations that share similar characteristics, such as populations served, service delivery system, goals, or issues.

For example, a therapeutic recreation specialist might network intraorganizationally (share information) with nursing staff, food service, and transportation to ensure the success of a community reentry outing. A therapeutic recreation specialist needs the cooperation of these support services to have consumers ready for the outing—medications given, meals concluded or perhaps prepared for the outing, and transportation provided. Through collaboration, all services contribute to the goal of quality service and care of clientele. A therapeutic recreation specialist might also share resources to assist another service unit, such as recruiting or scheduling volunteers for a fund-raiser or recruiting carnival booths and games from community parks and recreation peers for the hospital's employee picnic.

On an interorganizational level, all therapeutic recreation specialists within a community, both clinically and community based, might work together to promote Therapeutic Recreation Week during the second week in July. They would not only work within their own agencies but also persuade the city council to make a proclamation and encourage the media to run stories focused on therapeutic recreation during the week. Another example would be for therapeutic recreation specialists to join their parks and recreation agency peers in visiting their state or federal legislative representatives. The goal would be to increase the lawmakers' awareness of the importance of the reauthorization of the Individuals with Disabilities Education Act and the inclusion of therapeutic recreation and recreation as a related service or of the need for increased Land and Water Conservation Fund appropriations.

Summary

Therapeutic recreation is a profession. Like other allied health professions, therapeutic recreation embraces the distinguishing key elements of a profession: a systematic body of knowledge, professional development, professional authority, professional credentialing, standards of practice, and a code of ethics. A therapeutic recreation specialist may provide treatment or educational services and recreation activities to people with disabilities or illnesses in health care settings or community-based delivery systems or through combinations or variations of both. Emerging professional career opportunities within therapeutic recreation will tend to be in one- or two-person work units, such as a therapeutic recreation specialist in the schools or emergency care intervention, or an inclusion specialist, rather than in a larger service department. A professional association often dictates the professional culture, provides professional development or continuing education alternatives and networking opportunities, and defines the profession for professional credentialing at the state or national level. Ultimately, therapeutic recreation specialists are committed to making a difference in the lives of those whom they serve through a continuum of care.

DISCUSSION QUESTIONS

1. When and why should a therapeutic recreation specialist begin addressing career resilience?

2. Does having a professional credential make a therapeutic recreation professional more qualified or a better practitioner? Why or why not?

3. What are the benefits of professional credentialing for the individual therapeutic recreation specialist? For the employer? For the consumer?

4. How does the therapeutic recreation profession determine, that is, define and measure, professional competence?

5. Maintaining client confidentiality is an ethical responsibility of the therapeutic recreation specialist. Is confidentiality absolute or situational? Why?

6. How does the professional (moral agent) contend with consumers' choices that are immoral in nature?

7. Why and how are professional organizations important to the vitality of the profession? How and why are organizations beneficial to the individual specialist?

4

Person-First Philosophy in Therapeutic Recreation

Mary Ann Devine | **Jessie L. Bennett**

LEARNING OUTCOMES

At the end of this chapter, students will be able to

- describe the person-first concepts related to people with disabilities,
- explain the role of person-first terminology as it relates to reflecting a person-first philosophy,
- discuss the issues of multidimensionality of barriers relative to a person-first philosophy,
- explain the role of attitudes toward people with disabilities as they relate to embracing differences,
- identify the factors that influence one's attitude toward people with disabilities, and
- understand various philosophical models of service delivery and their relationship to therapeutic recreation.

Our differences make us interesting, but our humanity makes us the same. This chapter will explore the differences between people with and without disabilities and challenge you to view these differences in a positive way. All too often, society places people with and without disabilities at opposing ends of a spectrum. This notion has led to a collective focus on how we are different from one another rather than on what we have in common. This emphasis on differences has led to stereotypes and stigmas about those with disabilities that have prevented their full participation in community life.

Therapeutic recreation specialists have often served as agents of change. By adopting an attitude that celebrates rather than discourages differences, we can continue to advocate for the rights and full participation of people with disabilities in our communities. This chapter will explore person-first, attitudinal, and service delivery aspects of disability. The emphasis will be on our perceptions and belief systems about those with disabilities and how those beliefs affect our profession. The chapter will conclude with a discussion about the role of therapeutic recreation relative to people with disabilities.

Who Is the Person With a Disability?

Over the years, people with disabilities have been stereotyped as limited in potential. This generalization is based on a comparison of them with people who do not have the same characteristic. Labels drive such stereotypes, and these labels can originate from several sources, some of which were originally intended for good. Labels referring to disabilities have been medically based, such as the labeling of a person as blind because he or she cannot see. Labels can be socially based. For example, a person who uses a wheelchair may be assumed to be disabled in ways that exceed his or her actual impairments. Labels can even be legally based and are often required for the provision of supportive services in school and recreation. For example, to qualify for certain special education services, a child must fall into specific diagnostic categories, such as autism or attention-deficit/hyperactivity disorder. Regardless of the mechanisms through which a person is labeled, the person with a disability is someone who has a limitation in some aspect of his or her functioning according to our social norms.

All people tend to be identified by and associated with characteristics that really are only superficial indicators of who they are. Society worships celebrities based solely on public personas that are crafted by Hollywood moguls and music industry executives. Likewise, society has a history of ridiculing and ostracizing those who do not meet these unrealistic standards. This superficial idea of perfection leads to judgmental standards built on trivial characteristics that have no relationship to the essence of a person. The labeling of people, and the stereotypical assumptions that we make based on those labels, discounts the true value of the person. In other words, labels and inaccurate stereotypes of society often overshadow the strengths, potential, and accomplishments of persons with disabilities.

To be fair, labels can serve a valuable purpose because they facilitate communication of the nature of a particular condition to others. This message in turn allows for the provision of appropriate care, access to resources or accommodations, and program enrollment. The danger of labels comes from people's misuse and misunderstanding of them as well as the tendency to generalize impairment of one particular area of functioning to the overall abilities of the person. An example of such a generalization would be assuming that a person has difficulty solving problems because he or she cannot hear. Even worse, we begin to focus so much on the disability that the differentiating characteristic overshadows the person.

According to the **Americans with Disabilities Act (ADA**, 1991), legally, a person with a disability is someone who

- has a physical, mental, or cognitive impairment that substantially limits one or more major life functions or activities;
- has a record of such an impairment; or
- is regarded as having such an impairment.

This legal definition requires the disability to result in a substantial limitation in one or more major life activities, such as walking, breathing, seeing, thinking, performing tasks, speaking, learning, working, driving, and participating in community life. Although this definition is clear, it goes beyond how well a person can function and the degree to which he or she can be independent. The spirit of the ADA also embraces a philosophy or belief system that the person should not be taken out of the equation. In other words, the person is much more than his or her disability. People with disabilities have the right to be treated as a person first, not as their disability. Beyond the individual's physical, mental, or cognitive limitations, the constant factor is his or her humanity (Bogdan & Taylor, 1992). Thus, the humanity should be our first consideration.

Each of the hundreds of disabilities has a differing degree of severity. Chapters 7 to 11 discuss characteristics and aspects of various disabilities from the perspective of disability-related characteristics and programs. Here, we will explore the idea of viewing a person with a disability as a person first, with the focus not on the person's limitations but on the individual as a person. This perspective is a key element in the prevention of handicaps. A handicap is a situation in which a person can be disadvantaged not by the disability but by other factors. These disadvantages may result from a preventable or removable barrier to performance of a particular activity or skill. Handicaps can include physical barriers but can also come from society's negligence or negative personal attitudes, beliefs, or knowledge. This

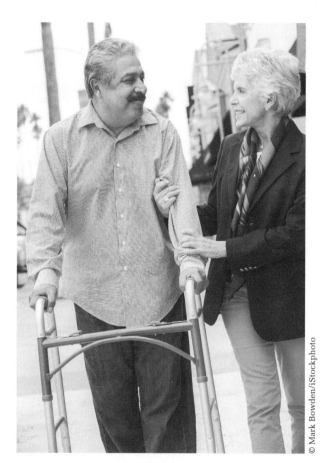

Each person is unique and has the potential to grow. Focus on this humanity rather than on marginalizing characteristics.

© Mark Bowden/iStockphoto

chapter focuses on the social issue of how society perceives and interacts with people with disabilities. In particular, we discuss person-first aspects of disability, the effect of negative perceptions of disability, and the role of therapeutic recreation relative to people with disabilities.

Person-First Philosophy

Considering our humanity first is predominantly the philosophy of therapeutic recreation. This philosophy means that we treat each other as unique human beings with the potential to grow and develop. We respond to each other first according to our human needs and second in terms of individual characteristics (Bogdan & Taylor, 1992). For instance, we address the person who has a cognitive impairment as a person first, not as a person who has trouble making decisions or recalling information.

The foundation of a person-first philosophy involves believing that each person is unique and that his or her uniqueness is a positive, not a negative, attribute. This philosophy is founded on the belief that each person is made up of many different qualities, such as possessing a sense of humor or being good at card tricks, not only his or her disability. A person-first philosophy embraces the belief that all persons have the potential to grow and develop as human beings. Regardless of his or her limitations, a person can learn new things, engage in activities, participate in reciprocal relationships, and have a fulfilling quality of life. We can embrace a person-first philosophy in several ways. One is through the terminology, or language, that we use when referring to, speaking to, or talking about people with disabilities. Another indicator of a person-first philosophy is an understanding of the multidimensionality of barriers that people with disabilities face.

Person-First Terminology

Words are powerful. They convey meaning, attitudes, philosophical beliefs, and personal perspectives. So being aware of words that we use when speaking with or about a person with a disability is important in embracing a person-first philosophy. **Person-first terminology** requires the use of respectful language when referring to those with disabilities. Specifically, terminology should focus on the person first, not the disability. For example, it would be more appropriate to state that "Joe is a child who has autism" rather than

"Joe is autistic." This distinction seems minor, but the former approach acknowledges Joe as a person first, whereas the latter does not. A broad example is in the preference for using "people with disabilities" instead of "disabled people," "the disabled," or "handicapped." Furthermore, it is important to refer to a disability only when relevant and necessary. Person-first terminology also requires us to avoid referring to someone with a disability as a "special child" or a "challenged person" because those terms focus on the disability as the identifying characteristic that makes someone unique. Terminology should reflect respect for the person by not referring to adults with disabilities as kids or referring to them in a childlike manner. Eliminating from our vocabulary words such as *imbecile*, *psycho*, *lunatic*, *moron*, *crazy*, *retarded*, and *spaz*, whether referring to someone or something, is another way to communicate respectfully.

Understanding the Multidimensionality of Barriers

To embrace a person-first philosophy, we need to understand that people with disabilities encounter barriers not only because they have functional limitations. We understand and view problems, limitations, deficits, boundaries, and constraints as resulting from a number of causal factors rather than simply a person's disability (Howe-Murphy & Charboneau, 1987). This perspective requires that constraints and limitations to participation in community life should focus not only on characteristics of disabilities but also on the design of programs, accessibility of buildings, and training of staff. For example, if a woman with a developmental disability is not participating in her community's recreation programs, the cause may be that the programs are beyond her financial means, inaccessible by public transportation, not designed with her abilities in mind, or unwelcoming to her. This principle requires looking beyond disabilities and considering environmental factors such as negative attitudes held by the public, accessibility of buildings, or program design.

Using Person-First Philosophy

Promoting a person-first philosophy means that we need to serve as change agents by modeling and insisting on actions that empower rather than demean people with disabilities (Dattilo, 2002). As a profession, we have an ethical responsibility to promote the dignity and rights of those whom we serve. By modeling person-first behavior, we demonstrate to others that we respect the uniqueness of each person and welcome differences between people. We provide opportunities that challenge myths and stereotypes that can reduce barriers to community involvement.

Therapeutic recreation specialists can play an important role in teaching skills to participants that help them to be more independent or interdependent in their leisure. Learning skills and new ways of thinking about leisure can empower those with disabilities and is a strong reflection of a person-first philosophy.

One service model that has been useful in delivering therapeutic recreation services has been the **leisure ability model** (Stumbo & Peterson, 2004). The components of this model are discussed more thoroughly in chapter 5. One component of this model is **leisure education**, a process based on the idea that people with disabilities can be taught how to make leisure choices; learn new recreation skills; and use community resources, such as parks and recreation services. A therapeutic recreation specialist can facilitate the examination of leisure values and attitudes to identify interpersonal barriers to leisure. By applying this model, a therapeutic recreation specialist can also teach new leisure-related skills, such as how to socialize in large groups, ski using adaptive equipment, or make decisions when faced with multiple choices. Framing services from the recreation engagement segment of this model, a therapeutic recreation specialist could refer people to accessible community services, assess a recreation program for inclusive participation with peers without disabilities, or implement an adapted recreation program.

Social Inclusion

Besides teaching skills and examining leisure values or attitudes, therapeutic recreation specialists can facilitate social inclusion in promoting a person-first philosophy. **Social inclusion** involves sharing common experiences, valuing the participation of all people, and providing support for participation (Devine, 2004; Goodwin, 2003). When a therapeutic recreation specialist facilitates social inclusion, he or she is concerned with more than the number of friends that someone with a disability may have. Instead, he or she focuses on creating a sense of belonging to a group, a feeling

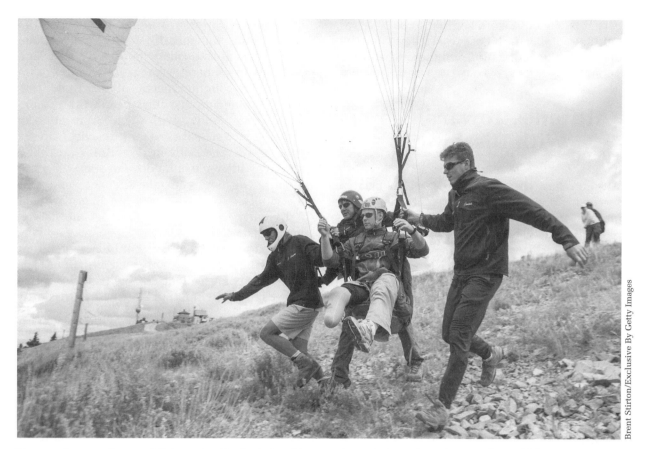

Therapeutic recreation specialists work with clients to achieve maximum independence in recreation and leisure.

that participation is valued. For instance, skills would not be ridiculed when they look different from those performed by peers without disabilities, the interests of participants with disabilities would be actively sought, and the atmosphere would be welcoming (Devine & Lashua, 2002).

Social inclusion is critical because lack of social acceptance in inclusive recreation environments is more constraining than are architectural or programmatic barriers (Bedini, 2000; Bedini & Henderson, 1994; West, 1984). Moreover, studies have found that people with disabilities take an emotional, social, and psychological risk when they choose to participate in inclusive rather than separate (i.e., disability only) recreation programs (Bedini & Henderson 1994; Devine & Lashua, 2002). Thus, social inclusion is a way to break down barriers so that people can feel comfortable and welcomed in a recreation environment.

Least Restrictive Environments

In promoting a person-first philosophy, therapeutic recreation specialists should create an environment that is least restrictive. These environments provide maximum support to people with disabilities for engagement in recreation or therapy without overreliance on adaptations if they are not necessary. **Least restrictive environments** are situations in which adaptations would be made only when evidence indicates that a person with a disability needs changes in order to function. The goal of a least restrictive environment is to make changes based on the person's individual strengths and limitations. Making changes or adaptations that are beyond the person's needs may actually make the environment more restrictive. As people learn and change, their skills and knowledge may change, eventually rendering adaptations no longer necessary (Dattilo, 2002).

Interdependence

When therapeutic recreation specialists foster interdependence among all participants, a person-first philosophy can develop. **Interdependence** implies relationships of cooperation and reciprocity among participants with and without disabilities as well as with the staff to accomplish tasks and achieve common goals. For example, participants could work together to paint a wall mural, with those who use wheelchairs painting the lower parts of the wall and those who do not painting the upper sections.

Attitudes Toward People With Disabilities

Attitudes have the power to create either positive forces for change or major barriers. Thus, our attitude toward differences between people is one point that distinguishes positive and negative interactions. Historically, society's attitude toward people with disabilities has been predominantly negative. This way of thinking has resulted in such actions as segregation (separating people based on a personal characteristic that is different) and discrimination (actions that devalue a person based on a personal characteristic).

Society at times has also treated those with disabilities as superhumans, resulting in perceptions that people must be extraordinary, that they must have capacities beyond those of typical humans, to live with a disability. After interacting with people who hold this attitude, some people with disabilities have felt that they have been treated as heroes simply because they have a disability.

Some people with disabilities experience a neutral attitude toward them, leaving them feeling invisible. One man who has a spinal cord injury described that neutral attitude as people looking past him or through him as though he were not present. What all of these ranges of attitudes have in common is their focus on the disability first, instead of the person first.

Influence of Society, Community, and Family

Our society as a whole is a strong influence on individual belief systems, attitudes, and perceptions toward people, events, language, and objects. Because most of us do not live in social isolation, our beliefs are a reflection of many variables.

Various institutions in society such as schools, governmental agencies, laws, and families play a role in shaping beliefs, attitudes, and perceptions of many things, including those related to people with disabilities. In particular, looking at our attitudes toward and perceptions of people with disabilities is important because they are a mirror to our beliefs about those with whom we will work.

As young children, we may have learned to avoid people who talk differently than we do or not to stare at someone who uses a wheelchair. Historically, schools segregated children with disabilities from their peers without disabilities, teaching students that their peers with disabilities did not belong with them. Segregation in schools sent a message that the difference between people with and without disabilities was not a positive difference but a devalued, negative difference. Our family members taught some of us to feel blessed or privileged to be born without a disability. Children were often taught that not having a disability was a stroke of luck or divine intervention and that we should be grateful for not having been born with such afflictions. The inadvertent consequence of such a belief is that it leads to the assumption that having a disability makes you less of a person.

During adolescence, our peer groups have a significant influence on our behavior because, by nature, we want to gain and maintain a sense of belonging (Witt & Caldwell, 2005). In this life stage, our peers influenced our attitudes toward those with disabilities by expecting us to go along with behaviors such as making fun of disability characteristics or name-calling each other using derogatory disability-related language. A perception of superiority can also hold sway in adolescence. For instance, one study that examined perceptions of youth toward inclusive recreation found that adolescents without disabilities felt that competing in sports or other recreation activities was unfair to their peers with disabilities because they were not as good at those activities as were those without disabilities (Devine & Wilhite, 2000).

In our play or leisure, we received the message from many sources that people with disabilities were less able and capable and inferior in their abilities to those of us without a disability. The loud message is that they are not like those of us without disabilities. The prevalence of segregated recreation options sends the message that only in these contexts can people with disabilities engage in recreation because their abilities are limited. Research has found that people without disabilities perceived that recreation participation with peers with disabilities would result in a watered-down experience that would be less challenging or enjoyable (Archie & Sherrill, 1989; Wilhite, Devine, & Goldenberg, 1999). We also have been taught that recreation skills must all look the same and skills performed differently are inferior and result in a less enjoyable experience.

CLIENT PORTRAIT:
PHOEBE'S LEAST RESTRICTIVE ENVIRONMENT

Phoebe is an 11-year-old girl with Prader Willi syndrome, a chromosomal disorder that results in **hypotonia** (low muscle tone), speech problems, and developmental delays. Like a typical 11-year-old, Phoebe has many recreation interests, such as painting, riding her bike, dancing, playing basketball, and spending time with friends. Phoebe has some cognitive delays that are not typical of an 11-year-old, such as difficulty remembering things, recalling sequences of tasks, reading, writing, verbally communicating her ideas, recognizing cause-and-effect situations, and problem solving. Her low muscle tone sometimes makes it difficult for her to control motor functions, such as grasping things and kicking actions, and she has low stamina for activities that require endurance.

As we learned, Phoebe likes to paint. Because of her cognitive impairment, she tends to forget what supplies she will need and how to prepare the area or herself for painting. The goal for Phoebe is to teach her to paint independently, with friends, or in a class. In keeping with the tenets of a least restrictive environment, a therapeutic recreation specialist would develop a way for her to remember what supplies she needs to gather, how to lay them out, and how to begin using them independently. Because Phoebe has difficulty reading, the therapeutic recreation specialist determines that pictorial charts would be a useful way to show her how to go about painting independently. Additionally, to address her problems of grasping and holding small objects, the therapeutic recreation specialist enlarges the handles of her paintbrushes with fabric and padded tape so that Phoebe will be able to use them more easily. Because Phoebe needs adaptations only for recall, sequencing, reading, and holding

small objects, these modifications will be the only ones made to this activity, in keeping with the principles of a least restrictive environment. The therapeutic recreation specialist develops one chart that has pictures of all the supplies that she needs and another chart that has step-by-step pictures that show Phoebe the sequence of preparing the area and herself for painting. The therapeutic recreation specialist first teaches Phoebe how to look at the chart and use a step-by-step process to gather items. She then teaches Phoebe how to use the pictures on the second chart to prepare herself and her area to paint. As Phoebe learns these skills, the therapeutic recreation specialist would stop assisting. Later, the charts can be withdrawn because Phoebe would no longer need them. Withdrawing modifications when they are no longer needed is the second principle of a least restrictive environment.

As Phoebe develops an interest in other recreation activities, she will need different modifications to meet her needs. This need is especially legitimate because she is at an age when she faces rapid changes emotionally, physically, cognitively, and socially even without added concerns of her developmental delays. Her therapeutic recreation specialist will watch for components of recreation participation that involve fine motor activities, reading, sequencing, short- and long-term recall, and problem solving and activities that require multiple pieces of equipment for which she may need an adaptation. When Phoebe needs these skills, adaptations will be made to help her. For example, if Phoebe wants to participate on a basketball team, frequent breaks will help compensate for her limited physical stamina. Activities that require problem solving, such as board games, may require modified rules to allow Phoebe to participate.

Clearly, what is being communicated is that a disability is a sentence to a poorer quality of life compared with the quality of life experienced by persons without disabilities. From this perspective, a disability is perceived as more than a loss of functioning resulting from impairment; it is disqualification from a full life as well as an enjoyable recreation experience (Devine & Sylvester, 2005).

Influence of Language on Attitudes

Another indicator of attitudes is language. As the example in the previous section indicates, the words that we use can create a vivid picture of our

stereotyped image of someone with a disability. Our language is a gauge of our beliefs about people with disabilities. For example, if we believe that a person with a disability is inferior to the rest of us, we may say, "He can't play checkers; he's retarded." We believe that the person cannot play the game because he is less intelligent than we are. If we believe that we should have pity for people with disabilities, we may say, "That poor woman is a victim of polio." Although some disabilities are more difficult to live with than others, referring to someone as a victim because he or she has a disability places the person in a helpless position.

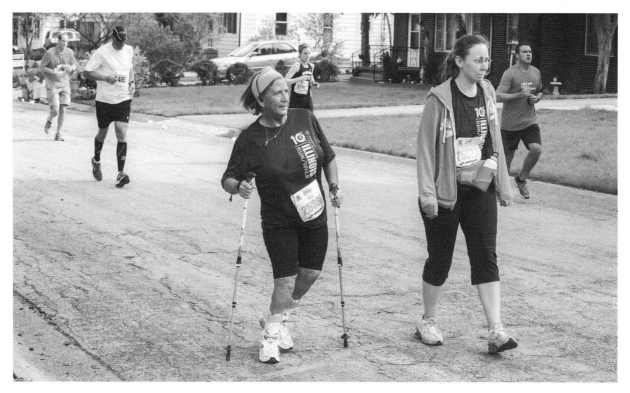

Disability is not a disqualification from a full life.

Some attitudes toward people with disabilities are reflective of them as objects. This viewpoint is evident when we use terms such as *the blind*, *the deaf*, or *the retarded*, words that place them in a category, reflecting an attitude that they are things, not people. Sometimes, people with and without disabilities are referred to as *them* and *us*. This distinction portrays an attitude that we are opposites; we are focusing on differences rather than similarities. The language that we choose to use is a mirror of our attitudes toward people with disabilities. Stereotypes or inaccurate reflections can create tension and lead to significant barriers for those with disabilities.

Influence of Laws on Attitudes

One mechanism for ensuring equity in leisure and life in general is the legal system and the associated laws that pertain to individuals and organizations within its jurisdiction. Clearly, the law enacted in the past 25 years that had the greatest effect on society as a whole as related to people with disabilities has been the ADA. This law requires private and public organizations to include people with disabilities in all aspects of services provided and amenities offered and to provide full and equal access to all services and programs.

Another law that has influenced services as well as attitudes is the Individuals with Disabilities Education Act (IDEA), which mandates that all children with disabilities have access to free and appropriate public education. Although laws mandate what recreation organizations and others can and cannot do when providing goods and services to people with disabilities, laws cannot mandate attitudes. Since the passage of the ADA and IDEA, an entire generation has been growing up in nonsegregated classrooms. The expectation of those with disabilities in this generation is to be included in all aspects of daily life, including recreation opportunities. An important question remains: What is the attitudinal response by society to the laws that govern goods, services, and programs and to the expectations of the next generation of people with disabilities regarding inclusion in community life?

Supporters and critics of the ADA appear to agree that since the adoption of this law, attitudes toward people with disabilities have advanced in some areas but regressed in others. The legal nature of providing services to people with disabilities is one concern. Specifically, the idea of being mandated or required by law to make changes and provide services to a statistically small percentage of the population has left some feeling resentful. They believe that providing

PATRICIA LaPLACE, RTC

Education: BS in Recreation Therapy, California State University at Long Beach
MPA, California State University at Dominguez Hills
Position: Lecturer
Organization: Department of Recreation and Leisure Studies, California State University at Long Beach

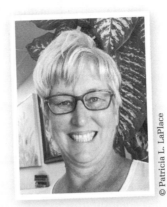

© Patricia L. LaPlace

My Career

I started my career as a recreation therapy aide in an acute psychiatric facility in Long Beach in 1975. At that time, there were a lot of changes in the mental health system delivery in California due to legislative mandates that required downsizing of the state hospital programs and moving toward more community-based treatment centers and programs. Unfortunately, this transition did not go smoothly, and monies were not available to provide the needed support and tools required to implement such programs. As a result, many institutionalized clients landed in private psychiatric facilities for short-term interventions with minimal supportive services in the community. This is where my passion in working in the mental health field began. I observed many consumers of mental health services being marginalized and stigmatized not only in the community and but also by service providers in the treatment process.

I was lucky to work in an environment that supported recreation therapy services, and I also learned advocacy and the recognition of quality of life and the right to self-determination with this population. Recreation therapy provided opportunities for mental health consumers to practice these rights as well as learn to control and manage symptoms through meaningful engagement in leisure and recreation activities.

I continued to work in acute psychiatric settings, including supervisory and management positions, until 2008; at that time I obtained the position of mental health coordinator for the City of Long Beach health department. In this position, I worked in the homeless services division serving this population and coordinating with other city entities and mental health providers to provide access and service connection. I found my therapy skills were a good fit for implementing and collaborating with various agencies and programs in terms of care coordination and system development. I was fortunate to lead a number of task forces and committees that evaluated and addressed various mental health issues and needs. This also included managing a large grant that provided outreach and engagement services for veterans experiencing homelessness in Long Beach along with the VA Long Beach Healthcare Center. As I had observed with mental health consumers in the late 1970s, I became aware of marginalization and stigma that existed with veterans experiencing homelessness; therefore, I had a renewed passion to try to make a difference with this population.

My career in higher education began in 1987 at California State University at Dominguez Hills as a part-time lecturer and proctor for their recreation therapy program. I continued to teach there part time, while working full time in the field, until the program closed in 2009. I had also been teaching part time at California State University at Long Beach (CSULB) since 1997, and I made the transition to teaching a full-time course schedule in 2015. I have found that my professional experience has assisted in my academic growth as an educator, and I feel blessed to have the opportunity to give back to the department of recreation and leisure studies at CSULB that planted the seed for my career. In addition to teaching, I serve on multiple boards and task forces for nonprofit agencies and community social service providers that offer services for mental health and veterans.

My Advice to You

I have loved everything about my jobs as a recreation therapist, an administrator, and now an educator. Recreation therapy provides such a holistic approach that it really makes a difference in someone's quality of life. I love sharing the passion of recreation therapy to students as well. It is a great honor to support future professionals and ambassadors. My advice to students and young professionals is this: Don't limit yourself. Take risks and think outside of the box. Develop your critical thinking skills and don't be afraid to fail. Not every task or endeavor you will encounter comes with an instruction manual. Your best lessons in life come from those experiences. Be an advocate and ambassador for the recreation therapy profession. Challenge the status quo and keep up to date on evidence-based practices. Engage in creativeness and imagination. Have good documentation and writing skills, and always remember the three Cs when constructing a document: clear, concise, and comprehensive. The most important thing to do for yourself is to have good self-care practices. We take care of others better when we take care of ourselves!

equal access is extremely costly and more trouble than it is worth. But research has shown that people with disabilities are among the most discriminated groups of people in our society (Burgstahler & Doe, 2006). Service providers face complications in complying with the ADA. In fact, some recreation service providers have felt unprepared to accomplish some of the more complex tasks related to meeting the mandates of the ADA, leaving them with a negative attitude toward the law (Devine & McGovern, 2001).

On the other hand, some feel that the ADA has empowered people with disabilities to seek a variety of recreation options and request inclusion in community life. Therapeutic recreation specialists have found that the law provides specific parameters for service provision, eliminating the guesswork of how to include people with disabilities in their communities. Although the jury may be out on specific influences on attitudes toward people with disabilities because of the ADA and IDEA, one way to judge the current attitude of society is through people's behavior.

Behaviors are observable and measurable acts or responses by people, and these actions tend to reflect attitudes. Historically, behaviors toward people with disabilities occurred in the form of stereotyping, discrimination, stigmatizing, segregation, and inaccessibility, to name a few. Earlier in this chapter, stigma and stereotypes were mentioned as being the opposite of a person-first philosophy. Behaviors can also reflect negative attitudes toward people with disabilities. One hope that people with disabilities had about the ADA and other laws was that they would feel less stigmatized and negatively stereotyped. Although attitudes cannot be subject to laws, behavior can. Thus, behaviors that may reflect negative attitudes, such as discrimination in recreation access, building of inaccessible parks, and segregation of people with disabilities in sports activities, can be subject to scrutiny under the ADA. By challenging stereotypes that may lead to segregation, the law can reshape people's attitudes. For example, the ADA mandates access to equal benefits of recreation participation. If people with disabilities have access to sports competitions, then the belief that they cannot be athletes may change.

Service Delivery

Therapeutic recreation has viewed people with disabilities in various ways over the history of the field. In the early years, therapeutic recreation took a social reform perspective whereby recreation was used to keep children who lived in poor and often unhealthy environments off the streets (see chapter 2; Duncan, 1991). Over the years, we have used medical, social, ecological, and biopsychosocial models along with a strengths-based approach to care, all recognizing and celebrating differences. Although therapeutic recreation has viewed disability with multiple models, the major ones are the medical model, the social model, the ecological model, and the biopsychosocial model.

Medical Model

The **medical model of disability** views disability as a variation from the physical norm that can disadvantage the person physically and in quality of life (Koch, 2001). This model of disability is based on a number of assumptions. One assumption is that disability is a physical condition in that something is physically different about a person as compared with the norm. This physical condition is less desirable than the norm and can be treated or changed through medical or therapeutic intervention. This model applies the idea that it is the responsibility of society to use resources such as therapies to try to cure disabilities, with the medical profession having the greatest responsibility (Devine & Sylvester, 2005). In addition, services received by people with disabilities must be prescribed by someone in a medically authoritative position. This model regards all services received by people with disabilities, including recreation participation, as therapy (Wehman, 2001). Barriers experienced by people with disabilities arise from individual functional limitations resulting from disability instead of social factors that limit individuals (Fine & Asch, 1988; Oliver, 1996).

Therapeutic recreation has applied this perspective in the treatment and functional improvement components of our service delivery models. The focus is on the illness or disability of the person to address limitations in coordination, endurance, mobility, strength, hand–eye coordination, emotional or social functioning, and cognitive limitations as well as sensory limitations. With this model, recreation is used in a prescriptive way to correct or improve negative effects of a disability.

Social Model

The **social model of disability** views disability as a result of social discrimination toward people who are different from the norm. Rather than being a problem with the individual, disability occurs when society does not accommodate physical, cognitive, social, or emotional differences (Koch, 2001). Society has prescribed a set of standards for and values of functional independence, capabilities, and social reciprocity. When people cannot function at those standards or they have a biological composition below those standards, they are assumed inferior and subject to social exclusion (Allen & Allen, 1995; Bogdan & Taylor, 1992; Hahn, 1988). For example, the fact that a person uses a wheelchair to ambulate tells little about his or her physical condition, but it offers a great deal of information about how buildings, curbs, and parks are designed and built to exclude people who use this equipment. As such, disability, or handicaps, arise out of society's failure to accommodate its members who have impairments.

Therapeutic recreation has long embraced the role of being advocates for the rights of people with disabilities. Advocacy involves commitment to a cause, taking risks, and challenging norms (Wolfensberger, 1977). This role reflects the social model of disability. Therapeutic recreation service models provide guidelines through leisure education services in promoting the teaching of skills and accessing of community resources. Some service models have embraced the social model of disability by viewing a person with a disability as someone who could have an active, healthy lifestyle (see chapter 5; Stumbo & Peterson, 2004; Wilhite, Keller, & Caldwell, 1999).

Ecological Model

The **ecological model of disability** is based on the idea that people and their environments are interconnected. That is, reciprocity and interaction occur among systems within which we live (Howe-Murphy & Charboneau, 1987). Systems can be defined as social organizations (e.g., family, schools, religious affiliations, or society) that people interact with directly and indirectly. The ecological model asserts that if a change occurs within the community, the change will affect not only that system but also individuals, directly or indirectly. In addition, if something occurs to an individual, a reciprocal influence will occur in another system (e.g., family). For instance, when the ADA was written into federal law, the change affected state and local governments, communities, families, and individuals with disabilities. On the other hand, when a person acquires a disability, this event affects his or her family, the school system, and the community by virtue of the person's changing needs.

Evidence of the ecological model can be seen in therapeutic recreation services. For instance, when a therapeutic recreation specialist consults a patient's family members, schoolteachers or employers, or other members of a therapy team or surveys the person's home and community environment when composing a discharge plan, then he or she is applying the ecological model. Some of the service delivery models have included this perspective by taking a person's life course (where a person is in his or her life span) into consideration when providing services and evaluating the parts of services and needs in the person's life (Wilhite, Keller, & Caldwell, 1999).

Biopsychosocial Model

The **biopsychosocial model** is an integration of the medical and social model. It is a holistic approach that takes into consideration multiple factors (i.e., biological, psychological, and social) influencing the individual's health or disability (Engel, 1977). The biological factors of an individual can include gender, disability, immune function, age, nutrition, and hormones. The psychological factors are related to the individual's ability to learn and his or her attitudes, personality, coping skills, emotions, and past trauma. The social factors can include the individual's social supports, family background, socioeconomic status, and education. The main focus of the biopsychosocial model is increasing functioning by determining the biological, psychological, and social factors that are affecting the person's health as a whole.

An example of a biopsychosocial model relevant to therapeutic recreation is the *International Classification of Functioning, Disability and Health* (World Health Organization, 2001; ATRA, 2005). The *ICF* framework was developed by the World Health Organization to determine someone's health based on more than just the individual's body functions and structures (i.e., medical model); it also includes his or her activity, participation, environmental factors, and personal factors (World Health Organization, 2002). The therapeutic recreation specialist can use the ICF framework to develop a patient-centered approach to care that is based on more than just the individual's diagnosis (i.e., medical model) or environmental factors (i.e., social model). Therapeutic recreation specialists can evaluate the *ICF* factors affecting an individual's health or disability and use this information for providing a strengths-based approach to care.

Strengths-Based Approach

A strengths-based approach to care involves developing programs and services based on people's strengths and capacities. Strengths-based care focuses on what people hope for, value, and are good at and what supports are in their environment. This approach helps individuals reach their goals and aspirations (Anderson & Heyne, 2012a). The strengths-based approach to care is a foundational element of therapeutic recreation and fully supports a person-first philosophy.

These strengths are both internal (e.g., abilities, talents, knowledge, aspirations, and interests) and external (e.g., community resources, family support, friendships, home resources, and high expectations; Heyne & Anderson, 2012). In addition, recreation is seen as both an internal and external strength. Not only is recreation a strength, but therapeutic recreation specialists use recreation as a modality to develop both internal and external strengths (Anderson & Heyne, 2012b; Heyne & Anderson, 2012). Facilitation of a strengths-based approach to care by therapeutic recreation specialists allows for a patient-centered holistic approach that supports a person-first philosophy (see chapter 5 for additional information on strength-based models of practice).

Summary

Society in general has been slow to respond to the rights of people with disabilities to participate actively in all that communities have to offer. By embracing person-first philosophies, being aware of their role as change agents, and knowing the various service delivery models of disabilities, therapeutic recreation specialists can become more informed and competent as practitioners. Person-first philosophy not only provides a framework from which to influence societal attitudes but also serves as an internal compass that helps professionals keep sight of the true potential of every client.

DISCUSSION QUESTIONS

1. How can labels be detrimental to people with disabilities?

2. What characteristics legally constitute a person with a disability according to the ADA?

3. A foundation of person-first philosophy is the belief that each person is unique and his or her uniqueness is a positive, not a negative, attribute. In your own words, describe what this means.

4. In what ways is social inclusion an important component of recreation participation for individuals with disabilities?

5. Identify and discuss the two primary components of a least restrictive environment.

6. In the story of Phoebe, you learned of two ways to make her environment least restrictive. Identify other ways that would reduce the restrictiveness of her environment.

7. What suggestions can you provide that could foster a positive attitude toward Phoebe's participation in her community?

8. What effect have the ADA and IDEA had on the inclusion of people with disabilities in community life?

9. How does the social model of disability differ from the medical model of disability?

10. How does the *ICF* support the biopsychosocial model?

11. How does a strengths-based approach to care promote a person-first philosophy, especially in therapeutic recreation?

Models and Modalities of Practice

Jamie Hoffman | Terry Long

LEARNING OUTCOMES

At the end of this chapter, students will be able to

- describe elements of predominant models of practice,
- identify philosophical and conceptual differences and similarities across such models,
- identify commonly used therapeutic recreation modalities,
- explain the basic principles of the *International Classification of Functioning, Disability and Health*, and
- justify potential applications of various modalities within specific client populations.

The authors gratefully acknowledge the significant contributions of Richard Williams and David Howard to this chapter.

Every college student will occasionally hear professors ramble on about "models," which can be right alongside "theories" when it comes to the least favorite topics that students think they want to hear about. In reality, models can be pretty cool, and daily life is full of them. Think about the maps that represent streets, the props used in anatomy class, or even the Harry Potter exhibit at Universal Studios. All these models are used to depict large, complex things in an understandable way. In therapeutic recreation, models serve the same purpose—to depict and help us understand and vicariously experience what therapeutic recreation practice really entails. Of course, there is no "right" model for therapeutic recreation, but some models are definitely better than others. The models presented here have been vetted at some level and have value when applied in the right context. The challenge is to become adequately familiar with these models, recognize when they have relevance and value, and apply the chosen model in a way that effectively guides therapeutic recreation practice.

Therapeutic Recreation Practice Models

Over the years, a variety of therapeutic recreation practice models have been developed, each model showing a different perspective on how therapeutic recreation services might be conceptualized and delivered. Several of these models are described in the following section. We encourage you to explore these models in detail by reading the publications in which they were originally presented or revised. The descriptions below are provided to highlight the general principles of a few select models, but a more detailed understanding of the models is necessary for use in practice. We also encourage you to learn about other models as well. There are many models in existence and new models are constantly being developed for use in practice.

Leisure Ability Model

The **leisure ability model** has been described in numerous publications, perhaps most fully in Peterson and Gunn's (1984) *Therapeutic Recreation Program Design*. More recently, Stumbo and Peterson (1998, 2009) have presented updated explanations of the theoretical foundations of the model, yet the essential elements of the model have remained unchanged through the years.

For therapists who use the leisure ability model, the ultimate outcome of therapeutic recreation is "improved ability of the individual to engage in a successful, appropriate, and meaningful independent leisure lifestyle, that, in turn, leads to improved health, quality of life, and well-being" (Stumbo & Peterson, 2009, p. 29). A leisure lifestyle is "the day-to-day behavioral expression of one's leisure related attitudes, awareness, and activities revealed within the context and composite of the total life experience" (Peterson & Gunn, 1984, p. 83). The model organizes therapeutic recreation services into three components: functional intervention, leisure education, and recreation participation (see figure 5.1). Depending on individual needs, clients might be engaged in only one of the components or all three of the components concurrently.

Functional Intervention

Therapeutic recreation services delivered in the **functional intervention (FI)** component focus on correcting functional deficits related to leisure-related activity in the physical, mental, emotional, and social domains. The general goal of FI services is the elimination of, improvement in, or adaptation to functional deficits that constrain participation in leisure. During FI, the therapeutic recreation specialist maintains a high level of control (e.g., assigning clients to programs), whereas client behavior is relatively constrained, dependent, and motivated by extrinsic rewards.

Leisure Education

Therapeutic recreation services delivered in the **leisure education** component focus on supporting clients in acquiring "leisure-related attitudes, knowledge, and skills" (Stumbo & Peterson, 1998, p. 89) and are organized into four subcomponents: leisure awareness, social skills, leisure activity skills, and leisure resources. A therapeutic recreation specialist who uses the leisure ability model might offer a single leisure education program that addresses elements from all four components of leisure education or separate leisure education programs for each element. Generally, the goal of leisure education services is to guide clients to understand the importance of leisure and learn ways to participate successfully in leisure.

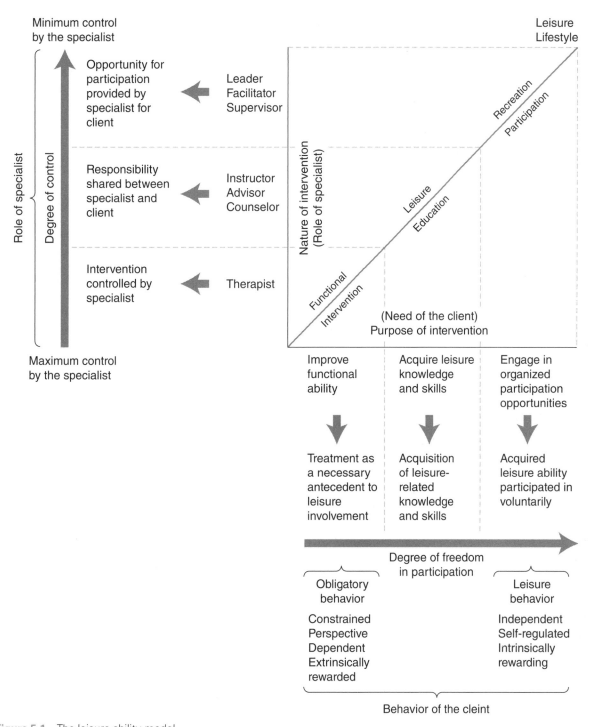

Figure 5.1 The leisure ability model.

Reprinted by permission from World Health Organization (WHO), all rights are reserved by the Organization.

Although therapeutic recreation specialists maintain some control during leisure education services and assume the roles of instructor, adviser, and counselor, clients have opportunities for choice and experience more freedom than they do during FI.

Leisure education can be an invaluable aspect of therapeutic recreation services across a variety of practice settings. For example, leisure education is a critically important element in corrections because positive leisure choices, understanding leisure motivation, and leisure awareness are at the forefront of facilitation techniques. With inmates who have been incarcerated for 20 or more years, understanding current leisure trends in society can influence their successful reintegration once paroled. This can allow inmates to establish a positive leisure lifestyle, therefore reducing recidivism and increasing their quality of life. Patients in rehabilitation benefit from lei-sure education in much the same way they adjust to any long-term effects of injury or illness. For those receiving mental health services, leisure education provides important information and skill development regarding emotional coping, self-care, and social adjustment.

Recreation Participation

The final component of the leisure ability model is recreation participation. The purpose of recreation participation is to "provide opportunities for fun, enjoyment and self-expression within an

CLIENT PORTRAIT: MR. NELSON

USING THE LEISURE ABILITY MODEL WITH MR. NELSON

Mr. Nelson was an 82-year-old man living in a skilled-nursing facility. His wife died 5 years ago, and after living independently in his home for 2 years, he began to experience symptoms of Alzheimer's disease. As his cognitive symptoms grew progressively more pronounced, Mr. Nelson had an increasingly difficult time caring for himself. Mr. Nelson recently agreed with his adult son and daughter-in-law that he should move into Tall Oaks Center, a long-term-care facility in his hometown. Marcy, a certified therapeutic recreation specialist (CTRS) at Tall Oaks, consulted Mr. Nelson's chart and then met with him to perform an assessment. After the assessment, Marcy and Mr. Nelson worked together to set goals and choose therapeutic recreation programs of interest that would help Mr. Nelson achieve his goals.

Functional Intervention

Mr. Nelson's past interests had included reading the morning paper with his wife at breakfast. The loss of his wife and his cognitive decline had limited his ability to engage in this cognitively stimulating activity. Marcy recommended that he attend the daily "coffee talk" session each morning following breakfast to allow him the opportunity to read, discuss interesting topics with others, and relate this information to long-term memories. In these sessions, residents and staff members sit around a table and discuss items related to the newspaper or other presented media. Topics of focus might include the date, season, weather, media-reported stories, and any memories that the discussion might trigger.

Marcy actively facilitates this discussion at a level appropriate for attendees. Newspapers and news magazines are made available to the clients, and a large marker board highlighting current events and recent topics of discussion helps orient clients to the discussion. The intent of the activity is to provide cognitive stimulation, maintain social engagement, and reinforce connectedness to the past and present. Additionally, because Mr. Nelson had gained a substantial amount of weight since the loss of his wife, Marcy recommended a low-impact exercise class to help him control his weight and become more physically active.

Leisure Education

Mr. Nelson's son and daughter-in-law came for occasional visits, but otherwise, he was socially isolated. To help him gain social support through other residents at Tall Oaks, Marcy recommended that Mr. Nelson attend a program called Circle of Friends, a daily support group facilitated by staff members and residents. Additionally, Mr. Nelson began to participate actively in the many community outings offered by Marcy and the other CTRSs. Both programs helped Mr. Nelson become more socially involved and prevented isolation.

Recreation Participation

Mr. Nelson had lived on a farm during his childhood, and he and his wife were avid gardeners. Since his wife's death, Mr. Nelson had quit gardening. When Marcy told him about the Tall Oaks residents' garden and small greenhouse, he immediately expressed interest in helping with the garden. Additionally, Mr. Nelson enjoyed attending occasional special events put on by the therapeutic recreation staff and others.

organized delivery system" (Stumbo & Peterson, 2009, p. 62). During these services, client behavior is intrinsically motivated, and therapeutic recreation specialists exert relatively little control beyond acting as facilitators. Recreation participation can vary from something that is sedentary, such as drawing or painting, to highly challenging activities, such as mountain biking or downhill snow skiing. The goal is to increase the client's use and knowledge of equipment and create an environment where safety, fun, and learning go hand in hand to allow the client to attain greater functional independence and a satisfying leisure lifestyle.

Health Protection/Health Promotion Model

Another therapeutic recreation model with historical significance is the **health protection/ health promotion** model (Austin & Crawford, 1996; Austin, 2011; see figure 5.2). Under this model, the goal of "recreational therapy" includes "(a). restoring health and assisting clients to cope with chronic conditions and disabilities and (b). helping clients to use their leisure in optimizing their potentials and striving for high-level wellness" (Austin, Crawford, McCormick, & Van Puymbroeck, 2015, p. 15). This model identifies that when people become healthier, they are able to attain control over their lives and truly experience leisure.

For therapists who use the health protection/ health promotion model, the patient must stabilize and protect his or her health, which then allows the therapist to provide therapeutic interventions that facilitate leisure experiences and, ultimately, contribute to self-actualization. The model is based on theories related to humanism, wellness, and self-actualization, with the goals of therapeutic recreation services being to assist clients in recovering from "threats to health (health protection)" and accomplishing "as high a level of health as possible (health promotion)" (Austin, 1998, p. 110).

The health protection/health promotion model is similar in structure to the leisure ability model in that it organizes therapeutic recreation services into three components: prescriptive activities, recreation, and leisure, but the model differs in that it more directly aligns with health care delivery models (Williams, 2008). The three components are referred to as "interventions," which reflect a continuum of services that move clients "from health restoration toward the achievement of high-level wellness" (Austin et al., 2015, p. 16). The health protection/health promotion model "reflects the full extent of RT [recreation therapy] practice," and clients can enter the continuum of services at any point based on their level of health.

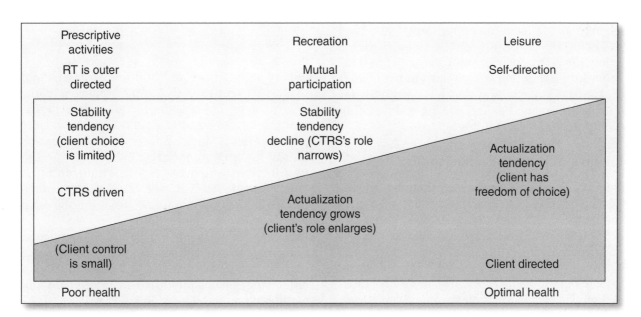

Figure 5.2 The health protection/health promotion model.

Reprinted by permission from D.R. Austin and M.E. Crawford, *Therapeutic Recreation: An Introduction* (Needham Heights, MA: Allyn & Bacon, 2001), 27.

Prescriptive Activities

According to Austin (1998), "When clients initially encounter illnesses or disorders, often they become self-absorbed. They have a tendency to withdraw from their usual life activities and to experience a loss of control over their lives" (p. 112). Thus, therapeutic recreation specialists may have to prescribe activities that will help clients regain control of their lives and begin progressing toward health and actualization. The therapeutic recreation specialist largely directs activity during this component, and one of the main goals of treatment is simply to help clients stabilize.

Recreation

As clients gain stability, begin to assume some control, and move toward health and actualization, they move into the recreation component of the health protection/health promotion model. Relying on the naturally restorative powers of recreation, therapeutic recreation specialists provide opportunities to gain valuable skills, knowledge, and values. As clients become healthier and more actualized, they take more control over their lives and health.

Leisure

The first two components of the health protection/health promotion model focus on health protection, but the third component focuses on health promotion. Through engagement in leisure, clients have the opportunity to become self-determined and ultimately, self-actualized. After threats to health have been largely eliminated in the first two components of the model, the third component provides the opportunity for clients to become healthier and begin reaching their potential.

Leisure and Well-Being Model

Over time, models portraying therapeutic recreation practice have become more systemic, ecological, and holistic. More detailed portrayals of key elements involved in human functioning, both internal and external, have been developed in these contemporary models. Furthermore, throughout the health care world, traditional medical model perspectives on treatment have been challenged. What it means to be well or to recover is no longer limited to removal of symptoms or absence of a medical condition.

The leisure and well-being model is an example of a therapeutic recreation model that provides an alternative to traditional medical models. The model is strengths based, meaning that it focuses on using one's intrapersonal and interpersonal capacities and external assets to achieve potential rather than overemphasizing symptoms and limitations (see figure 5.3; Carruthers & Hood, 2007; Hood & Carruthers, 2007). Within this model, enhancing leisure and developing resources are emphasized as focal points for therapeutic recreation services. Five specific approaches to enhancing leisure experiences are identified and include

- savoring leisure,
- authentic leisure,
- leisure gratifications,
- mindfulness leisure, and
- virtuous leisure.

Equally important is the development of psychological, cognitive, social, physical, and environmental resources. According to the model, enhancing these resources and providing opportunities to engage in the five elements of leisure will improve an individual's well-being (see figure 5.4; Carruthers & Hood, 2007).

Flourishing Through Leisure Model

One of the more radical departures from the traditional medical model is the flourishing through leisure model (Anderson & Heyne, 2012a; see figure 5.5). Like the leisure and well-being model, this model also targets participants' leisure experiences and building strengths and resources, within both the participant and the environment. The creators, however, describe the model as an "ecological extension" of the leisure and well-being model. This **ecological approach** affirms the importance of considering the person within the context of his or her surrounding environment. As such, the flourishing through leisure model provides a very strong emphasis on strengths-based intervention and expands on the influence of environmental factors on therapeutic outcomes. To accomplish this, the model expands on the strengths, resources, and mechanisms for enhancing leisure identified in the leisure and well-being model (Carruthers & Hood, 2007). As a result, the model is one of the most practical and practice-friendly frameworks for therapeutic recreation practice developed thus far.

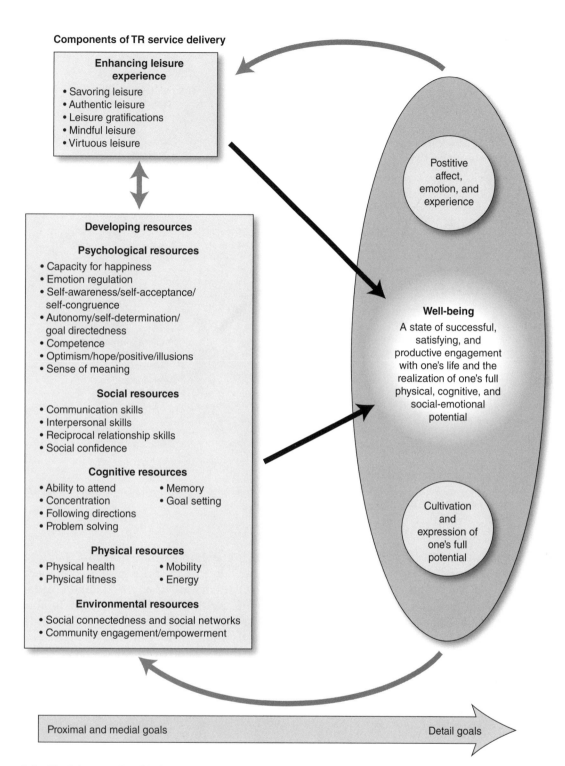

Figure 5.3 The leisure and well-being model.

Reprinted by permission from C. Hood and C. Carruthers, "Enhancing Leisure Experience and Developing Resources: The Leisure and Well-Being Model, part II," Therapeutic Recreation Journal 4l, no. 4 (2007): 298-325.

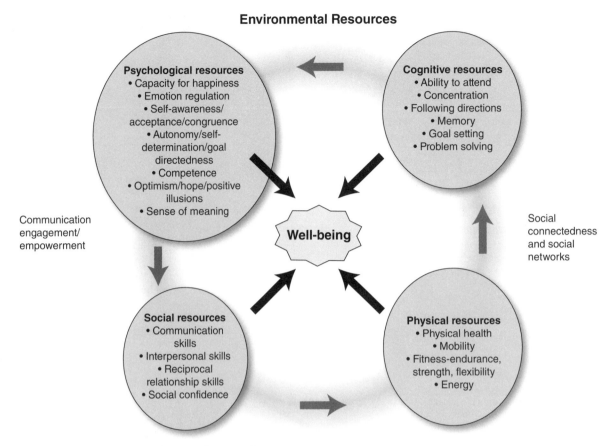

Environmental Resources

Psychological resources
• Capacity for happiness
• Emotion regulation
• Self-awareness/
acceptance/congruence
• Autonomy/self-
determination/goal
directedness
• Competence
• Optimism/hope/positive
illusions
• Sense of meaning

Cognitive resources
• Ability to attend
• Concentration
• Following directions
• Memory
• Goal setting
• Problem solving

Communication
engagement/
empowerment

Well-being

Social
connectedness
and social
networks

Social resources
• Communication
skills
• Interpersonal skills
• Reciprocal
relationship skills
• Social confidence

Physical resources
• Physical health
• Mobility
• Fitness-endurance,
strength, flexibility
• Energy

Figure 5.4 The resource development framework.

Reprinted by permission from C. Hood and C. Carruthers, "Enhancing Leisure Experience and Developing Resources: The Leisure and Well-Being Model, part II," Therapeutic Recreation Journal 4l, no. 4 (2007): 298-325. © Sagamore Publishing LLC.

Look at figure 5.5, and note that the left side of the model depicts "what the therapeutic recreation specialist does." Specific focal points for facilitating strengths and resources are identified for each of five dimensions of well-being (psychological, cognitive, social, physical, and spiritual). Successful facilitation contributes to "a flourishing life." The upper left box depicts focal points for facilitating leisure experiences, which are inherent in all aspects of therapeutic recreation services.

The flower image located on the right portion of the model depicts the outcomes that can be experienced as a result of therapeutic recreation: physical, cognitive, psychological/emotional, social, spiritual, and leisure-related outcomes are each represented by a flower petal. The pot supporting the flower represents the environmental resources and personal strengths that contribute to "a flourishing life."

It is also important to note that the flourishing through leisure model is grounded in the upward spiral theory of lifestyle change (Anderson & Heyne, 2016; Frederickson, 2015). In short, this theory says that behavior change lasts only when positive emotions persist. Positive emotions provide the motivation necessary for behavior to continue on, and leisure experiences have the potential to drive positive emotions. Simply put, the key to keeping a behavior going is to find ways to make it pleasant, enjoyable, or just plain fun.

Broader Models of Practice

The models presented thus far have been designed specifically for therapeutic recreation practice. It is important to note other broader conceptual-

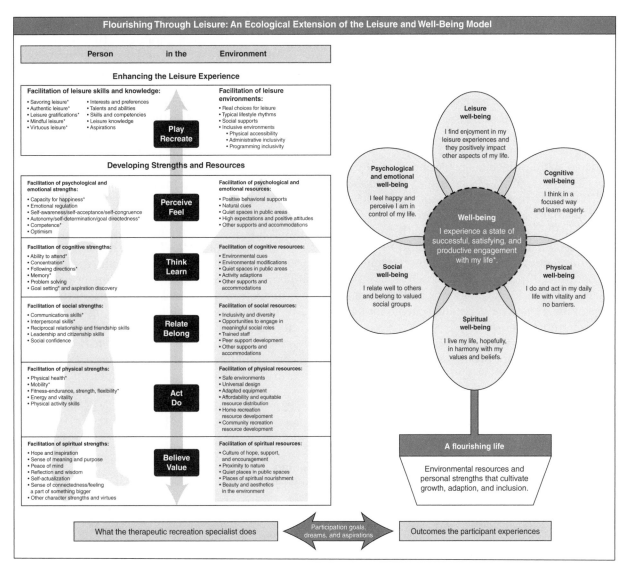

Figure 5.5 The flourishing through leisure model.

Reprinted by permission from L.S. Anderson and L.A. Heyne, "Flourishing Through Leisure: An Ecological Extension of the Leisure and Well-Being Model in Therapeutic Recreation Strengths-Based Practice," *Therapeutic Recreation Journal* 46, no. 2 (2012): 129-152.

izations of health care and wellness that can be useful not only in providing therapeutic recreation services but also in aligning these services with national and global perspectives on health and wellness. In this section, we explore two such examples that have the potential to provide a framework for practice that aligns not only with the work of other professionals within the treatment team but also with models designed for a broader audience that can provide guidance in aligning therapeutic recreation practice with more comprehensive perspectives.

WHO, the *ICF*, and Implications for Therapeutic Recreation

The World Health Organization (WHO) was formed by the United Nations in 1948. That same year, the WHO established a definition for health that is still being used today. By defining **health** as "a state of complete physical, mental and social well-being and not merely the absence of disease or infirmity," the WHO set in place the ideal of a **holistic** approach to health. In an effort to further describe this concept of holistic health and to make possible a worldwide system of standardized communication and collaboration in health care, the WHO published the *International Classification of Functioning, Disability and Health*. Commonly referred to as the *ICF*, this document was the result of 7 years of work and collaboration with health professionals in more than 60 countries (WHO, 2001).

The overall aim of the *ICF* is "to provide a unified and standardized language and framework for the description of health and health-related states" (WHO, 2001, p. 1). This aim manifests through four primary goals: (a) to provide a scientific basis for the consequences of health conditions; (b) to establish a common language to improve communications among health professionals; (c) to permit comparison of data across countries, health care disciplines, services, and time; and (d) to provide a systematic coding scheme for health information systems.

One key characteristic of the *ICF* is that it requires health care professionals to use an integrative approach rather than focus on a medical or social model. This method entails considering all factors that interact to influence a person's health, including the importance of recreation, leisure, and play. This approach is different from the traditional health care paradigms that focus solely on **etiological** causality and the linear progression of a person's disease or disability.

By offering a framework to consider the context in which people live instead of just the person (see figure 5.6), the *ICF* further empowers therapeutic recreation specialists to create and enhance communities that support positive free-time choices and experiences. The *ICF* is also intended for application across cultures as a universal model without reliance on Western concepts, encouraging our discipline to use the diversity within our clientele as a positive for all people.

The concepts of the *ICF* and its terminology are compatible with therapeutic recreation practice. Therefore, therapeutic recreation practitioners, educators, and researchers can further their discipline by being attentive and willing to participate in efforts to align health care and the therapeutic recreation discipline with the *ICF* as a global conceptualization of health. The *ICF* should be a critical piece of every therapeutic recreation specialist's professional training and skill set. The following sections describe basic concepts and mechanisms used in the *ICF*.

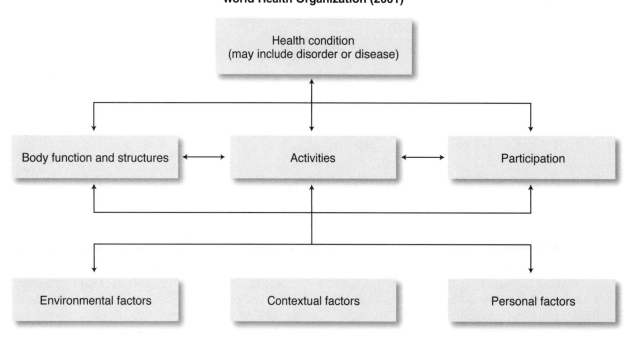

International Classification of Functioning, Disability, and Health (ICF)
World Health Organization (2001)

Figure 5.6 The *ICF* is an interactive model that illustrates the relationship between the concepts of a person's health condition, body structures and functions, activities and participation, and environmental and personal factors (WHO, 2001).

Health Condition

The use of the term **health condition** refers to the current health status of each person regardless of whether a disease, disorder, or trauma exists. The *ICF* does not classify or code disorders or diseases, deferring that function to another of the WHO's family of classifications, the *International Classification of Diseases*, or *ICD*. The *ICD* had its origins in the 1850s and now exists in its 11th edition. A useful simplification is to view the *ICD* as a manual that codes the various ways in which people experience disease or disorder and die, and the *ICF* as a manual that describes and codes the way in which people live.

Body Structures and Functions

Body structures and functions are identified in eight sections: (1) the nervous system and mental functions; (2) related structures of the eyes, ears, and sensory functions (including pain); (3) structures involved in voice and speech and corresponding functions; (4) cardiovascular, immunological, and respiratory systems and related functions; (5) digestive, metabolic, and endocrine systems and corresponding functions; (6) genitourinary and reproductive systems and corresponding functions; (7) structures related to movement and neuromusculoskeletal functions; and (8) structures and functions related to the skin. The term **impairment** is used when a significant deviation, loss, or problem in a body function or structure is present (WHO, 2001).

Activity and Participation

The features of the *ICF* that are of greatest salience to therapeutic recreation are probably the **activity** and **participation** sections. The *ICF* describes activity as being able to execute and complete tasks (e.g., reading, thinking, walking, dressing, voiding, solving problems, engaging in basic interpersonal interactions, and making decisions). **Activity limitations** are difficulties experienced when attempting to perform tasks.

Participation is defined as involvement in meaningful life situations (e.g., going shopping, spending time on a hobby, dating, completing work tasks, volunteering, or attending a sporting event). Participation restrictions include any and all elements or situations that interfere with participating in meaningful life events. Within the *ICF* book, activities and participation make up nine chapters: (1) learning and applying knowledge; (2) general tasks and demands; (3) communication; (4) movement; (5) self-care; (6) domestic life areas; (7) interpersonal interactions; (8) major life areas; and (9) community, social, and civic life. This last chapter includes descriptions of recreation and leisure with separate definitions of play, sports, arts and culture, crafts, hobbies, and socializing (WHO, 2001).

Contextual Factors of the ICF

Within the *ICF* are two types of contextual factors—environmental and personal. Environmental factors are classified within five groups: (1) products and technology; (2) natural and human-caused changes to the environment; (3) services, systems, and policies; (4) support and relationships; and (5) attitudes. Personal factors include characteristics that have a role in health and disability, such as gender, race, age, fitness, lifestyle, behavioral patterns or habits, upbringing, coping styles, social background, economic circumstance, education, profession, past and current experience, individual psychological and personality traits, and other such characteristics. Personal factors are not classified or given codes as are the other parts of the *ICF* because of the large social and cultural variations associated with them (WHO, 2001).

ICF's Schematic Coding Scheme

Within the *ICF* is a schematic coding scheme that allows body functions, activities and participation, and personal and environmental factors to be given a numeric code. A generic 5-point qualifying scale (from no problem, coded as 0, to complete problem, coded as 4) can be used with each code. Use of qualifiers allows further description of what a person is or is not able to do. For example, in coding activity and participation components, a **performance qualifier** (what a person does in his or her current environment) and a **capacity qualifier** (a person's highest probable level of functioning) can be indicated and differentiated depending on whether activity and participation are occurring with or without assistance. Body structures are coded based on (1) the extent or magnitude of impairment, (2) the nature of the change to the body structure, and (3) the location of the impairment (e.g., left or right, front or back, proximal or distal; WHO, 2001).

How codes are created using the *ICF* coding scheme deserves a brief introduction. Codes always begin with a letter that designates part of the *ICF*—body structure (s), body function (b),

KARALEE WHITE, CTRS

Education: BS in Parks, Recreation and Tourism–Therapeutic Recreation, University of Missouri Columbia
Position: Recreation Therapist
Organization: KidsTLC, Kansas City, Missouri

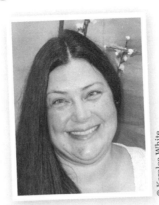

© Karalee White

My Career

Originally, I set my sights on a career as an adventure therapist, but halfway through my undergrad experience, I was in a five-car accident that left me in traction for several months with a wishbone injury to my pelvis and a broken sacrum. In rehab, it was the recreation therapist who was able to reach through to me in my uncertainty and depression, changing the course of my career and ultimately my life. Once back on my feet, I pursued adventure therapy through the lens of therapeutic recreation. I worked in northwest Arkansas as a CTRS and supervisor at an inpatient psychiatric residential treatment facility for children and adolescents. Because much of the state of Arkansas is a national forest, I was able to continue my pursuit of adventure therapy experiences with low- and high-ropes courses, day and weekend hiking trips, camping, caving, kayaking, and canoeing.

After eight years, I returned home to the Kansas City area to work at Marillac, an acute care psychiatric hospital for children and adolescents. In 2006, my focus shifted to trauma-informed care as breakthroughs in brain science research began to reveal a picture of the actual damage caused by trauma, neglect, or even attachment wounds. In 2012, I moved to Shelterwood Academy, a therapeutic boarding school with a brain balance learning center located on the campus. Once exposed to sensory motor integration interventions, my focus shifted to neurological behaviors as a result of developmental trauma. When I moved to KidsTLC in 2016, I was able to bring that focus and pair it with the remediation properties of healthy relational attachments in my therapeutic recreation and wellness programming.

KidsTLC contains one of the few psychiatric residential treatment facilities in the state of Kansas. KidsTLC works to provide children and families with a broad continuum of care through programs that focus on autism, outpatient behavioral health, intensive outpatient care, parent support programs, and street outreach for homeless teens. The services provided are centered around evidence-based therapies and trauma-informed care with a focus on family wellness and preservation.

"To bring joy and to be joy" is my unofficial job description. Officially, I am tasked with developing and implementing therapeutic recreation programming that supports an organizational value of "connection before correction." I focus on relationship building and developing intersubjectivity, a brain-based concept of developmental dyadic psychotherapy that highlights the importance of surrounding children and adolescents with acceptance, empathy, and curiosity as they work through their traumatic experiences. I also design shared recreational experiences that create unity and build community on our campus through a variety of themed activities, events, and camps.

I have to say that it warms my heart to create therapeutic events that bring the entire campus together in creative pursuits such as coffee house talent shows, black light escape rooms, and battleship clue games. To see the kids in service learning settings, giving back to those around them, is healing. The growth of my team of kids and staff alike is very meaningful to me, and I am blessed to witness the culture shift to inclusion and acceptance. I love those breakthrough moments when kids and staff feel safe enough to work through hard things together. Watching a kid relax into hope, as they move through brain and wellness integration plans that strengthen their abilities to cope and interact with their world successfully, allows me to celebrate with them. I love that it is my role to bring the joy that is the counterbalance to the sorrow they have experienced.

My Advice to You

A degree in therapeutic recreation leads you to so many worthwhile endeavors. Don't be afraid to focus on developing heartfelt relationships with your clients; genuine connection with a stable, caring human is what changes lives, because it is directly linked to healthy brain development and function. Have clear, strong professional boundaries in all areas, and have healthy boundaries that show care for yourself. Healed people heal people.

activities and participation (d), and environment (e). The remaining digits of the code are numbers that refer to the level of classification. The first number corresponds to the *ICF* chapter. For example, b2 refers to a body function, more specifically sensory functions and pain, which is the second chapter of the body function section of the *ICF*. More precise levels of classification describe this portion of a person's health condition, such as seeing functions (b210), quality of vision (b2102), and contrast sensitivity (b21022).

Recovery Model

The recovery model is another example of a more contemporary perspective that challenges the traditional medical model and is widely used in mental health and addiction programs. Often referred to as an approach rather than a model, the recovery model, emphasizes hope, empowerment, peer support, and self-management as contributing factors to recovery. Recovery, as

conceptualized within this approach, is more about resilience, symptom management, and quality of life than it is about complete removal of symptoms (Jacob, 2015). The model has been embraced by therapeutic recreation specialists as a means to influence individuals to manage and overcome their given disease or symptoms; create a stable and safe place to live; create purpose and meaningful daily activities; and establish a community, including relationships and social support systems (Duckworth, 2015).

Therapeutic recreation specialists use this model to engage clients in owning their own recovery through multiple interventions that should emphasize values clarification and leisure education. Providing opportunities for personal growth and empowerment supports the focus of the recovery model. Like other models presented earlier, considering the surrounding environment and focusing on strengths are important elements. This is apparent when considering the four dimensions of recovery as defined by the

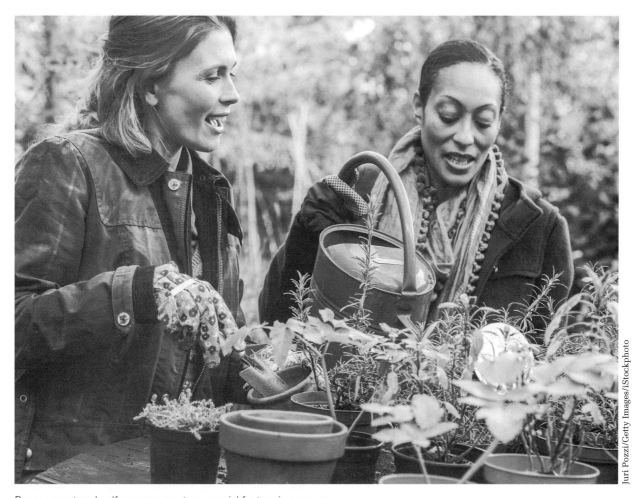

Peer support and self-management are crucial factors in recovery.

Juri Pozzi/Getty Images/iStockphoto

Substance Abuse and Mental Health Services Administration (2018).

- *Health.* Overcoming or managing one's disease(s) or symptoms—for example, abstaining from the use of alcohol, illicit drugs, and nonprescribed medications if one has an addiction problem—and for everyone in recovery, making informed, healthy choices that support physical and emotional well-being
- *Home.* A stable and safe place to live
- *Purpose.* Meaningful daily activities, such as a job, school, volunteerism, family caretaking, or creative endeavors, and the independence, income, and resources to participate in society
- *Community.* Relationships and social networks that provide support, friendship, love, and hope

Each of these models, whether specific to therapeutic recreation or part of a broader representation of health care, can be used to create a framework for purposeful and goal-oriented facilitation of therapeutic recreation. The models presented here are just a selection of the many models that can provide a framework for practice. It is the expectation that the therapeutic recreation specialist will consider the given environment and population when selecting a practice model. Doing so will help ensure that the many unique client needs align with whatever framework is being used by the CTRS to implement his or her daily practice. Utilizing the appropriate model, the CTRS can then apply the therapeutic recreation process in a manner that allows for effective and efficient goal achievement.

Therapeutic Recreation Treatment Modalities

Therapeutic recreation specialists use the term **treatment modality** to describe recreation or other activities used to help clients meet therapeutic goals (Austin, 2001). Considering the wide variety of settings in which therapeutic recreation is practiced and the equally broad spectrum of desired client outcomes, therapeutic recreation specialists must become proficient in using many interventions. The ability to select the most appropriate modality for a client is equally important. Thus,

using evidence-based practice (EBP) is essential for ensuring that the modalities used in practice are effective. EBP requires the use of research findings to critically examine the effectiveness of any modality to be used for client care. The outcome of such practice is that the practitioner is able to maximize the quality of client. Stumbo and Peterson (2009) have noted, "Evidence-based practice is the process of applying the results of outcome research to improve the day-to-day therapeutic recreation service to clients" (p. 229). Simply put, EBP requires that therapeutic recreation specialists avoid the temptation to "go with what they've always done" and instead, use the most recent research-based evidence to select interventions that are best for clients.

EBP requires that practitioners constantly reconsider the approach taken when applying the therapeutic recreation process; however, there is some benefit in examining the more common modalities used in practice. Examining trends can enhance one's understanding of what professionals do on a daily basis and what they find to be most effective with their clients. In addition, examining modality trends over time can provide insight into how the field has evolved. A comprehensive list of therapeutic recreation modalities was developed by Shank and Coyle in 2002 and is provided in table 5.1 with modifications as a starting point for describing modalities that can be used in therapeutic recreation programs. Note that the modalities in this table are placed into categories indicating the nature and focus of the intervention and related client or participant populations. The suitability of any one of these methods will depend on the nature of the clientele and the targeted goal area. The therapeutic recreation specialist must identify potential modalities, ensure that they are appropriate for client goals, ensure that there is evidence of their effectiveness, and implement them in a competent manner.

Games and Parties

Kinney, Kinney, and Witman (2004) noted that although therapeutic recreation specialists commonly use games and parties, not all modalities need to be taught to therapeutic recreation students. Most games are relatively simple to learn, and therapeutic recreation students will have played many of them before enrolling in college. Instead, therapeutic recreation students would make better use of their time and tuition by learning about the therapeutic processes relevant

Table 5.1   Examples of Modalities Falling Within Shank and Coyles' (2002) Intervention Categories

Modality	Modality category (Shank & Coyle, 2002)	Mechanism for change	Possible client populations or conditions	Possible client goal areas
Aquatics	Physical activity	Buoyancy, increased resistance, and water temperature facilitate participation and goal achievement.	Arthritis, cerebral palsy, multiple sclerosis, limb deficiencies	Learn to swim, strength, balance, endurance, physical activity
Exercise	Physical activity	Education and participation programs provided to clients	Senior populations, mood disorders, substance abuse, physical rehabilitation	Strength, mobility, endurance, and physical and psychological health
Sports	Physical activity	Skill development and organized sport programs	All disability groups, with opportunities for inclusive participation	Sport skills, psychomotor skills, and self-concept social skills
Tai chi	Mind–body	Various styles utilize movement sequences for physical and mental development.	Senior populations, anxiety disorders, physical rehabilitation, and intellectual disabilities	Balance, coordination, stress, anxiety, and physical activity
Sensory stimulation	Mind–body	Senses stimulated with pleasurable or meaningful stimuli, such as home videos	Clients with limited or no responsiveness (coma) or with advanced dementia	Increased arousal and responsiveness to stimuli
Medical play	Mind–body	Play is used to help children cope with fears and anxieties about medical care.	Children receiving medical care	Educate child about his or her condition and reduce related fear and anxiety
Dance and movement	Creative–expressive	Utilizes physical, social, and emotional expression through dance	Intellectual disability, psychiatric care, and physical disability	Social interaction, self-expression, and psychomotor skills
Storytelling	Creative–expressive	Oral narratives read, created, and presented by clients as meaningful to personal goals	Family counseling; psychiatric care; and coping with change, hardship, or abuse	Creativity, memory, social anxiety, and self-expression
Arts and crafts	Creative–expressive	Clients are taught skills related to art or crafts; both process and product are applied to therapy goals.	Substance abuse, physical disability, psychiatric care, and intellectual disability	Self-expression, leisure-skill development, self-efficacy, and personal achievement

(continued)

Table 5.1 *(continued)*

Modality	Modality category (Shank & Coyle, 2002)	Mechanism for change	Possible client populations or conditions	Possible client goal areas
Adventure/ challenge	Self-expression and discovery	Adventure/challenge experiences are related to client goals.	Psychiatric care, substance abuse, victims of abuse, and youth at risk	Courage, empowerment, problem solving, and relationships
Reminiscence	Self-expression and discovery	Past memories evoked by prompts are discussed to reaffirm self-worth.	Late life transitions and terminal illness	Self-worth, dignity, and come to terms with past life issues and mortality
Values clarification	Self-expression and discovery	Writing tasks, worksheets, and discussion of personal value system	Substance abuse, family counseling, career planning, and youth and adult criminal offenders	Identify values and examine choices and actions in light of value system
Assertiveness training	Social skills	Group work built around games, role-play, and rehearsal	Intellectual disability, victims of abuse, and family counseling	Social aggression, social passivity, and self-advocacy
Anger management	Social skills	Thinking strategies are learned, rehearsed, and applied in social situations.	Violent offenders, family counseling, and various mental conditions	Expressing and coping with anger in acceptable manner
Reality orientation	Social skills	Environmental cues and verbal reminders used to reorient client	Disorientation from stroke, traumatic brain injury, or Alzheimer's disease	Reduce disorientation, confusion, and resulting distress
Animal-assisted therapy	Nature based	Utilizes animals to enhance goal areas	Autism, orthopedic injury, and depression	Depression, initiative, balance, coordination, and personal care
Horticulture	Nature based	Utilizes gardens/ plants to enhance goal areas	Stroke, traumatic brain injury, and intellectual impairment	Endurance, coordination, concentration, planning, and decision making
Assistive technology training	Education based	Education about assistive devices available to clients	Physical or communication-related disabilities of all types	Eliminate barriers to communication and participation
Community reintegration	Education based	Education about and practice of activities in the community	Physical rehabilitation, psychiatric care, and substance abuse	Identify resources and barriers, make adaptations, and maximize participation

to client change and the ways in which games and parties can activate or enhance such mechanisms. Furthermore, simply facilitating a game or planning a party does not fit within the scope of **active treatment**. To serve our clients in the best way possible, be taken seriously as practitioners, and gain access to the resources readily available to similar professionals (e.g., occupational therapists), therapeutic recreation specialists must be sure that the activities they use purposefully target measurable outcomes that address the therapeutic needs of clients.

To be sure, games can be used as an effective treatment modality, but therapeutic recreation specialists must be sure that therapeutic outcomes of a particular game can be clearly documented and meet the goals of the client. For example, many educational games can be used to teach community skills, such as the use of money. Additionally, therapeutic recreation specialists frequently adapt commercially available and familiar games (e.g., Jenga and Uno) to help clients reach therapeutic goals. For instance, children can learn colors and numbers playing Uno. Jenga might be used to assist people in achieving a variety of goals (e.g., improved frustration tolerance, attention, problem solving, social skills, or motor skills). As such, therapeutic recreation specialists

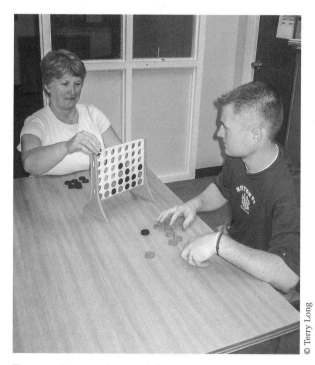

© Terry Long

Therapeutic recreation specialists can use commercially available and familiar games to help clients reach therapeutic goals.

should consider and choose games and parties based on their potential to affect client goals and have a therapeutic outcome.

Community Reintegration Outings

Therapeutic recreation specialists and other health care practitioners frequently use community reintegration outings with clients who have acquired life-altering disabilities, such as spinal cord injuries, and with clients who have been institutionalized for a long period. As reported by Kinney et al. (2004), community reintegration outings were the most commonly used therapeutic recreation treatment modality in physical rehabilitation settings.

Typically, community reintegration outings are planned visits to local businesses (e.g., restaurants) and public facilities (e.g., museums and post office). The risk management issues associated with outings are too numerous to cover, but outings clearly require extensive planning to ensure the safety of clients. For instance, when facilitating such an outing, therapeutic recreation specialists must determine the appropriate ratio of health care personnel to clients and recognize that this ratio will vary greatly depending on the nature of the outing and the characteristics of the clients.

The purposes of community reintegration outings include (a) reducing the stigma associated with an acquired disability, (b) practicing in a real-world setting the skills that have been learned in treatment, and (c) gaining familiarity with community resources. There is a need for further research on the effectiveness of community reintegration outings, but many therapeutic recreation specialists have found the modality to be an effective treatment option for a variety of clients, including people with physical disabilities, addictions, and psychiatric disabilities and older adults.

Creative Arts

Participation in creative arts activities provides clients with a medium for self-expression. Learning skills such as painting or needlework can lead to continued, meaningful participation in these activities outside treatment. For clients who are unable or unwilling to express themselves verbally, creative activities provide an important outlet. Manipulating paintbrushes, clay, and other art supplies can help clients develop fine motor skills. Additionally, successfully completing projects can contribute to the self-esteem, self-image, and overall psychological well-being of a client. From a practical perspective, many therapeutic recreation specialists value arts and crafts because the supplies needed are relatively inexpensive and easily stored and the activities are often popular with clients. Using creative arts as a modality allows clients the opportunity to communicate and express themselves sometimes more than they could independently or verbally.

Therapeutic recreation specialists can use group creative arts projects such as murals to facilitate appropriate social skills such as sharing, turn taking, and teamwork. Although many group activities (e.g., sports and games) rely on competition, which can cause undue tension among participants, group art projects often facilitate cooperation and prosocial communication as well as a collaborative therapeutic process.

Self-Esteem Activities

Therapeutic recreation specialists use a variety of programs to facilitate enhanced self-esteem and self-image of clients. Almost any recreation activity that provides the opportunity for success and self-exploration can be used to address goals related to self-esteem. Clients often list self-esteem as a goal without the proper context. Remember that people develop a positive opinion about themselves when they have accomplished something. Poor self-esteem results from failure. Thus, to facilitate self-esteem, therapeutic recreation specialists must create programs that provide an opportunity for clients to succeed. It is important to provide alternatives to competitive activities, such as sports and winner-take-all games, and cooperative activities are particularly effective at helping clients develop positive self-esteem. Although success is an important aspect of increasing self-esteem, it is also important to allow clients the opportunity to fail, regroup, and then succeed. Winston Churchill once said, "Success is not final, failure is not fatal: it is the courage to continue that counts." This is an important thing to remember when working with individuals because we need to provide opportunities for growth and development as we work toward achieving targeted therapeutic outcomes.

Adventure programming entails many types of cooperative activities that therapeutic recreation specialists and others have successfully used to promote self-esteem. These activities include wilderness activities, such as camping, rafting, rock climbing, and hiking. Other activities within this category include challenge courses, also sometimes called ropes courses. Therapeutic recreation specialists structure these activities so that clients must depend on and cooperate with one another to succeed in progressively more difficult tasks. As the group meets with success, people gain confidence, and ultimately, their self-esteem increases.

Exercise

Considering the well-documented physical and psychological benefits of exercise for practically all people, it is no surprise that exercise is a common treatment modality in therapeutic recreation practice. Benefits of exercise include improved cardiovascular fitness and strength, increased bone density, decreased incidence of connective tissue disorders (e.g., arthritis), and improved mood.

Despite the benefits, many therapeutic recreation clients are hesitant to engage in exercise for a variety of reasons. For instance, people from different generations and cultures have different beliefs about appropriate behavior. Although practically no population could reap more benefits from resistance training than older women because of its positive effects on bone density, connective tissue, and muscle mass, some older women resist such exercise because they were reared at a time when many forms of exercise were considered unladylike. Other clients may resist engagement in exercise because of concerns about how they might appear or unpleasant past experiences with exercise. Therapeutic recreation specialists must help clients understand the benefits of exercise and use some creativity to help clients find a form of exercise that they can enjoy. A particular client may not enjoy lifting weights, but he may enjoy other activities that can provide similar benefits, such as a water aerobics class or gardening. As with any strenuous activity, therapeutic recreation specialists should carefully consider any medical restrictions or general limitations that a client may have.

For clients with physical disabilities, adapted sports are a common and effective intervention used by therapeutic recreation specialists. Adapted sports such as wheelchair basketball, wheelchair tennis, or quad rugby offer the opportunity for clients to engage in physical activities that may have been an important part of their lives before they acquired their disability. Others who acquire their disabilities early in life or at birth can benefit from early opportunities to master adapted sports skills. Almost any sport can be an adapted sport. Although the list is far from complete, people with disabilities commonly engage in adaptations of the following sports: snow skiing, water skiing, rock climbing, horseback riding, golf, tennis, basketball, rugby, scuba diving, archery, and even hunting. Therapeutic recreation specialists must consider the interests and abilities of clients when programming adapted sports and be creative to facilitate active participation.

Summary

Therapeutic recreation services are offered in many types of facilities and to a wide variety of clients. As a result, the services delivered can vary greatly from program to program. Fortunately, existing models for therapeutic recreation services are available to help therapeutic recreation specialists organize the programs they offer, and all high-quality therapeutic recreation programs have certain features in common. Perhaps most important, high-quality therapeutic recreation services are designed to provide active treatment based on the needs of individual clients. The many modalities available provide the opportunity for therapeutic recreation specialists to create programs that help clients gain knowledge; increase skills; and ultimately, improve quality of life and functional independence. It is with the goals of safety, fun, and learning that a therapeutic recreation specialist can deliver programs and services in multiple environments utilizing numerous interventions.

DISCUSSION QUESTIONS

1. What commonalities and differences have you noticed among the presented models?

2. What are the pros and cons of having so many different models in therapeutic recreation?

3. Identify the pros and cons of each of the presented models. Which do you like best and why?

4. With the large number of therapeutic recreation treatment options available, how does a therapeutic recreation specialist choose which interventions to use with his or her clients?

5. What is the difference between the implementation of a therapeutic recreation intervention such as arts and crafts and a client's choice to do a crafts project in his or her free time?

6. Which modalities would you be most comfortable facilitating? Which ones would you find difficult to implement and why? What can you do in the near future to overcome these difficulties?

Potential Areas
of Practice

The Therapeutic Recreation Process

Terry Long

LEARNING OUTCOMES

At the end of this chapter, students will be able to

- identify the four parts of the therapeutic recreation process,
- identify basic assessment methods and potential applications of each,
- identify critical considerations for planning therapeutic recreation programs,
- conduct activity analysis, task analysis, and activity modification,
- differentiate between comprehensive program planning and specific program planning,
- identify planning and implementation considerations related to technical skills and counseling skills,
- identify and explain various aspects of briefing and debriefing therapeutic recreation–based experiences, and
- identify appropriate techniques and applications of client and program evaluation.

The **therapeutic recreation process** consists of four parts: assessment, planning, implementation, and evaluation. **Assessment** involves identification of the client's current level of functioning as it relates to therapeutic recreation services. **Planning** includes developing a plan of care for the individual client, placing the client into appropriate therapeutic recreation programs, and structuring those programs in a manner that best addresses targeted goals. **Implementation** involves delivery of planned programs and facilitation of related experiences before, during, and after the program. **Evaluation** comes in many forms, but the ultimate purpose is to document client progression or regression. Gathered information can then be used to fine-tune various aspects of the ongoing therapeutic recreation process.

The therapeutic recreation process, at first glance, may appear to involve a linear progression through the four stages, but this is not the case. After conducting initial assessment and engaging the client in the therapy process, each of these four stages can occur and reoccur. Recently, scholars and experts in the field have advocated that documentation be specified as a fifth major element of the therapeutic recreation process, which further illustrates the importance of understanding the process from a nonlinear perspective. As such, it is common to see this process referred to as both "APIE" and "APIED". Documentation is critical at every phase when working with clients, from day 1 to departure. An overview of the therapeutic recreation process is shown in figure 6.1.

In short, mastery of all aspects of the therapeutic recreation process is critical to competent professional practice. A therapeutic recreation professional must continually consider the need to revisit assessment, revise treatment goals, alter program delivery, and evaluate outcomes, all while documenting the details along the way. The therapeutic recreation process maximizes program effectiveness through best practices and avoids the pitfall of becoming locked into "old-school" programming approaches that are outdated, ineffective, and misaligned with the needs of clients. Thus, understanding how the therapeutic recreation process works is a fundamental skill that all practicing therapeutic recreation professionals must master.

Assessment

An endless number of definitions have been provided for assessment, most of which are fancy ways of saying the same thing. Put simply, assessment is the information-gathering process that starts when clients enter the therapeutic recreation program and continues until departure from the program. The nature and use of this gathered information will vary based on the purpose of the program. In most cases, this information is used to identify wants and needs of the client (current level of functioning and goals for the future) as well as any information relevant to the process of addressing those needs (e.g., personal strengths, financial limitations, or family support).

Stumbo (2002) provided a more formal conceptualization of assessment by classifying the purposes of therapeutic recreation assessment into four areas.

- To gather client information in order to establish a baseline for client functioning and monitor and summarize client progress
- To determine overall program effectiveness
- To communicate with other professionals inside and outside of therapeutic recreation
- To meet the requirements for assessment by administrators and external agencies such as the Centers for Medicare & Medicaid Services (CMS), the Joint Commission on the Accreditation of Healthcare Organizations (JCAHO), and the Commission on Accreditation of Rehabilitation Facilities (CARF), agencies that oversee issues such as financial reimbursement (CMS) and agency accreditation (JCAHO and CARF)

The basic information gathered for each of these purposes may be the same, but it is used in different ways, all of which are directed toward providing the best service possible to clients. Assessment is the starting point for therapeutic recreation services, whether clinical in nature or more community focused. All actions of therapeutic recreation professionals should be grounded in some form of assessment. As noted in the American Therapeutic Recreation Association (ATRA) standards of practice, assessment is a critical skill for all therapeutic recreation professionals and a necessary component of the therapeutic recreation process (see chapter 3).

Assessment Methods

When dining at a nice restaurant, choosing a dish is a critical part of determining how enjoyable the

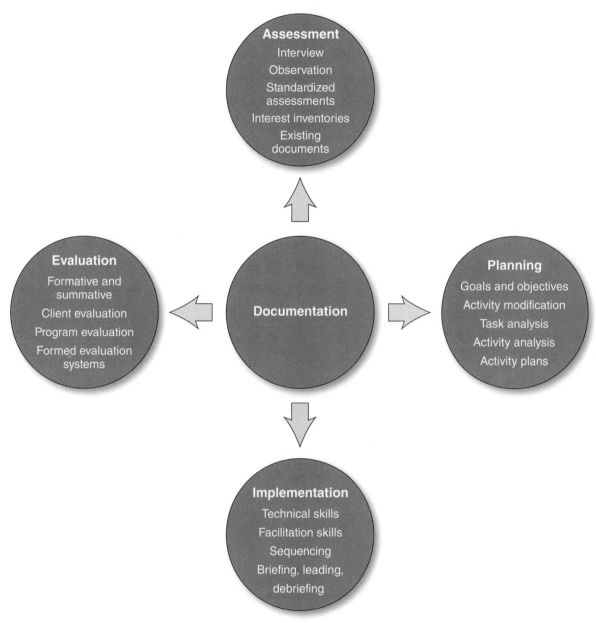

Figure 6.1 The therapeutic recreation process.

evening will be. In making this choice, there are many factors to assess. Reading each menu item carefully, asking for the specials, thinking back on past meals, asking other people for their opinions, and even looking at plates being served at other tables are all valuable sources of information that can be used to devise a plan for ordering a quality meal. Conducting an assessment is similar to ordering a meal in that multiple sources of information are used to devise a plan for helping the client. The more that can be learned about the client's current situation and ambitions for the future, the greater the potential to assist him or her.

Several specific data-gathering strategies are available to ensure a true and complete understanding of the client's situation. Methods include existing documents, standardized assessments and interest inventories, interviews, observation, and registration forms. Selection of one or more of these methods depends on various situational factors including the functional level of the client, the purpose of the program, and available resources such as time and money.

Existing Documents

The most useful existing document is typically the intake **assessment report**. This document comes from a **psychiatrist**, **psychologist**, **social worker**, doctor, or other approved professional who is responsible for identifying and developing a plan to address the client's needs. This report will contain a substantial amount of information including the presenting problem, related history, precautions or standing orders from the lead doctor, results from various assessment procedures, and a summary that includes the overall goals and objectives for the client. When therapeutic recreation specialists conduct a therapeutic recreation assessment, they will create a similar report that pertains specifically to therapeutic recreation goals and objectives. Reviewing the intake assessment helps identify appropriate lines of questioning for interviews and ensures that already available information isn't needlessly gathered (although some instances might require verification of facts). This process also helps ensure that therapeutic recreation goals are congruent with the overall treatment goals of the client, as specified by the lead doctor. Clients' long-standing charts or medical histories can also be useful in gaining an understanding of their issues. These charts often include periodic case summaries that are helpful in identifying critical issues in what may otherwise be an overwhelming collection of information.

The following list represents commonly reported information that should be noted when reviewing intake information in preparation for assessment and planning a program for a client. This list is not all inclusive, and some items may be irrelevant in certain settings.

- General information such as name, age, and family members
- Presenting problem or reason for referral
- Results from previously conducted assessments (e.g., intellectual functioning)
- Any reported leisure-related interests, skills, strengths, attitudes, behavior patterns, or barriers
- Limitations regarding physical activity
- Medication precautions
- Dietary requirements
- Any other standing orders (requirements) from the lead physician
- Facility restrictions and privileges, such as requirement to be in a secured ward

- General behavioral patterns, such as self-injurious behaviors, aggression, and sexual behaviors
- General client goals

In community settings, the therapeutic recreation professional is likely to be the lead service provider; therefore, a general assessment conducted by a doctor typically will not exist. Registration forms generally take the place of a general intake assessment as the primary source of existing information. Quality registration procedures and paperwork can help focus therapeutic recreation services and identify any need for additional assessment. Records from ongoing or past programs, such as incident reports or other forms of documentation, may also be useful in understanding client needs. Although not present in every case, information may also be provided by medical professionals regarding the nature of a particular client's condition. For example, the therapeutic recreation program might require medical clearance for certain known medical risks, such as **atlantoaxial instability** (a condition involving instability of cervical vertebrae that sometimes coexists with Down syndrome).

Regardless of the setting or clientele, confidentiality of information from historical documents should always be maintained. When gathering this information from existing documents, be sure to monitor these files appropriately and return them as quickly as possible. Always keep in mind that information pertaining to an illness or disability should not be disclosed to parties outside the immediate treatment team or service providers without client or guardian permission. In addition, it is critical to confirm the accuracy of information from historical documents.

Standardized Assessments and Interest Inventories

Various standardized instruments have been developed for use in therapeutic recreation settings. Burlingame and Blaschko (2010) provided a comprehensive review of therapeutic recreation assessments in the "Red Book," including details pertaining to the development, psychometric properties, and intended use of each assessment. These instruments are too numerous to discuss individually, but mentioning a few of the more commonly used assessments will be helpful. One of the older, most well-developed assessments is the Leisure Diagnostic Battery (LDB), created by Witt and Ellis (1989) as an indicator of perceived freedom in leisure and leisure barriers.

This instrument can be administered through pencil-and-paper or computerized procedures, producing five subscale scores for perceived freedom (perceived competence, perceived control, needs, depth of involvement, and playfulness) and three subscale scores for leisure functioning (barriers, leisure preferences, and knowledge of leisure opportunities).

Another therapeutic recreation–specific instrument is the Leisure Competence Measure, or LCM (Kloseck & Crilly, 1997). The LCM measures current levels of functioning in eight leisure domains.

- Leisure awareness
- Leisure attitudes
- Leisure skills
- Community integration skills
- Community participation
- Cultural and social behaviors
- Interpersonal skills
- Social contact

Each domain is rated based on the therapeutic recreation professional's observations. The client's level of functioning within each domain is rated with a 7-point rating system that is modeled after the functional independence measure (FIM). Scores range from 1 (complete dependence) to 7 (complete independence) and are individually developed to represent a continuum of independence within each leisure domain. The original FIM is a standardized rating procedure implemented in various health care settings, most notably physical rehabilitation; therefore, the LCM is especially useful because of its consistency with agency-wide assessment procedures.

A third frequently used assessment tool is the Comprehensive Evaluation in Recreational Therapy (CERT). The CERT comes in two versions (see Burlingame & Blaschko, 2010). The CERT–Psych/R is designed to determine one's ability to integrate successfully into society through social interaction, and the CERT–Physical Disabilities examines functional abilities related to leisure skills. Both scales are formatted to allow the certified therapeutic recreation specialist (CTRS) to track changes over time. The CERT–Psych/R assesses social interaction skills across 25 items scored on a scale of 0 to 4, based on the observations of the CTRS. The CERT–Physical Disabilities consists of 50 items related to the following functional domains.

- Gross muscular function (9 items)
- Fine movement (4 items)
- Locomotion (4 items)
- Motor skills (5 items)
- Sensory (6 items)
- Cognition (11 items)
- Communication (5 items)
- Behavior (6 items)

Besides assessments developed specifically for the therapeutic recreation setting, several

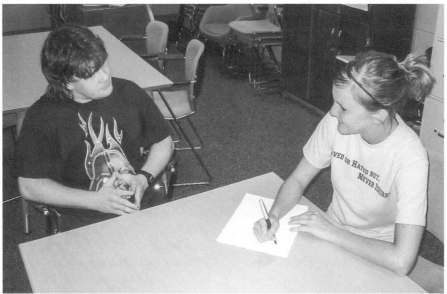

An interview will help you gauge the client's interests and identify therapy goals.

general assessment systems used in certain health care systems or settings are important. Because therapeutic recreation professionals are part of treatment teams within these systems, they must be aware of how these assessments function. The first assessment is the Inpatient Rehabilitation Facility–Patient Assessment Instrument (IRF–PAI). This instrument is used in inpatient rehabilitation settings to assess client functioning in domains such as self-care, locomotion, communication, and social cognition. The CMS requires that this assessment be completed for all patients receiving fee-for-service **Medicaid** funding (part A). The IRF–PAI rates the client's level of functioning with the earlier-mentioned FIM system. A simple decision-making tree is used to determine the score for each rated functional area.

The second system-specific assessment is the Resident Assessment Instrument–Minimum Data Set (RAI–MDS). The RAI–MDS is a computer-based assessment designed by the CMS for use in long-term-care facilities. A team of care providers works to complete the assessment based on observation of the client's functional level. Section N of the RAI–MDS covers activity pursuit patterns and is particularly relevant to therapeutic recreation services. Information relevant to this area is often provided by therapeutic recreation professionals and relates to issues such as time awake, average time involved in activities, and preferred activities. Gathered information is entered into a computer, which then generates guidelines for appropriate treatment plans and determines cost of care.

Both the RAI–MDS and the IRF–PAI are comprehensive assessments that are, at most, only partially completed by the therapeutic recreation specialist, but the results of these assessments can still influence the nature of provided services. As noted earlier, such assessments can be valuable sources of information when developing individualized program plans for therapeutic recreation services (treatment plans). In the case of the IRF–PAI, the LCM can be integrated into the assessment process to ensure that recreation and leisure needs are addressed. Likewise, the RAI–MDS consists of domains directly relevant to leisure and can serve as a major source of information when establishing therapeutic recreation goals and objectives.

Interviews

Interviewing clients is a critical part of the assessment process. Questions should focus on leisure functioning (leisure interests, behaviors, desires, barriers, and resources) as well as physical, social, emotional, cognitive, and spiritual considerations related to this area of function. Understanding the relationship between leisure and other aspects of functioning is a critical competency for therapeutic recreation professionals. When conducting interviews, the therapeutic recreation specialist who has this knowledge can ask the right questions, identify areas that need further questioning, and determine the importance or meaningfulness of responses. See the Client Portrait: Assessing Huyen in this chapter for examples of questions that an interviewer might present to a client.

The quality of the interview depends heavily on preparation. Reviewing available existing documents and results from standardized assessments can be tremendously helpful in appropriately focusing the interview content. Equally important is allotting adequate time for the interview and conducting the interview in a location without distractions. To ensure preparation, the therapeutic recreation specialist should address the following questions before conducting the interview.

- What documents should I review before the interview?
- Have I arranged for needed space and time?
- How should I start the interview?
- What behaviors should I be watching for during the interview?
- What questions do I want to ask related to the reason for seeking services?
- What questions do I want to ask related to recreation and leisure?
- When do I want to ask these questions (beginning, middle, or end of the interview)?
- When I'm finished questioning, how will I close the interview?

The first of these questions has already been addressed, but it is listed here because reviewing documents will help identify information pertinent to the rest of these issues. The second and third questions, related to how to open the interview, are equally important. Goals for opening the interview should include informing the client about the purpose of the interview and therapeutic recreation in general. The therapeutic recreation professional should also introduce himself or herself and explain his or her role within the organization. If the interviewer is an intern, he or she should not hide this fact if it comes up. The intern should be honest with the client, inquire about any apprehensions the client has, and assure the client that more-experienced professionals are also part of the team.

This initial conversation is also critical to establishing some level of rapport with the client. Casual conversation can be used to relax the client and inform him or her of the interviewer's intentions. A casual (but still professional) tone should be carried into the early stages of the interview, meaning that questioning should be oriented toward nonthreatening topics and information that is not too personal. As the interview progresses, the interviewer can move to higher levels of intimacy regarding the topics being discussed. Bringing discussion back to casual conversation before ending may also be necessary, especially if the conversation is emotionally challenging for the client.

In closing, the interviewer should provide the client with information pertaining to the next step. When will the interviewer be back? What does the interviewer intend to do with all the information that the client has provided? What will the interviewer and the client do next time? The interviewer should address these questions before leaving the client.

One question listed earlier that has yet to be addressed is related to observing behavior during the interview. The level of orientation of the client should be noted because it is relevant to a variety of presenting problems (e.g., dementia, traumatic brain injury, or stroke) as well as the validity of information gathered during the interview. Orientation refers to whether the clients know what day, month, and year it is (time), where they are (place), and who they are (person). Time disorientation is usually the first orientation lost. More severe disorientation will progress to place and then person. The interviewer should note the client's posture, eye contact, tone of voice, and overall demeanor because those observations may also be relevant to client condition, assessment results, and appropriateness of certain activities.

Interviewing is a skill that takes practice. There are basic elements of conducting interviews that students should learn, such as avoiding leading questions or questions that solicit yes or no answers when needing more information. Even well-posed questions can be problematic if the interviewer fails to recognize significant informa-

tion within the client's response. A talented interviewer will be able to ask follow-up questions that reveal critical details. Ultimately, knowing how therapeutic recreation services can help clients and then recognizing information relevant to this process during an interview is a key component to effective services. When conducted effectively, the interview is one of the most powerful tools available to the therapeutic recreation professional.

Observation

Observation is a useful assessment tool during the interview, but it can be used in a variety of other ways. One of the major benefits of observation is that it documents actual behavior. Interviews, on the other hand, may be misleading when it comes to differentiating between what people say they do, what they desire to do, and what they actually do. The second major advantage to observation is that it does not depend on the client's communication skills. Many illnesses, injuries, or disabilities may not allow effective interviewing or use of standardized, self-report assessments (although parents, partners, siblings, or friends can serve as information resources). Likewise, some clients may not wish to cooperate with interviews; therefore, observation provides an alternative source of information. In some cases, observation is combined with a standardized assessment, such as the case with the two versions of the CERT. Note that observation cannot measure **constructs**, or internal states, such as motivation, depression, or intelligence. Rather, observation focuses on documenting behavior patterns.

Therapeutic recreation professionals should closely examine the quality and intended purpose of any assessment procedure that they are considering for use in practice. In particular, evidence that a particular assessment strategy is producing reliable (consistent) information and allowing for valid (accurate) assumptions about the client should be considered. This information should also be directly relevant to the client's presenting problem and the potential service areas of the therapeutic recreation program. Assessing areas of function that are irrelevant to either the client's needs or the corresponding intervention or program will result in information that is not usable. Valid, reliable, and usable assessment results are the foundation for developing goals and objectives for the client, and any threat to assessment legitimacy can compromise the entire therapeutic recreation process.

Huyen is a 47-year-old woman who is receiving treatment in a residential drug and alcohol treatment facility. After a recent DUI arrest and conviction, Huyen was sent to the 8-week program by the courts as part of her sentence.

Historical Documents

The intake assessment report conducted by Huyen's lead counselor reported that this was her third DUI and that her life has been significantly affected by drinking over the past 10 years. Most notably, she has lost custody of her 9-year-old daughter, who now lives with Huyen's parents. Huyen also took part in an outpatient counseling program after her divorce. A summary from these counseling sessions (referred to as a chart summary) indicated that Huyen was drinking heavily at the time, but the summary also stated that her husband left because he "didn't want to be a father." Huyen also indicated that her drinking at the time was temporary and her way of coping with the divorce. Despite a previous diagnosis of alcohol dependence, Huyen denied during the intake interview that she had any problem with drinking. As part of the intake assessment, Huyen had completed the Substance Abuse Subtle Screening Inventory (SASSI), which produced results that supported the previous diagnosis. Huyen's explanation for her current situation was that she "just liked to have a good time" and she "wasn't even drunk this time, the alcohol limits are just set low to trap people." Huyen did indicate a strong desire to participate in the 8-week program because she wanted to make the judge happy and regain custody of her child; however, she did not see the program as being useful to her.

Standardized Assessments

Huyen's therapist had her complete the LDB, which suggested that Huyen had high levels of perceived competence in leisure but reported limited perceived control in leisure. Results from the LDB also indicated barriers related to money, opportunities, time, and decision making.

Interview

With the information from the historical documents and the standardized assessments in hand, Huyen's therapist constructed the following questions for an interview with Huyen.

- Tell me about yourself.
- What goals do you have for the future?
- How do you like to spend your free time?
- With whom do you typically spend your free time?
- Have you always done these things, or have your interests changed over time?
- What about when you were a kid, in high school, or even before? Were you into sports, drama, hanging out?
- How would you describe a perfect day for you?
- You've mentioned your daughter and your desire to regain custody. Can you tell me about your relationship with her? Do you currently have any contact with her?
- When you are with her, what do you two like to do?
- What about your parents? How is your relationship with them? What kinds of things do you do with them?
- Let's go back to your current interests and pastimes. You mentioned that you like to hang out at Joe's Pub and to play softball. How often do you hang out at the pub?
- When you play softball, do you drink then too? Does everyone on your team drink, or are there some who don't?
- Why do you think that alcohol is such an important part of hanging out with friends?
- What negative consequences have you experienced as a result of your drinking?
- Would you consider drinking to be a problem for you? Please explain further.
- Do you have any friends who don't drink? What do they say about your drinking?
- What activities do you enjoy that don't involve drinking?
- What activities would you like to try that you don't currently do? How about with your daughter?
- What keeps you from doing these things?
- What things in your life make you happiest?
- On whom do you depend when you are in a jam or need someone to talk to?
- What strengths do you have when it comes to recreation? Social relationships? Family? Life in general? Can you think of anything else related to our conversation that you can tell me?

Although Huyen reported during both her intake interview and therapeutic recreation assessment interview that drinking alcohol was not a problem, her therapist observed that she was, in fact, experiencing problems related to persistent drinking during free time. With the answers from the documents, standardized assessments, interview, and careful observation, the therapist was able to form a more accurate picture of Huyen and her needs so that a plan could be formed to help her reach her goals. Note that during the interview, the line of questioning focused specifically on how Huyen's leisure choices both fed into and were being driven by her drinking, but also encouraged her to express her own goals for leisure and life. Huyen's therapeutic recreation program would most likely focus on these choices and the importance of finding alcohol-free activities and friends as well as how making better choices could help her regain access to her daughter. Also, note that the interviewer attempts to understand the strengths and resources available to Huyen, which can serve as a foundation for building a sober and resilient lifestyle.

Planning

Planning occurs at multiple levels in therapeutic recreation. The broadest form of planning is called comprehensive program planning (see Stumbo & Peterson, 2009). This process refers to the development of the overall therapeutic recreation department, program, or agency. Developing a mission statement, setting goals for the comprehensive program, and identifying specific programs to be implemented within the comprehensive program are all part of this process. The second tier of planning is specific program planning, which involves the detailed planning of the chosen specific programs to be implemented within the department. Individual clients may require different programs, so a comprehensive program or agency typically has several programs. The third tier of planning relates to planning for the individual client. Because comprehensive and specific program planning are a major focus of other courses and corresponding textbooks, this section focuses primarily on planning for the individual client. The concepts presented are, however, analogous to many of the tasks associated with the other planning realms, and the lines drawn between these three tiers are less apparent in real practice.

After a therapeutic recreation assessment has been conducted, the resulting information is placed into a therapeutic recreation–specific assessment report and **individualized program plan (IPP)**, which complement the general assessment report and treatment plan (remember that a doctor typically conducts the general assessment, and in community settings, such documents may not be available). The assessment report refers to a summary of results from the assessment, whereas the IPP is a statement of the client's strengths, limitations, goals, and objectives. Although the therapeutic recreation assessment report and the IPP are developed as separate documents, they are often integrated into a single report. No standardized procedure for reporting assessment results is used across all therapeutic recreation departments or programs, but every organization should require some form of standard assessment report and plan. In addition, the IPP may be referred to by many other names, including treatment plan or individualized intervention plan, but they all serve essentially the same purpose. This purpose is to specify appropriate client goals and objectives based on assessment results, which provide a starting point for the planning process.

Planning Goals and Objectives

Therapeutic recreation **goals** are the general accomplishments that the client strives to achieve through participation in the therapeutic recreation process. Goals should be directly tied to the assessment results and developed in collaboration with clients whenever possible. In fact, thorough assessment reports are like the trail of bread crumbs that Hansel and Gretel left to find their way home. Every goal listed in the treatment plan should be detectable in both the raw data from the assessment and the assessment report. Likewise, any significant need identified through the assessment process should be addressed in client goals and objectives. Essentially, a trail of evidence should support each stated goal and objective throughout the assessment report and IPP.

Objectives are specific, measurable behaviors that indicate when the broader goal is being met. A correctly written objective typically consists of four parts, referred to as condition, behavior, criterion, and time. The condition refers to the circumstances under which an objective is intended to be achieved (e.g., while with peers, during non-work hours, or when requested by a parent). Condition is important because performance can vary based on circumstances. For instance, singing in front of an audience can be much more anxiety provoking than singing in the shower, making the task more difficult. The behavior specifies the measurable behavior to be performed and is represented by an action verb and associated noun (e.g., throw a ball, balance the body, greet a stranger, or identify coping strategies). The criterion specifies the measurable indicator of goal achievement (e.g., at least 75 percent of the time, three out of five times, or meeting 8 of the 10 criteria). Time refers to the expected time frame in which the objective will be achieved (e.g., by June 1 or within 20 days). To illustrate the elements of an objective, consider the goal and objective in the sidebar Anatomy of Goals and Objectives. This example is typical of what might be included in the IPP of a 12-year-old child with cerebral palsy who is participating in a sports day-camp program.

Because goals are generally broad, several objectives (three to five) are typically listed under each of the client's goals. Notice in the example in the sidebar that the objective addresses only one element of the goal. In practice, additional objectives would be necessary to adequately address this goal. In addition, goals should be prioritized. The potential goal areas that might arise during an assessment are often broad. Identifying where the majority of time and resources should be dedicated helps focus therapeutic recreation services on goals that are most critical to the client.

Various models have been presented for establishing and writing goals and objectives. Another common approach is to use SMART goals. SMART stands for strategic, measurable, attainable, results oriented, and time bound. SMART goals are particularly popular in education but are utilized in therapeutic recreation as well. Because goals and objectives are relevant to both planning and evaluation, a more detailed description of SMART goals is provided later, in the evaluation section of this chapter; however, please be aware that SMART goals can be used as an alternative format for writing client objectives and some agencies may prefer one framework over another. Essentially, both models provide a framework for defining targeted client outcomes and also a framework for evaluating those same outcomes during and after participation in a therapeutic recreation program.

Placement of Clients

After establishing goals and objectives for a client, the therapeutic recreation specialist must then determine the best way to help the client achieve these goals. Besides considering the client's goals, the professional must also be concerned about program goals. These are the goals of the various programming options available to clients (e.g., leisure education, social skills group,

ANATOMY OF GOALS AND OBJECTIVES

Sample Goal

Improve motor skills related to throwing, kicking, and catching

Sample Objective

By June 1, the client will overhand toss a 6-ounce (170-g) beanbag into a 3-foot (1-m) diameter hula hoop from a distance of 10 feet (3 m) on four out of five attempts for 3 consecutive days.

Condition, Behavior, and Criteria

- Condition: Using a 6-ounce beanbag, from a distance of 10 feet, into a 3-foot hula hoop.

- Behavior: Overhand toss a beanbag
- Criteria: On four out of five attempts for 3 consecutive days.
- Time: By June 1

Considerations

What part of the goal does the objective address, and what parts still need attention?

What elements of the objectives could be further specified?

How could you alter the objective once it has been met, and why would this be important?

self-esteem, problem solving, **strength training**, adapted aquatics, and so on). Such programs are usually delivered in separate sessions or groups that the therapeutic recreation specialist implements throughout the day. Establishing a match between client goals and specific program goals ensures that the client is placed in or signs up for appropriate programs.

The overall therapeutic recreation program (sometimes a therapeutic recreation department) will typically provide a variety of programs (whether participatory, educational, or therapy oriented) designed to address a certain set of outcomes that are commonly beneficial to the agency's clientele. No one program can address every client need. For example, a social skills group for adults with intellectual impairment is unlikely to adequately address fitness-related goals. The therapeutic recreation professional's job is to match clients with specific programs that address their personal goals. This means that

- not every client needs to participate in every program,
- the groups that a client participates in should provide outcomes consistent with his or her goals, and
- therapeutic recreation specialists are likely to be planning several specific programs at the same time.

The third bulleted item is notable because therapeutic recreation specialists must be careful not to abandon this purposeful philosophy for a "whatever is easiest" approach. To prevent this from happening, planning must be seen as a necessary aspect of every group, session, or activity.

Other Considerations for Planning

Program planning is a complex responsibility. Working with multiple clients with diverse needs and an array of ongoing programs designed to address those needs presents a challenging work environment. Therapeutic recreation specialists typically work to plan programs for the long term, but daily planning for each session of a program based on various client factors and environmental factors is also necessary. These challenges make it easy to lose sight of the therapeutic recreation process and the importance of developing programs that consistently address client goals.

Stumbo and Peterson (2009) made several recommendations related to activity selection that can help address this challenge. These authors emphasized the importance of developing therapeutic recreation programs that will produce predictable and replicable outcomes among clients. This approach is consistent with the concept of purposeful intervention, which was presented in chapter 1 as a key component of the definition of therapeutic recreation.

Considering that Stumbo and Peterson (2009) advocate outcome-driven planning, it is not surprising that the first area they identified for consideration when selecting activities is "activity content and process." Stumbo and Peterson used the term *activities* to describe "the methods by which therapeutic recreation specialists help clients change their abilities, knowledge, and attitudes" (p. 213). Some important considerations related to activity content and process include the following.

- "Activities must have a direct relationship to the client goals" (p. 213).
- Activity characteristics can influence successful activity implementation and related outcomes.
- Clients should be able to place the activity in the context of overall therapeutic recreation goals (outcomes).
- Activities should be interesting and engaging as well as enjoyable for the client.

At the beginning of this list is the concept of purposefully selecting activities that inherently align with client goals. This concept has been repeatedly mentioned, starting with chapter 1 of this book. Stumbo and Peterson (2009) offered more specific suggestions pertaining to this goal and specifically noted that activities related to functional intervention and leisure education involve a purpose that goes beyond participating for the activity's sake.

The second bulleted item pertains to how the characteristics of an activity or the surrounding environment can affect outcomes. Examples of characteristics that might support successful completion of an activity include factors such as client-to-staff ratio, the physical environment, and the presence or absence of skills necessary to participate successfully in the activity. Conducting an activity in a distracting environment or at a level that is above the developmental level of clients will negatively affect outcomes regardless of whether the initial intent of the activity was directly tied to targeted outcomes.

The third bulleted item in the list refers to the need for clients to understand why they are being asked to participate in an activity. Some therapeutic recreation modalities or activities involve

EXEMPLARY PROFESSIONAL

SANDRA K. NEGLEY, MTRS, CTRS

Education: BS in Leisure Studies (Emphasis in Therapeutic Recreation), University of Utah
MS in Recreation and Leisure (Emphasis in Therapeutic Recreation), University of Utah
Positions: Assistant Professor and Director of Recreational Therapy Program, University of Utah
Private Consultant, Trainer, and Public Speaker
Special Awards

* Exemplary Alumni, University of Utah Department of Recreation and Leisure (1994)
* Exemplary Professional, American Therapeutic Recreation Association (1993)
* Presidential Award, American Therapeutic Recreation Association (1998)
* Distinguished Teaching Award, University of Utah College of Health (2007)
* Distinguished Fellow Award, American Therapeutic Recreation Association (2015)

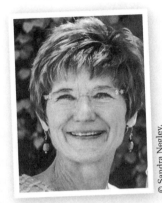
© Sandra Negley.

My Career

I have worked primarily in the area of behavioral health my entire career. In 1977, immediately after graduation, I began my first job in psychiatry. In 1986 I was hired by the Western Institute of Neuropsychiatry (WIN) as the director of activities therapy (AT). The AT program grew from three recreation therapists to 17 full-time expressive therapists. Through the support of the hospital and staff, I founded and directed the Self-Esteem Institute and a challenge course program called ROPES, and I later became the director of adolescent services. The University of Utah purchased WIN and renamed the hospital the University of Utah Neuropsychiatric Institute (UNI). In 1996 I was given the rare opportunity to do the two things I enjoy most: teach and practice recreational therapy. For the following 10 years, I

had a full-time appointment directing the expressive therapies program at UNI and teaching as a clinical instructor in recreational therapy for the department of parks, recreation, and tourism.

I was then offered the position of program coordinator of the therapeutic recreation program, and in 2016 that program moved to a degree program in recreational therapy in the department of occupational and recreational therapies. This is an administrative appointment that requires the oversight of the BS/BA degree program and development of the MS degree program. I teach the clinically based and management courses, and I serve on master's student committees. Contribution to the university and profession—through research, scholarship, presentations, and involvement in professional organizations—is expected. Throughout my career, I have also served in a variety of service and leadership roles through organizations such as the Utah Recreation Therapy Association, the National Association of Recreation Therapists, and the American Therapeutic Recreation Association (ATRA). I am a past president of ATRA.

My Advice to You

Recreational therapy is a health and human service profession that provides a unique, holistic approach to improving the overall quality of life of the individuals we serve. Believe in what you do! Advocate for individuals with disabilities and their rights to equitable services. Embrace the profession of recreational therapy and get involved by joining professional organizations and educating others about recreation therapy. Advance the profession through evidence-based practice and providing quality services. Always remember to create balance in your life between your work, your relationships, and your leisure.

extensive problem solving on the part of clients, so the therapeutic recreation specialist should not be overly helpful during these activities. This guidance does not mean that professionals should hide the targeted outcome from clients. Presenting a task without adequate explanation of its purpose and watching clients wallow in confusion and failure is counterproductive. The activity may be counterproductive even if clients succeed because they may not associate the activity with the targeted outcomes. Therapeutic recreation specialists should fully inform clients about how the activities pertain to their therapeutic recreation goals and objectives. This task relates to planning in that it reinforces the need to plan activities oriented toward client needs and to be prepared to deliver such activities in a useful way.

The fourth bulleted item is associated with the critical second aspect of therapeutic recreation (see chapter 1), which was an inherent relationship with recreation and leisure. When describing the need for interesting, engaging, and enjoyable activities, Stumbo and Peterson (2009) suggested that the planning process should identify activities that clients would participate in even if they were not part of treatment or rehabilitation. In other words, programs should provide activities that reflect clients' recreation and leisure preferences. For this to happen, therapeutic recreation specialists should collaborate with the client as much as possible. When clients are unable to take part in the planning process, family involvement can help ensure that the IPP is consistent with the clients' needs and interests (Shank & Coyle, 2002).

Tools for Planning

Besides describing activity content and process, Stumbo and Peterson (2009) also pointed out that client characteristics and available resources need to be considered. The following section describes several procedures or tools that the professional can use to identify and organize relevant factors related to client characteristics, required activity skills, and the potential application of various resources (e.g., equipment and number of staff needed).

Two commonly used tools for planning activities in therapeutic recreation include the **activity analysis** and the **task analysis**. Sherrill (2004) described these terms as being interchangeable, with activity analysis more commonly used in

therapeutic recreation and task analysis more commonly used in education. Stumbo and Peterson (2004), however, assert that the two tools are inherently different and useful in different ways.

Task Analysis

Task analysis first involves breaking down a specific skill into its component parts. How basic, or precise, these parts need to be depends on how one uses the task analysis. As an example, bending over to pick up a ball off the floor is a behavior that could be task analyzed. The task analysis might look something like this.

- *Step 1.* Flex the neck into the downward position.
- *Step 2.* Visually locate the ball.
- *Step 3.* Position the body so that the ball is next to the foot, directly below the hand.
- *Step 4.* Bend at the knees, keeping the back straight until the hand touches the floor.
- *Step 5.* Grasp the ball.
- *Step 6.* Rise to a standing position.

More-detailed steps or elements of the task could be added if necessary, but for the sake of this discussion, the example is sufficiently comprehensive. Note, however, that the gaps between steps must not be too large or overlook critical aspects of the behavior.

After the elements of a task have been identified, the chronological list of steps is used as a checklist to identify which elements a person can or cannot perform. For example, step 4 in the above example, "bending at the knees", may be difficult for a person who has difficulty with balance. The task analysis serves as an assessment tool that specifies where difficulties are occurring and helps identify necessary focal points for intervention or adaptation. For example, the balance issue mentioned above could be addressed by teaching the client to use a cane for support while bending over, which would allow objects to be picked up from a standing position. Task analysis can also be used to identify appropriate increments of skill or information when teaching complex behaviors in incremental steps.

Activity Analysis

Activity analysis examines an activity as a whole, systematically identifying the skills within each

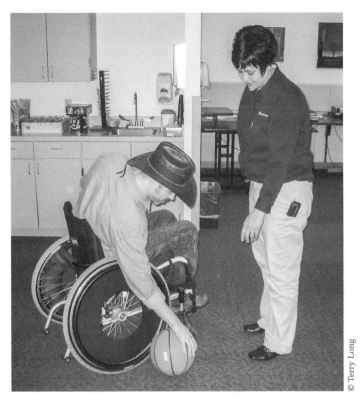

This certified therapeutic recreation specialist uses task analysis to evaluate basic activity skills and identify necessary interventions or adaptations.

commonplace in everyday life, and many everyday products and services cater to commonly needed modifications. Video games offer varying difficulty levels, car seats adjust to accommodate individual differences in height, and sporting equipment comes in all shapes and sizes to fit individual needs. The game of golf is one massive modification system. A golfer can walk or ride, tee off from various distances to meet his or her ability level, and even use oversized clubs and "far-flying" golf balls to turn an average drive into a 300-yard (274-m) monster. Golf is one big adjustable mechanism for finding an appropriate balance between skill and challenge, which is a critical element of any modification.

In therapeutic recreation, activity modifications circumvent barriers to participation. These modifications often come in the form of specialized equipment but can also involve adjusting rules, the surrounding environment, procedures, or the technique used to perform an activity. A softball with a beeper inside, a bowling ball with a retractable handle, a rule change that allows two bounces in tennis, a reduction in the size of a soccer field, or the use of a "sip and puff" device to play a video game are all considered modifications. In any case, modification should allow participation while minimizing the effect on the inherent nature of the activity. Modifications should be made only when necessary. As mentioned in chapter 4, removing modifications that are no longer needed is also important, although some modifications will be permanent. Enabling independent and successful participation is the primary goal. As long as the client is engaged in the activity in the most rewarding, normalized, and independent manner, the modification is appropriate.

functional domain that are necessary for participation. Generally, activity analysis considers physical, social, cognitive, and emotional elements of an activity as well as administrative or environmental factors that relate to the activity. The comprehensive approach of an activity analysis can provide further insight into the results of a task analysis by further exploring the skills necessary for each sequential step of an activity. For example, activity analysis can isolate the reason that a client may have difficulty bending down during an activity. What might appear as poor balance at first glance may actually be a flexibility limitation or a vestibular disturbance (dizziness when tilting the head). Task analysis alone does not provide such details.

Activity Modification

Task analysis and activity analysis allow for appropriate activity modifications. Activity modifications involve adjusting the activity or activity environment to meet the ability characteristics of the client. Activity modifications are

Activity Plan

Whenever possible, professionals should develop an activity or session plan that outlines exactly what will occur during a particular therapeutic recreation program. The activity plan helps address logistical concerns that should be considered during the planning process and is critical to successful programming. Key issues to be addressed include

- equipment needed,
- safety precautions,

- targeted program and client goals,
- rules and procedures,
- potential modifications, and
- activity time line.

Whether the activity plan is a formally written document or just a checklist for planning, the professional should consider each of these issues. The last bulleted item, activity time line, should include a rough estimate of how long each aspect of the activity will take. The time line should not only cover the actual activity but also any discussion that might be necessary (briefing, leading, and debriefing are described later in this chapter).

Activity plans are often developed and kept on record for future sessions but should be reviewed and considered within the context of the current client or group of clients. What may have been appropriate for last year's group of clients may not be suitable for the current group. Within an overall group, individual clients may require certain safety precautions or a change in the manner in which the professional presents or discusses an activity.

Evidence-Based Practice

Evidence-based practice (EBP) is a decision-making framework that can be used by all therapeutic recreation specialists to identify the most efficient and effective approaches to therapeutic recreation service provision. When implementing EBP, the therapeutic recreation specialist makes practice-related decisions by

- closely consulting with the client about their preferences regarding care or services,
- reviewing the most recent research related to the modalities or programs they plan to implement, and
- utilizing past experiences and current expertise to make decisions in the context of client needs and the current literature.

These three considerations allow for best practices to be identified while still honoring the wishes of the client and the wisdom of the practitioner. The ability to engage in EBP is a "must" in contemporary healthcare and has value across all realms of therapeutic recreation. Not only does it pertain to planning interventions and programs, but it is also useful when identifying assessment strategies, determining best practices for facilitation or implementation, and selecting program evaluation strategies. For the aspiring therapeutic recreation student, it is critical to develop a basic understanding of how to find, interpret, and analyze literature pertaining to therapeutic recreation. Working professionals must also be diligent in ensuring they can practice EBP effectively, and should encourage their colleagues to implement an EBP approach in their existing programs.

Implementation

Mental health professionals often describe counseling as a profession that is as much art as it is science. Although therapeutic recreation and counseling are not the same, this artistic aspect of counseling is definitely present in some therapeutic recreation situations. Ask any intern what it was like to facilitate a group experience with real clients for the first time, and he or she will tell you that no predetermined list of questions or activities can ensure that the professional will "say the right thing."

Developing this artistic element of helping others takes practice. A thorough knowledge of theoretical frameworks and practical facilitation skills is necessary, but just as a person doesn't become a great painter from painting by numbers, no one becomes a great therapeutic recreation professional solely from reading a book. Effectively interacting with clients is the most difficult part of working in a helping profession. Genuine therapeutic moments occur when what the professional says (or doesn't say) significantly affects a person's experience, day, month, or lifetime. These moments can range in context from figuring out how to get a camper out of his wet sleeping bag without embarrassment, to persuading a client to recognize the potential effect of her risky behavior, to responding to a physical rehabilitation patient with a severe injury who says, "Why should I play a stupid game when my life is ruined?" Intimidating situations such as these present the professional with an opportunity to have either a positive or a negative influence on clients.

Facilitating such experiences is a skill that is critical to client success, but equally important is preparedness. Therapeutic recreation specialists who have adequately prepared for an activity can focus on the experience of the client rather than dealing with distractions, such as a last-minute search for equipment or stumbling through an unfamiliar activity during a group session. Implementing a program without preparation is like coaching a sport without knowing the rules. Mastering the "nuts and bolts" of any therapeutic recreation program is critical to successful implementation and often involves the development of technical skills.

Technical Skills

Technical skills, sometimes referred to as hard skills, include physical tasks and procedures associated with job responsibilities. Examples include completing paperwork or electronic chart notes, using and maintaining equipment correctly, planning sessions, and demonstrating an activity skill correctly. **Facilitation skills**, sometimes called soft skills, are related to the interpersonal interactions that therapists have with clients. Facilitation skills are maximized when technical skills are mastered and performed in a competent manner. To put it bluntly, if the "professional" pulls a random activity out of a book 20 minutes before a session, fails to understand activity rules and prepare for equipment needs adequately, and neglects to think through how the session relates to the current needs of clients, he or she will almost certainly fail to facilitate beneficial activities or sessions. Adequate preparation and practice, on the other hand, allow the professional to focus on the one thing that he or she should be thinking about during the group: how to facilitate therapeutic growth. As such, the ability to use technical skills successfully during a session depends on whether related technical considerations were addressed in the planning stage (and included in the activity plan).

One important technical skill related to both planning and implementation that can significantly increase the likelihood of success in any therapeutic recreation environment is sequencing. The sequence of activities should be specified in the time line portion of the activity plan. **Sequencing** is arranging the elements of a session or series of sessions in an order that facilitates successful performance. Everyone benefits from sequencing when learning new tasks. A small child learns to walk a balance beam that is extra wide and 6 inches (15 cm) off the ground. As skills develop, the beam becomes higher and narrower. This appropriately graduated difficulty encourages

early success, builds confidence, and provides a consistently attainable goal for the client. The experience of succeeding can itself be therapeutic, especially among those who lack self-confidence or have been discouraged in the past. Such individuals are sensitive to failure, and creating a few simple, early successes can greatly affect confidence as well as their willingness to participate and take appropriate risks.

Sequencing can be planned ahead of time, but the therapeutic recreation specialist must also be able to identify appropriate times to move to the next level of participation and modify activities in midstream to meet the client's needs. When this happens, sequencing is as much a soft skill as a hard skill. It requires on-the-fly adjustments to facilitate a successful experience. Progression through sequential stages can occur over several months or within a few minutes. The issue for the therapeutic recreation specialist is to provide the appropriate level of challenge that both engages the client and allows improvement. Sequencing is a planned element of any activity but also reflects the "art" aspect of therapeutic recreation—the ability to recognize necessary adjustments as they arise and improvise accordingly.

Another important skill associated with implementation is the ability to monitor all clients at all times. This responsibility includes staying in tune with not only what clients are doing but also how they are doing. In some cases, therapeutic recreation specialists monitor from an outside perspective, observing and facilitating the activity without participating. In other cases, they may participate in an activity with clients. Active involvement can sometimes increase the ability to facilitate successes (note that success does not mean performing a skill or creating a solution *for* clients), but this approach can also be a distraction for professionals who focus on their own game instead of monitoring and facilitating the experience of the client. Professionals must never lose sight of their purpose. Maintaining this awareness also represents a transition from technical skills to facilitation skills. Being an excellent glassblower (a technical skill) is much more valuable in a therapeutic environment if one is also an excellent listener, teacher, and facilitator.

Facilitation Skills

Facilitation skills are what create and maximize a therapeutic relationship or experience. They

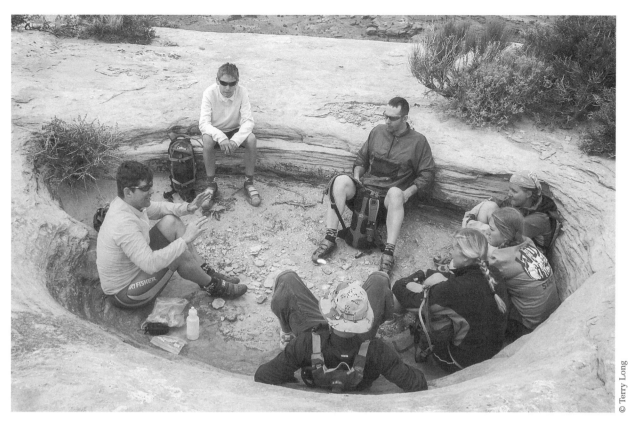

Skilled facilitation empowers clients to reflect upon and understand the meaning of therapeutic experiences.

represent the humanistic side of therapeutic recreation. Observation skills, active listening, and counseling skills all work together to enable personal growth. Because facilitation occurs within the context of technical tasks, the following section will present a mixture of the two. Specifically, three stages of implementation will be discussed. The professional should address these stages during the planning stage, but also be ready to react to events as they occur. In reading this section, keep in mind that sequencing should be present across and within the stages.

Briefing

Briefing involves informing clients of what is about to happen, describing associated behavioral expectations, and establishing goals related to the session activities (Schoel, Prouty, & Radcliffe, 1988). Briefing can occur many days before a session or immediately before the session starts. Whenever possible, clients should be involved in establishing session goals. Two types of goals are used in therapeutic recreation. **Activity goals** focus on the task-at-hand during a therapeutic rec-

reation session or program. For example, activity goals might include successfully completing a challenging group activity, dancing the two-step, or painting a self-portrait. **Spiral goals** go beyond the immediate activity and relate to the Individualized Program Plan and other broader aspects of the client's life. Examples of spiral goals might include controlling anger, overcoming social anxiety, or increasing self-esteem.

Briefing is also a time to maximize client interest in the activity. Through briefing, the therapeutic recreation professional can begin to engineer an experience that is engaging but not overwhelming. Many factors can influence this balance, including clearly defined expectations, appropriate levels of novelty, verbal persuasion, and appropriate use of modeling (demonstration). Appropriate briefing focuses clients on goals and creates motivation and arousal levels that optimize performance.

Leading

When leading a session, the therapeutic recreation specialist works consistently to ensure that the events that take place relate to the targeted goals. Leading involves tasks such as encouraging clients to exercise choice in activities or to continue participating in an especially challenging task. It might also involve the use of skilled questioning that encourages clients to independently consider alternatives and choose a plan of action. Obviously, this "facilitation" of experiences involves decisions and actions that occur in real time and require real time responses from the practitioner. Many inexperienced therapeutic recreation specialists struggle with this skill. Asking leading questions such as "What would happen if you made a net out of the rope and then carried Joe across the gap?" provides solutions that clients should be allowed to discover independently. Another common mistake involves growing impatient with clients and providing hints or other forms of assistance that make the activity too easy. Maintaining balance between too little and too much assistance is just one of many important skills necessary for leading sessions. In working to develop this talent, the therapeutic recreation specialist should consider the following questions after facilitating therapeutic recreation sessions:

- What role was I playing during the session?
- Where was I physically? How did my location and movement affect the group?
- Where was I emotionally? Was I nervous, frustrated, impatient, or distracted?
- How was I communicating (verbally or nonverbally)? Listening? Directing? Facilitating?
- Was I anticipating problems such as victimization or isolation?
- What were my successes and mishaps? Did I facilitate any specific successes? Did I help too much?
- Was I monitoring goal achievement and making adjustments?
- Did I take notes? Mentally or written? What were they, and what was their relevance?

Therapeutic recreation specialists who answer no to this last question will probably be unable to answer any of the previous ones. Failure to take note of significant events is a problem because the facilitator will be unable to process the experience appropriately. As such, the ability to facilitate a group while identifying and remembering significant events that occur during the session is a critical skill.

Debriefing

Debriefing therapeutic recreation sessions, otherwise known as processing, includes reviewing the events that occurred during the session, the experiences and emotions of clients, the progress made toward session goals, and the relevance of this progress to overall therapy goals (spiral goals when relevant). Many structured techniques have been developed for processing experiences. One of the most widely used is the "What, So What, and Now What" approach, often referred to as the Outward Bound approach (Schoel, Prouty, & Radcliffe, 1988). The *What* involves reviewing concrete events that occurred during the session. This discussion helps clients remember what occurred and encourages open discussion by focusing on comfortable topics. The *So What* involves reviewing activity goals that were established for the session as well as emotional reactions to the events that occurred and the effect on the individual or group. The concrete nature of activity goals makes them easy to discuss. This discussion primes the group to talk about related emotions that may have occurred, and how the activity relates to spiral goals. The *Now What* consists of relating the content of the session to issues outside the therapy environment (i.e., spiral goals related to the real world). Questions such as "How is your unwillingness to help the group similar to the challenges that you have faced with your parents?" would be useful during this stage. It focuses on how experiences related to the activity can translate to the client's spiral goals. The *Now What* discussion is the most personal and difficult to facilitate. When there are multiple phases to a program or session, the *Now What* discussion might also address how the experience is related to the next session and how the therapeutic recreation process will continue. As one session ends with debriefing, there is a transition into briefing for the next session.

A more directed processing strategy developed by Jacobson and Ruddy (2004) involves five stages of questioning. According to these authors, the five questions follow the natural processing tendencies of the human mind, easing the movement from stage to stage and the resulting insight of clients. The first question is "Did you notice . . . ?" followed by "Why did that happen?" "Does that happen in life?" "Why does that happen?" and "How can you use that?" The similarity between the two techniques is not coincidental because both are meant to achieve similar results, but there are also differences.

One of the most notable differences is the fact that the first of the five questions, "Did you notice . . . ?" is not open ended, requiring the facilitator to refer to a significant observation made during the leading stage. Jacobson and Ruddy believed this to be critical in setting up the rest of the discussion and avoiding large gaps between what has happened and what can be learned. In contrast, the *What* stage might offer less guidance for participants about appropriate discussion content and relies on the facilitation skills of the professional. Jacobson and Ruddy's process provides a more open-ended approach for the final four questions, but they are still much more specific in nature than the questions asked in the Outward Bound approach.

Important in both approaches is the sequencing of discussion from the immediate experience to the overall therapeutic goals of the client. The therapist must determine how simplistic, complex, directed, or open ended this discussion should be for any particular client or group. For more information on specific debriefing skills and strategies, refer to Jacobson and Ruddy's (2004) affordable book *Open to Outcome*.

These two approaches are general guidelines for processing therapeutic recreation sessions, so not all parts will be relevant in every situation. For example, a leisure education program for adults with intellectual impairment may focus on reviewing events and reinforcing lessons learned with "What would you do if?" questions, demonstrating learned skills, and offering positive reinforcement for successes. In any case, therapeutic recreation specialists should think about the processing strategy before the session ever starts and adjust accordingly to fit the clientele.

Besides the general format for processing described here, several strategies that are more specific have been developed. These methods focus more on how to ask rather than what to ask and can typically be used in conjunction with the two approaches presented earlier. A brief description of some of these strategies is provided in table 6.1.

Table 6.1 Commonly Used Debriefing Techniques

Technique	Description
Go Around	Each client contributes a descriptive sentence or word regarding the activity or a portion of the activity. ("Can each of you share an emotion you experienced during the session?")
Whip	Similar to Go Around, but each client completes a sentence stem presented by the facilitator. Examples include "One thing we did well today was . . ." or "I feel good about . . ."
Memory Game	Clients recall the events of a session in chronological order, with each client taking up where the previous one left off. The facilitator indicates when to pass off the story to the next person.
Gestalt	The client closes his or her eyes, recalls an event, and describes it as if he or she were actually going through the event again. Essentially, the client mentally relives the experience. The facilitator questions the client about the experience when appropriate. "What do you see as you stand in front of the group?"
Props	Props can be used to stimulate discussion, including "talking sticks," playing cards, and other commercially produced processing products.
Artifacts	Physical items created or related to the experience can be used to stimulate discussion. Examples would include T-shirts, medals, craft projects, and self-assessments such as the colors personality test.
Videos or photographs	Videos, photos, or audio recordings made during a session can later be used as a prompt for recollection and discussion of the experience.

Regardless of the technique used, the therapeutic recreation specialist should be facilitating the discussion rather than lecturing clients. In fact, clients should do most of the talking. The role of the facilitator is to ensure that discussion stays focused on targeted goals or other relevant concepts and help clients make connections between the session and their goals. In addition, the facilitator works to ensure constructive discussion and addresses attacking or avoidant comments.

Regarding programs that are more participatory in nature, extensive debriefing may not be necessary or appropriate. Still, discussion should occur about the extent to which activity goals are being achieved with the client, even if the goal is simply to have fun.

Evaluation

As with the other three aspects of the therapeutic recreation process, evaluation techniques vary based on clientele and setting. This section will briefly summarize some of the general concepts of evaluation.

Stumbo and Peterson (2004) defined evaluation as "the systematic and logical process of gathering and analyzing selected information in order to make decisions about the quality, effectiveness, and/or outcomes of a program, function, or service" (p. 364). Everybody wants to see quality documented in therapeutic recreation programs. Insurance companies, government funding programs, accreditation agencies, professional therapeutic recreation organizations, and internal administrators all request documentation of outcomes. This documentation justifies the cost of services by demonstrating outcomes, which in turn justifies the value of therapeutic recreation.

The group most entitled to quality assurance and accountability is the client population. Cost is important to this group, but what they really want is quality care. For the individual professional (and for the organized profession), this should be the motivating factor in meeting demands for quality evaluation. As such, the first aspect of evaluation to be considered is client evaluation.

Client Evaluation

One of the big challenges in conceptualizing an evaluation protocol (procedure) is determining what outcomes should be measured. Logic suggests that evaluating an individual client's progression or regression should be built around his or her preestablished therapeutic recreation goals and objectives. If the client's goal was to participate successfully in an adapted ski program, evaluation should focus on associated skills and participation rates. If the client's goal was to remove leisure barriers, evaluation should focus on the presence or absence of these barriers. Data can be collected in an ongoing manner (formative evaluation), which allows for changes to be made as necessary. Data can also be gathered at the end of the program (summative evaluation). Summative evaluation does not help identify needed midstream program changes, but it is cleaner in terms of documenting the outcomes of a specific treatment protocol or program. Fortunately, the therapeutic recreation process allows clients with similar needs to be placed in similar programs. Because clients within these programs are likely to have similar goals, the data collected to evaluate these goals can be pooled. This approach allows for the overall evaluation of specific programs.

Program Evaluation

Evaluation of a specific program can involve information sources other than pooled outcomes of multiple clients. Financial reports can be combined with outcome data to analyze the cost-to-benefit ratio. Various reporting forms can be used to track the nature and content of individual activity sessions. This type of form is helpful in ensuring that professionals are planning and implementing sessions in a manner that is consistent with client goals and objectives.

Besides looking at specific programs, the evaluation process should review the overall comprehensive therapeutic recreation program. Individual client evaluation and specific program evaluation usually are conducted internally, but internal or external parties can mandate comprehensive program evaluations. Most notably, insurance providers and accreditation agencies may mandate certain evaluation procedures. External agencies, such as the CMS and JCAHO, regularly audit health care agencies to ensure quality of care and accountability. These audits include verification that the health care provider is following appropriate assessment, documentation, and evaluation procedures. In addition to external evaluation requirements, the agency should ensure there is an internal evaluation of the overall program. Such evaluations help document quality programs and justify requests for funds from public or private funding sources.

Evaluation Tools

Before considering specific strategies for evaluating clients, a review of what areas should be evaluated will be useful. Attendance and participation are two of the easiest areas to evaluate but are probably the least informative. Simple checklists typically can be used to record this information, possibly with notations about the level of involvement. Another outcome to consider is participant satisfaction levels. This item is most commonly targeted in participatory programs, but it is relevant to all therapeutic recreation settings. This information can be gathered from participants, spouses, guardians, or parents. The third major area is, again, client goals (targeted outcomes). These goals might focus on client behaviors, emotional states, attitudes, knowledge, or skills and abilities. Methods for measuring each of these areas will vary, but procedures should allow for documentation of outcomes that were targeted earlier. Interviews; observation; standardized assessments and interest inventories; and existing documents can all provide useful, evaluative information and will often be the same tools used for the initial assessment of clients. Evaluation also frequently involves the use of surveys or interviews to gather information after programs have ended or the client has departed.

Even in settings that do not involve clinical intervention, all aspects of the therapeutic recreation process should be implemented. Adjustments must be made to make the process responsive to client needs. The processes of assessment, planning, implementation, and evaluation in a community-based, inclusive recreation program will be much different from those that occur in physical rehabilitation or mental health settings, as will the mechanism for documenting the therapeutic recreation process. This reality does not change the fact that the therapeutic recreation process is necessary to ensure that services produce the desired outcomes. Moreover, therapeutic recreation professionals must have a thorough understanding of how this process works, how it relates to different client groups, and how it interacts with other aspects of the overall therapeutic recreation agency or department.

Evaluation Systems

Many systems have been developed to provide a structured mechanism for evaluation. Two creative approaches worth mentioning here are goal attainment scaling (GAS) and SMART goals (Conzemius & O'Neill, 2002). GAS was first described by Kiresuk and Sherman (1968) as a general method for evaluating the outcome of mental health treatment. It takes a measurable objective and establishes various levels of achievement. The client is then scored based on his or her level of achievement. This scoring system provides a consistent mechanism for evaluating agency effectiveness in achieving individual or program goals.

The creators of GAS provided a system that allows clients to be compared with one another, even when the targeted goals are different (Kiresuk, Smith, & Cardillo, 1994). The current author has used GAS on several occasions as an evaluation tool for a therapeutic recreation camping program for adjudicated youth (referred to as the Empower Me program). The example in table 6.2 illustrates how five goal areas were operationalized into different levels of attainment.

Various sources of documentation from the Empower Me program were used to determine the extent to which these goals had been met. In this case, the same goals were used for all participants, but the system can be tailored to use goals of the individual client. For stage 2 of the Empower Me program (which occurred after camp), clients worked with counselors to establish individual goals under each goal area. One of the most attractive characteristics of GAS is that the evaluation of an overall program can be based on the unique goals of individual clients.

SMART goals provide another method of evaluation. As noted earlier, SMART goals are established as part of the planning process for individual clients but can also be used to evaluate outcomes at the client and program levels. The acronym SMART refers to goals that are specific and strategic, measurable, attainable, results oriented, and time bound. Tree diagrams are used as a tool for operationalizing SMART goals (see figure 6.2). This approach is less complex than the GAS approach but can be equally useful in ensuring that individual and departmental goals and objectives are being developed and evaluated.

Table 6.2 GAS Worksheet and Scoring for the Empower Me Program

Level	Scale 1 Self-concept	Scale 2 Social competence	Scale 3 Planning and decision making	Scale 4 Constructive use of time**	Scale 5 Activity skills***
Much less −2 than expected	Regression in self-esteem.	Average score on CC* social ratings was less than 2.5.	Average score on CC* ratings was less than 2.5.	Appropriately participated in one Empower Me bonus opportunity.	Average score on activity ratings was less than 3.0.
	Three or fewer completed journal entries.	Five or more behavioral violations.			
Somewhat less −1 than expected	Self-esteem scores improved by less than 5%.	Average score on CC* social ratings was 2.5-2.99.	Average score on CC* ratings was 2.5-2.99.	Appropriately participated in two Empower Me bonus opportunities.	Average score on activity ratings was 3.0-3.49.
	Four completed journal entries.	Four behavioral violations.			
Expected level 0 of outcome	Self-esteem scores improved by 5-7.5%.	Average score on CC* social rating was 3.0-3.49.	Average score on CC* ratings was 3.0-3.49.	Appropriately participated in three Empower Me bonus opportunities.	Average score on activity ratings was 3.5-3.99.
	Five completed journal entries.	Three behavioral violations.			
Somewhat more +1 than expected	Self-esteem scores improved by 7.6-10%.	Average score on CC* social rating was 3.5-3.99.	Average score on CC* ratings was 3.5-3.99.	Appropriately participated in four Empower Me bonus opportunities.	Average score on activity rating was 4.0-4.49.
	Six completed journal entries.	Two behavioral violations.			
Much more +2 than expected	Self-esteem scores improved by more than 10%.	Average score on CC* social rating was 4.0 or greater.	Average score on CC* ratings was 4.0 or greater.	Appropriately participated in five Empower Me bonus opportunities.	Average score on activity ratings was 4.5 or greater.
	Seven or more completed journal entries.	One or no behavioral violations.			
Score					
Comments					

*CC refers to challenge course ratings conducted by counselors that corresponded to the goal area.

**Empower Me bonus activities were free-time choices made by the campers.

***Every camp activity involved a 1 to 5 rating of the level of camper engagement.

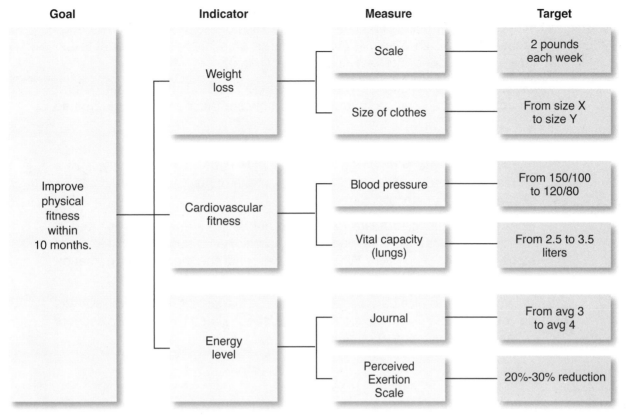

Bill's SMART Goal Tree

Goal	Indicator	Measure	Target
Improve physical fitness within 10 months.	Weight loss	Scale	2 pounds each week
		Size of clothes	From size X to size Y
	Cardiovascular fitness	Blood pressure	From 150/100 to 120/80
		Vital capacity (lungs)	From 2.5 to 3.5 liters
	Energy level	Journal	From avg 3 to avg 4
		Perceived Exertion Scale	20%-30% reduction

Figure 6.2 This tree diagram helps operationalize SMART goals.

© Terry Robertson

Summary

Up to this point, the duties associated with the therapeutic recreation process have been presented in regard to helping individual clients achieve their therapeutic recreation goals. Note that therapeutic recreation specialists are also responsible for developing the comprehensive therapeutic recreation program. This responsibility includes developing the overall mission and goals of the therapeutic recreation department as well as the specific programs mentioned earlier. Clients can then be introduced to specific programs that fit their needs.

In most cases, specific therapeutic recreation programs are already in place, but the professional should always be looking to make adjustments and upgrades. There is no guarantee that an existing program is adequately aligned with the needs of the agency clientele. Development of comprehensive and specific programs is somewhat beyond the scope of this book, but gaining an understanding of how the therapeutic recreation process functions within the context of organized frameworks is important.

All professionals, regardless of where or with whom they work, must be competent in delivery of the therapeutic recreation process. Lack of skill and knowledge in any one of the four areas can threaten the well-being of clients. In truth, the therapeutic recreation specialist has an ethical responsibility to master these skills to the best of his or her ability. At this point, the prospective professional should start to think about being the best therapist possible rather than just getting through college. The foundation of being an outstanding therapeutic recreation specialist lies in making a personal decision to master the therapeutic recreation process. Your personal commitment must be not only to academic preparation but also to the individual people whom you will one day serve.

DISCUSSION QUESTIONS

1. What pros and cons do you see regarding each of the assessment methods presented in this chapter (existing documents, standardized assessments and interest inventories, interviews, and observation)?

2. Discuss the relationship between assessment and planning. What does it mean to target a particular outcome, and how are these outcomes identified or established?

3. How can task analysis assist a therapeutic recreation specialist in determining appropriate sequencing for an activity? Perform a task analysis of a recreation-related behavior, and give an example of how the activity could be sequenced for a particular client group.

4. How does sequencing relate to the two debriefing strategies presented in this chapter? What might happen if a therapeutic recreation specialist skipped stage 1 of either approach? What might happen if the therapeutic recreation specialist failed to proceed past stage 1 of either approach?

5. What is the difference between assessment and evaluation? What similarities do you see? How is writing goals and objectives related to these two aspects of the therapeutic recreation process?

Therapeutic Recreation and Mental Health

Melissa D'Eloia | Keith Fulthorp | Terry Long

LEARNING OUTCOMES

At the end of this chapter, students will be able to

- communicate the role of a therapeutic recreation specialist in psychiatric care,
- understand how therapeutic recreation professionals interact and collaborate with other mental health professionals to provide services,
- demonstrate knowledge of various mental disorders described in the *DSM-5*,
- apply theoretical frameworks for treatment of mental disorders to therapeutic recreation programming,
- identify appropriate therapeutic recreation modalities for use with specific mental disorders or symptomology, and
- recognize the influence of positive psychology and related paradigms on therapeutic recreation practice.

Many therapeutic recreation professionals work with clients whose therapeutic goals are oriented toward psychological well-being. In fact, mental health centers often employ an entire department of therapeutic recreation specialists who work with clients who are receiving psychiatric care. These clients may be facing a variety of challenges, including depression, anxiety, eating disorders, drug-related issues, schizophrenia, or personality disorders. Beyond these clinical settings, many individuals in our communities struggle with mental health on a daily basis. Community-based therapeutic recreation programs provide another layer of support and assistance for those who have difficulty with mental health.

Because leisure is a major domain of functioning that can both affect and be affected by mental health, the therapeutic recreation specialist can play a significant role in both treatment and prevention of mental disorders. Therapeutic recreation programs designed to target psychological well-being are not limited to traditional mental health treatment facilities. Community-based support groups, after-school or summer programs, wilderness-based programs, and challenge-course programs all can be designed to address issues such as self-concept, sobriety, self-confidence, resilience, values, attitudes, and behavior.

Every therapeutic recreation specialist should have a basic understanding of psychological functioning and associated mental health concepts regardless of the setting or clientele associated with his or her work. As pointed out in chapter 1, psychological well-being of the client should always be considered. This chapter will first discuss the role of therapeutic recreation in the treatment of psychiatric disorders and its application to several diagnostic groups. Second, it will identify various psychological concepts that are relevant to all people regardless of disability presence and type. Finally, specific therapeutic recreation interventions that have relevance to mental health outcomes will be presented. Regardless of where a therapeutic recreation specialist works, this chapter is important to his or her success as a professional.

Components of a Healthy Mind

What does it mean to be mentally healthy? Therapeutic recreation specialists should understand that mental health is one component of the more complex concept referred to as psychosocial health. This concept views a healthy mind as having four components: mental health, emotional health, social health, and spiritual health. A psychosocially healthy person has a positive self-image, gets along well with other people, is able to deal with the stress of everyday life, responds appropriately when experiencing negative emotions, and has a positive outlook on life. Additionally, psychosocially healthy people value all people and have a sense of how they fit into the world. Achieving psychosocial health is a lifelong process. Many factors influence a person's psychosocial health including heredity, the environment, family life, personality, patterns of daily life, self-efficacy, self-esteem, and level of optimism. Various factors can cause a person's psychosocial health to deteriorate. Physical problems, extreme stress, or environmental factors can result in problems that affect a person's ability to function in everyday life. In extreme cases, mental illness or a mental disorder may occur.

What Is a Mental Disorder?

Mental disorders are described as "a syndrome characterized by clinically significant disturbance in an individual's cognition, emotion regulation, or behavior that reflects a dysfunction in the psychological, biological, or developmental processes underlying mental functioning" (American Psychiatric Association, 2013, p. 4). The American Psychiatric Association further explains that mental disorders are typically "associated with significant distress or disability in social, occupational, or other important activities" and should not be confused with socially deviant behaviors or socially appropriate responses to stress and significant loss (e.g., unemployment or death of a friend). This definition offers a guiding framework for determining what constitutes a mental disorder and warrants inclusion in the *Diagnostic and Statistical Manual of Mental Disorders* (*DSM*). Further discussion about the *DSM* follows in this chapter as well as some of the more common diagnoses seen in therapeutic recreation clients and potential techniques or modalities for providing services to them.

The *DSM* is a handbook published by the American Psychiatric Association that psychiatrists, psychologists, and other qualified mental health professionals use to assess, diagnose, and classify

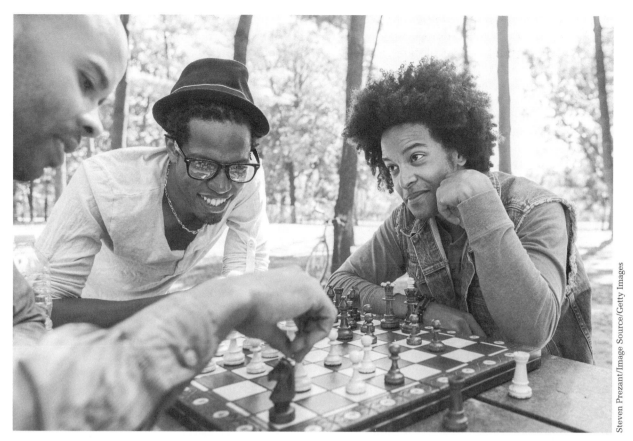

A psychosocially healthy person has a positive self-image, gets along well with other people, is able to deal with the stress of everyday life, responds appropriately when experiencing negative emotions, and has a positive outlook on life.

Steven Prezant/Image Source/Getty Images

mental disorders in the United States. By providing a diagnosis for a client's symptoms, mental health practitioners can develop fully informed treatment plans that meet the unique needs of the individuals they serve. The first edition of this manual was published in 1952 and has since undergone five major revisions, the most current of which is the *DSM-5*.

Released in 2013, the *DSM-5* presented major changes in organizational structure and diagnostic classification. One of the goals for these changes was to align the *DSM* with the World Health Organization's *International Classification of Diseases* (*ICD*) to improve the clinical utility of the classification system and ease of conducting quality scientific research. The alignment of the *DSM-5* with the *ICD-10* was achieved by creating a shared organizational structure as well as harmonized numerical coding system. Significant changes to the organizational structure of the *DSM* were made, most notably the removal of the multiaxial system. In the previous *DSM-IV-TR* edition, there were five specific axes clinicians used to assess and understand a client's current level of mental

health functioning. In the *DSM-5*, the multiaxial system was replaced with a dimensional approach where mental disorders are categorized based on shared features such as symptoms, biomarkers, family traits, and neurological functions. Each diagnostic grouping constitutes its own chapter, which is organized in sequence with the developmental life span, actively addressing age and development as part of the diagnosis. Disorders commonly diagnosed during childhood are discussed first, followed by conditions diagnosed during adolescence, adulthood, and later in life. The overarching goal of these changes was to promote research across the diagnostic categories and gain an enhanced understanding of how various mental disorders are related.

There are currently 20 diagnostic categories, each of which has an identifying statistical code that medical agencies use for billing and data collection purposes. For each primary diagnosis, there is a set of **subtypes** and/or **specifiers** that mental health clinicians use to more clearly define a client's diagnosis. Subtypes are specific subgroups within a diagnosis that are mutually exclusive (e.g., bipolar disorder, type I). Specifiers communicate characteristics of the diagnosis (e.g., major depressive disorder, with seasonal pattern), course of prognosis (e.g., early onset or in partial remission), and severity (mild, moderate, or severe). Social and environmental factors that affect a client's treatment are addressed through additional clinical notations and a series of **V codes** contained in the *ICD-9* and the new **Z codes** contained in the *ICD-10*. The *DSM-5* presents over 130 V codes/Z codes, some of which include psychological abuse, problems related to current military deployment status, insufficient social insurance or welfare support, social exclusion or rejection, and victim of terrorism or torture. An example of a nonaxial diagnosis is presented below.

F32.1 Major Depressive Disorder, recurrent, moderate severity, with mixed features

- V15.59 (Z91.5) Personal History of Self-Harm
- V61.10 (Z63.0) Relationship Distress with Spouse or Intimate Partner

With the new edition of the *DSM* came additional changes that practicing recreation therapists should be aware of. For example, the diagnosis mental retardation was replaced by intellectual disability (intellectual developmental disorder); schizophrenia is no longer broken down into specific subtypes (e.g., paranoid, disorganized, or catatonic); and hoarding disorder, once identified as a specific form of obsessive-compulsive disorder, is designated as a distinct form of mental illness. There were also changes made to the diagnosis associated with autism, which are currently facing criticism from various professional and community-based groups. Prior to the *DSM-5*, there were three specific diagnoses associated with autism: autistic disorder, Asperger's disorder, and pervasive developmental disorder. These specific disorders are no longer identified in the *DSM-5* and have been replaced by one umbrella term: autism spectrum disorder.

Lastly, the *DSM-5* presents several changes to how diagnoses are categorized. For example, substance abuse and dependence are no longer

EXEMPLARY PROFESSIONAL

RON TANKEL, CTRS

Education: BS in Therapeutic Recreation, University of Missouri
Position: Therapeutic Recreation Specialist
Organization: Truman Medical Centers, Kansas City, Missouri

My Career

Following graduation in 1974, I started working as a recreational therapist in a state hospital. In the early 1990s, I decided to obtain my CTRS certification. I now have 40 years of combined experience in both inpatient and outpatient behavioral health settings with adolescent, adult, and senior clients. I've never considered what I do as a job or as work. Each day is exciting, unpredictable, and different. I have really enjoyed my involvement with the American Therapeutic Recreation Association (ATRA). Highlights have included serving as behavioral health section co-chair for two years, presenting at several conferences, contributing to ATRA newsletters, and publishing two articles in the *American Journal of Recreation Therapy*.

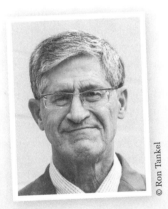
© Ron Tankel

I currently work as a therapeutic recreation specialist in the New Frontiers outpatient behavioral health program at Truman Medical Centers in Kansas City, Missouri. Truman Medical Centers is a 388-bed acute care medical center with two locations, 188 long-term care beds, and inpatient and outpatient behavioral health services. The New Frontiers program is based on a "clubhouse" model that provides a day setting with structured psychosocial rehabilitation groups that provide support and programming for mental health recovery. My role is to plan and implement therapeutic recreation interventions within the facility to enhance physical, cognitive, social, and affective development and to facilitate daily living and community functioning skills.

My Advice to You

Don't be afraid to try something new. Explore, create, and innovate. Live a healthy lifestyle and you will be a role model for those whom you serve.

differentiated and are represented by the broader diagnosis of substance use disorder. Major depressive disorder and bipolar disorder are now separated into two distinct diagnostic groups: depressive disorders and bipolar and related disorders. Finally, the anxiety disorders category no longer includes obsessive-compulsive disorder or posttraumatic stress disorder because they are now separately categorized under obsessive-compulsive and related disorders and trauma and stressor-related disorders.

Role of Therapeutic Recreation in Treating Mental Disorders

Therapeutic recreation specialists typically work as part of a cross-disciplinary team to address the general treatment goals of the client. In mental health settings, this team might consist of psychiatrists, psychologists, psychiatric nurses, **art therapists**, case managers, teachers, vocational rehabilitation professionals, and various other specialized service providers and support staff members. These people work together to identify and address the needs and strengths of clients under their care. One of the primary roles of the therapeutic recreation specialist is to communicate with this group by sharing information that might help others work with the client and gathering information relevant to ongoing therapeutic recreation services. This sharing takes place through formal **progress notes** (charting), daily or weekly team meetings, and direct communication.

Another major responsibility is to provide services to clients that follow the therapeutic recreation process (assess, plan, implement, evaluate, and document; see chapter 6). To understand the context in which this process takes place, consider the general manner in which clients enter into mental health care.

Clients entering a mental health treatment program typically take part in a general intake assessment immediately after being admitted. A psychiatrist, psychologist, or master's-level therapist or social worker conducts this assessment. The intake assessment is designed to identify the client's current level of functioning and establish general treatment goals. Results of assessment are typically accompanied by a general treatment plan that is implemented by the cross-disciplinary team of professionals.

The therapeutic recreation specialist uses this information when implementing the therapeutic recreation process. Therapeutic recreation assessment in mental health settings typically starts with a review of results from the intake assessment. This document, as well as any other historical sources of client information (e.g., client portfolio or chart), provides a basic description of the client's **presenting problem**, which can then be used to develop therapeutic recreation assessment strategies. In most cases, therapeutic recreation assessments in mental health settings involve some form of client interview. The interview usually focuses on leisure interests, attitudes, barriers, and functioning (past and present behavior), although nonleisure information is often gathered when relevant to aspects of the client's presenting problem that can be addressed through therapeutic recreation. Other sources of information include observation and standardized assessments, such as the Leisure Diagnostic Battery (LDB), Functional Skills Assessment–Rehabilitation (FSA–R), the World Health Organization's Quality of Life Brief (WHOQOL-BREF), or the Comprehensive Evaluation in Recreational Therapy (CERT). (See chapter 6 for a more detailed description of specific assessment instruments.)

After assessment results have been summarized in a therapeutic recreation assessment report and used to develop an **individualized program plan (IPP)**, or therapeutic recreation treatment plan, the client is placed in therapeutic recreation groups or programs that will address the identified goals. At the same time, the therapeutic recreation specialist works to evaluate the progress of other clients already participating in these programs. Essentially, all four elements of the therapeutic recreation process are performed at once, as well as the emerging fifth element, which is documentation. Furthermore, an individual client may cycle back through the process. For example, if ongoing evaluation indicates that a client is not responding as expected to a particular therapeutic recreation group, additional assessment and planning may lead to a change in how therapeutic recreation goals and objectives are being addressed.

The nature and content of the groups or programs that clients might take part in depend on the needs and abilities of the clientele served by the agency. Specific therapeutic recreation programs should be developed based on client needs and skills, and placement into programs should follow the same logic. Later sections of this chapter will elaborate on various therapeutic recreation modalities commonly used in mental health settings.

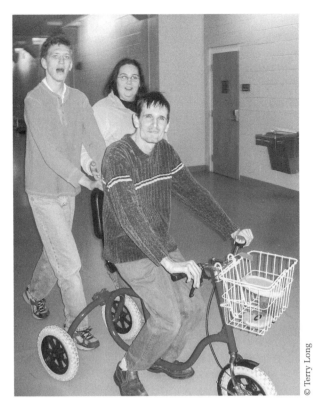

Clients should be matched with appropriate groups or programs based on their individual needs and abilities.

© Terry Long

treatment and residential programs may coexist in the same facility, and clients can move from the residential program to the day program when appropriate. The most independent level of care that exists within this continuum is **outpatient care**. Clients who receive outpatient care come in up to several times a week to participate in therapy groups.

In some cases, mental health facilities are designated as **forensic**, meaning that the facility houses people who are under the care of the judicial system. A forensic unit may serve convicted criminals or people who have been declared incompetent to stand trial as a result of mental status. The exact nature of a forensic unit or facility and the clients served will vary from facility to facility. Because mental illness often coexists with substance abuse, drug and alcohol rehabilitation programs are often part of the mental health care system. Some facilities are primarily geared toward treating substance disorders, whereas other agencies provide drug and alcohol rehabilitation as part of a broader range of mental health services. As with mental health service providers, drug and alcohol treatment programs vary in intensity from outpatient care to residential programs.

Levels of Care in Mental Health

Mental health organizations exist in a variety of forms in both private and public settings. Because therapeutic recreation professionals may work in any of these facilities, a description of several specific levels of care that can be provided will be useful. Clients may move through this continuum of services or receive services at only one level. The most supportive level of care would be **crisis care**, in which clients receive supervision 24 hours a day for a short time, typically for 30 days or less. This level of care is appropriate for people who are at high risk of harming themselves or others. Clients who are more stabilized but still in need of extensive therapy services may seek **residential care**. Although extended stays are less common because of trends away from institutionalization and funding limitations, residential facilities can provide services for several months or even years in some cases. Those who require less support may attend **day treatment** programs, in which clients spend part or all of the day in therapy and then return home. In some cases, day

Diagnostic Categories

The following sections present several of the more common diagnostic classes and some specific diagnoses and symptoms related to each class. A brief description of how therapeutic recreation relates to each diagnostic class is also provided.

Schizophrenia Spectrum and Other Psychotic Disorders

The term *psychotic* is one of the most misunderstood concepts associated with mental health. Society often associates any bizarre or dangerous behavior with the term. This tendency not only mislabels behaviors that may be associated with other conditions but also reinforces stereotypes of people with schizophrenia. The most common misperception is that schizophrenia always indicates some sort of risk to society. The truth is that you have likely sat in a college classroom with one or more people with schizophrenia. Although some people who have schizophrenia can at times be dangerous to themselves or others, this is by no means a defining characteristic of a psychotic disorder.

Definitions of the word *psychotic* vary, and a variety of other conditions or disorders (such as drug use) may cause the same symptoms used to diagnose psychotic disorders. The *DSM-5* (American Psychiatric Association, 2013) describes psychotic disorders as a group of conditions characterized by some or all of a particular group of symptoms. Some of these symptoms include delusions, hallucinations, disorganized speech, catatonic behavior, and flattening of affect. **Delusions** are false beliefs related to the perceptions or experiences of the client, whereas **hallucinations** are perceived sensory experiences that do not really exist. Auditory hallucination, such as hearing voices, is the most common type, but hallucinations can occur in any sensory modality. Disorganized thinking is often reflected in the inability to maintain purposeful conversation. The speaker may jump from topic to topic, answer questions with unrelated responses, or speak in completely nonsensical phrases. Catatonic behavior can take many forms (rigid and unusual postures or purposeless movements) but typically represents some type of disturbance in reactivity to the environment.

Various psychotic disorders are listed in the *DSM-5*, including schizophrenia, schizophreniform disorder, schizoaffective disorder, and delusional disorder, but all psychotic disorders involve some variation in the type, severity, and duration of the described psychotic symptoms. The first line of treatment for psychotic disorders is typically medication, but counseling and ancillary services such as therapeutic recreation can address functional deficits after more severely incapacitating symptoms have been partially or fully managed.

For example, people with schizophrenia may have difficulty adjusting socially or partaking in purposeful activities even after they have ceased to experience hallucinations, delusions, or thought disturbances. To put it simply, jumping into daily life can be difficult when you have spent a significant portion of your life hearing voices, seeing people who do not exist, or struggling to communicate with the outside world. Paranoid delusions can make it difficult to trust even the ones you love the most.

Persons with schizophrenia vary widely in their level of functioning; therefore, services appropriate for this group vary widely. Still, several specific programmatic implications should be mentioned, most of which fall under the realm of leisure education. For people who are not yet ready to function in highly social situations, expressive and creative programs (such as painting or model building) can help develop leisure skills that serve as expressive media and coping strategies but do not require immediate socialization. Programs that develop social skills are also common and can range widely in complexity. Goals may range from being able to maintain appropriate eye contact to integrating into crowded social settings that produce high levels of anxiety. As such, social skills programs can involve both functional intervention and leisure education.

Exploring leisure awareness, identifying leisure resources, and developing activity skills are also relevant to therapeutic recreation programs for people with schizophrenia, specifically under the realm of leisure education. Besides determining appropriate levels of socialization during programming, the therapeutic recreation specialist must consider the client's ability to organize thoughts and participate in complex behaviors. These factors will determine the appropriate content for a particular therapeutic recreation program.

Depressive Disorders

Depression is one of the most common mental health disorders in the United States, affecting over 16.2 million adults a year (National Institutes of Health, 2016). Disorders related to depression are categorized in the *DSM-5* as depressive disorders, including major depression, disruptive mood dysregulation disorder, and persistent depressive disorder. Previous to this change, these diagnoses were categorized as mood disorders, which included other diagnoses such as bipolar disorder. Bipolar disorder is characterized by an instability in mood where an individual cycles between depressive and **manic** states (American Psychiatric Association, 2013). However, the current edition of the *DSM* separates bipolar disorder from depressive disorders and places it into a new category: bipolar and related disorders.

Common among all these diagnoses included in the depressive disorders grouping are intense feelings of sadness, emptiness, and irritability, which have measurable effects on an individual's ability to engage in daily life tasks (e.g., work, social relationships, leisure, and family). Differentiating the diagnoses from one another are issues pertaining to the duration and timing of the symptoms in conjunction with the known causes

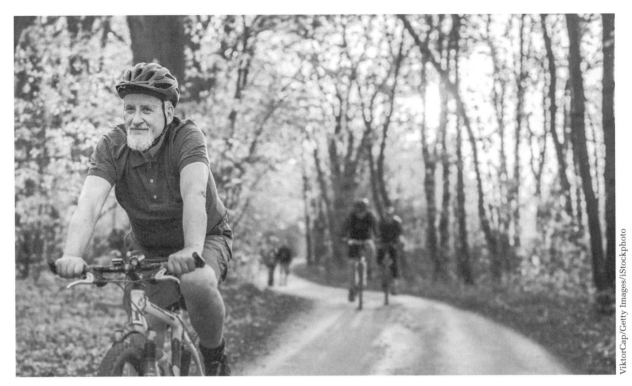

Physical activities help stabilize mood and can release endorphins that naturally enhance mood states.

ViktorCap/Getty Images/iStockphoto

of each condition. Major depressive disorder, one of the most prevalent diagnoses within this category, is characterized by episodes of depressed mood, diminished interest in pleasure, significant weight gain or loss, major disruptions in sleep, fatigue, and feelings of worthlessness.

One popular therapeutic recreation intervention for people with depressive disorders is **physical activity**. Physical activities such as dance, biking, and aerobic exercise help stabilize mood and can release endorphins that naturally enhance mood states. Coping skills can also be addressed through therapeutic recreation. The focus should be placed on issues such as decision making, problem solving, assertiveness training, and self-concept (e.g., self-esteem, self-efficacy, and learned helplessness). These issues can be addressed through leisure education, experiential activities such as challenge courses, and appropriately facilitated recreation experiences in both clinical and community environments. Stress management is another potential therapeutic recreation intervention for people with depression or anxiety disorders.

Anxiety Disorders

Anxiety disorders are often characterized by one of two general symptoms. The first anxiety disorder, agoraphobia, occurs when a person develops anxiety about and often avoids places that he or she may not be able to escape from when panic symptoms occur (American Psychiatric Association, 2013). The second anxiety disorder is the presence of panic attacks. A panic attack is "an abrupt surge of intense fear or intense discomfort that reaches a peak within minutes, accompanied by physical and/or cognitive symptoms" (American Psychiatric Association, 2013, p. 190). Examples of physical symptoms include shortness of breath, palpitations, chest pain, smothering sensations, and nausea. Cognitive symptoms include fear of losing control or fear of dying. These conditions may coexist with specific phobias toward objects or situations (riding in elevators or taking the car on a long trip). Essentially, people with anxiety disorders may have limited recreation and leisure lives. Panic attacks or the fear of having one can lead to isolation and avoidance.

Specific anxiety disorders included in the *DSM-5* include panic disorder, social anxiety disorder (social phobia), separation anxiety disorder, and generalized anxiety disorder. As stated earlier, stress management can be a critical part of treatment, as can be teaching specific techniques for relaxing in anxiety-provoking situations. Panic attacks (a primary symptom of panic disorder) typically involve physiological reactions such as accelerated or pounding heart, chest pain, shortness of breath, and dizziness (American Psychiatric Association, 2013). These physiological reactions often escalate into extreme levels of anxiety and psychological distress. Teaching clients relaxation techniques that focus on physically counteracting the early signs of a panic attack is a common intervention.

Therapeutic recreation interventions for anxiety disorders may also be built around behaviorist-driven strategies such as **systematic desensitization**. Such techniques are intended to allow the broadening of potential leisure behaviors into social environments that might otherwise provoke excessive anxiety. Systematic desensitization can be especially useful in clients who are experiencing agoraphobia. Agoraphobia involves anxiety related to the fear of having a panic attack in a place where escape or help would be impossible. Persons with agoraphobia often avoid leaving the safety of their homes. They use extreme measures to ensure their safety when they do leave home (e.g., by locating all police stations along the travel route). Gradually traveling farther from home, for longer periods, in increasingly crowded public places would be an example of how to apply systematic desensitization to agoraphobia.

Obsessive-Compulsive Disorder and Related Disorders

Obsessive-compulsive disorder and related disorders is a new grouping of mental disorders added to the *DSM-5*, which includes obsessive-compulsive disorder (OCD), hoarding, and body dysmorphic disorder. As described in the *DSM-5*, obsessive-compulsive disorder is characterized by the presence of obsessions and/or compulsions. **Obsessions** refer to "persistent thoughts, urges, or images that are experienced, at some time during the disturbance, as intrusive and unwanted, and that in most individuals cause marked anxiety or distress," whereas **compulsions** are "repetitive behaviors or mental acts performed in response to an obsession" and/or "to prevent or reduce anxiety or distress" (American Psychiatric Association, 2013, p. 237). Compulsions often occur as a means of relieving distress from a related obsession, although they are not connected in a realistic way.

Techniques consistent with behavior therapy and cognitive-behavior therapy are highly effective when working with this client group. A case study conducted by Sheldon and Mendenhall (1995) illustrated how therapeutic recreation specialists can successfully use behavior therapy techniques. The child in the case study demonstrated compulsive behaviors related to cleanliness. He avoided participation in any activity that was "messy," persistently cleaned surfaces in his personal space, and avoided touching messy foods when eating. To address this issue, the certified therapeutic recreation specialist (CTRS) made several initial activity adaptations that closed the gap between required behavior and client capabilities. These adaptations included offering all campers a washcloth during activities and providing alternative methods for painting during finger-painting activities. These adaptations were faded out as the client became more comfortable with the presented activities. For example, the washcloth was moved from the client's immediate possession at all times to a nearby area where it was available on request. This strategy demonstrated the use of systematic desensitization because the child gradually moved toward an anxiety-provoking activity. Also demonstrated is the concept of fading temporary adaptations, here accomplished by gradually removing the washcloth and offering alternative painting techniques. Fading is a technique regularly used to limit dependence on various types of prompts (reminders). Finally, the CTRS was careful to make adaptations for the child available to all campers, which minimized public attention toward his difficulty with "messiness."

Therapeutic recreation specialists have also turned to complementary and alternative medicine techniques, such as yoga, tai chi, and meditation, when working in mental health settings. Yoga, in particular, has been associated with a variety of health-related outcomes, such as improved mood, reduced stress, and decreased anxiety. Research investigating yoga-based interventions for people with OCD have tied yoga participation to improvement in OCD-related symptoms (Bhat, Varambally, Karmani, Govindaraj, & Gangadhar, 2016) and a reduction in the antianxiety medications many people with OCD take (Shannahoff-Khalsa & Beckett, 1996).

Trauma and Stressor-Related Disorders

Many people will experience trauma in their lives. Recent reports suggest that 60 percent of males and 50 percent of females will experience at least one traumatic event in their lifetime (National Center for PTSD, 2018). Many of them will go on to develop posttraumatic stress disorder (PTSD). Although PTSD can occur at any age and in any population, a common misperception of PTSD

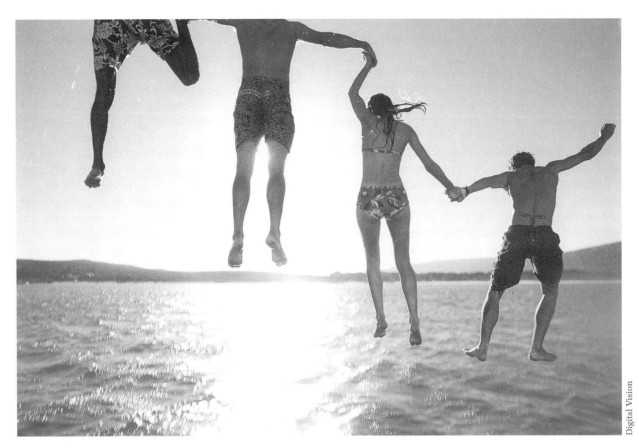

Recreation activities that connect people to natural environments can have significant impacts on mood, attention, social connection, and spiritual growth.

is that people must experience physical harm or injury as a result of the traumatic event. This, however, is not the case because PTSD can result when people experience, witness, or learn about a traumatic event. Symptoms of PTSD include angry and emotional outbursts; intense guilt or worry; recurrent nightmares; flashbacks; and intrusive, distressing memories of the traumatizing event (American Psychiatric Association, 2013).

The primary focus of therapeutic recreation interventions is to help people with PTSD develop effective coping skills and learn how to use leisure-time activities to reduce anxiety and promote community participation and psychological well-being. Outdoor recreation and nature-based activities, such as gardening, hiking, backpacking, surfing, and climbing, are innovated approaches that have demonstrated success, especially when working with the veteran population. Recreation activities that connect people to natural environments, even for short periods of time, can have significant effects on mood, attention, social connection, and spiritual growth.

Eating Disorders

The two most common eating disorders are anorexia nervosa and bulimia nervosa. The public usually associates bulimia with bingeing and purging and anorexia with refusal to eat and overexercising. These features, however, are not the characteristics used to distinguish these disorders from one another. Bulimia and anorexia may or may not involve bingeing, self-induced vomiting, and other inappropriate behaviors intended to prevent weight gain. What separates the two disorders is that people with bulimia do not experience significant weight loss, whereas anorexia involves significant weight loss, which in some cases, is life threatening.

Some people believe that societal norms and images in the media encourage eating disorders, whereas others believe that a psychological need for personal control is the cause. In all likelihood, both factors as well as various other environmental and personal factors contribute to the development of eating disorders. In selecting the treatment modalities to put in place, the therapeutic recreation professional should consider the underlying nature of a person's condition and the theoretical principles that drive treatment. This is accomplished by consulting with the treatment team.

Regardless of these factors, certain types of activity should be avoided when working with this population. Namely, aerobic forms of exercise are counterproductive to the goals of treatment. In addition, professionals must be conscious of other inappropriate behaviors that clients may exhibit. Eating disorders are hidden disorders, and those who have them are good at hiding associated behaviors. Community outings or other free-time activities are times when these behaviors may occur. Professionals must be aware of client tendencies and monitor appropriately.

Specific therapeutic recreation interventions for eating disorders generally work to provide choice and empowerment through appropriate leisure activities. Enhancing the client's sense of control and self-concept is a goal that will generally be in line with overall treatment goals. Interventions might include participation in self-esteem groups and leisure education programs geared toward developing a leisure lifestyle that enhances coping skills and encourages the client to exercise choice and experience control through healthy means.

Adjustment Disorders

Adjustment disorders are psychological responses to significant stressors in a person's life. People who react normally to traumatizing events can be diagnosed with an adjustment disorder if their symptoms significantly impair their functioning. Other cases of adjustment disorders involve a severe reaction that, based on the nature of the stressor, is not warranted (American Psychiatric Association, 2013). Adjustment disorders can involve anxiety, depression, and changes in behavior that cause significant impairment in function.

Working with people with adjustment disorders in the therapeutic recreation setting can involve techniques aimed at improving coping skills, enhancing self-concept, and exercising personal control. Various therapy approaches can be used to help the client improve his or her means of reacting to difficult situations. One approach is to encourage the client to examine his or her cognitive interpretations of the situation (cognitive-based approach). Another approach is to foster awareness, expression, and resolution of feelings toward the self and others (client-centered approach). These approaches refer to broad counseling paradigms, but they can be relevant to therapeutic recreation services delivered within the broader therapy program.

For example, Northwest Missouri Psychiatric Rehabilitation Center, in Saint Joseph, Missouri, uses a cognitive-based therapy approach in treating all clientele. The therapeutic recreation specialists who work with these clients implement problem-solving and decision-making groups that are built around these concepts. When these professionals use their challenge course, briefing and debriefing of the experiences might focus on concepts associated with how clients think through problems and experiences, how their thought processes affect emotions, and how thinking in absolute terms limits options.

If agencies do not align with a particular counseling paradigm, there may still be opportunities to integrate particular counseling frameworks into programs. Note, however, that counseling or talk therapy is not the purpose or the primary method of therapeutic recreation programs. Any such scenario would likely exceed the professional capabilities of the typical therapeutic recreation specialist (unless he or she also had adequate training in a counseling profession). Still, using counseling skills and concepts from a particular framework can be useful and is sometimes required in therapeutic recreation practice. Therapeutic recreation specialists must stay within the bounds of their training and seek professional development if their assigned job tasks begin to exceed their professional capabilities.

Theoretical Considerations

When providing therapeutic recreation services, daily work with clients should be aligned with theoretical models designed to provide guidance in the therapy process. A theory is like a lighthouse. The professional uses a theory to direct therapy efforts in a certain direction. To provide consistent and competent intervention, therapeutic recreation specialists can use the following theoretical concepts. As noted earlier, some agencies or settings may adhere to specific theoretical frameworks. Those entering the therapeutic recreation profession should be familiar with all the presented concepts and keep in mind that they will need a comprehensive understanding of one or more of these theories in the future.

Person-Centered Approach

Person-centered therapy, initially developed by Carl Rogers, is a basic theoretical guideline for therapy environments. Rogers identified three critical elements to a successful therapy relationship. The first element is **unconditional positive regard (UPR)**. UPR refers to the philosophy that all people are inherently good and only behavior is bad. Consequently, judgment is directed toward behaviors, not individual character. The therapist must have UPR toward the client, and the client must perceive the therapist as accepting him or her as a person, unconditionally. The second element of person-centered therapy is congruence, or simply put, genuineness. The client must believe that the therapist is genuine in his or her concern and projects his or her true self. Last, the therapist must work to develop accurate, empathetic understanding of the client's situation.

According to Rogers, these three elements are necessary for a productive therapy relationship. Although some people would argue that more is necessary, most people would support the idea that Rogers' concepts are critical elements of therapy relationships. Of course, simply caring about people is not enough. A critical part of this approach is the development of basic communication skills, such as active listening, paraphrasing, summarizing, and confronting (see table 7.1). By fostering expressive communication from the client, the therapist facilitates the therapy process. For the therapeutic recreation specialist, these concepts are invaluable. They allow the development of trust and provide a basic framework for communicating with clients within the therapeutic recreation specialist's scope of practice.

Table 7.1 Active Listening and Related Communication Skills

Skill	Steps
Active listening	1. *Receive.* Focus attention, make eye contact, face the client squarely, and open your arms. Use verbal and nonverbal feedback to let the client know that you are listening. 2. *Process.* Think about the message and ponder its meaning. Consider biases and blind spots that may cause you to miss meaning. 3. *Send a message, either verbal or nonverbal.* Use paraphrasing, reflecting, clarifying, summarizing, and other communication and counseling skills.
Paraphrasing	Rephrase the content of the client's statement as you've heard it: "So since you married your husband, you have taken on the house and childcare responsibilities and given up your free time with friends" (look to client for confirmation).
Reflecting	Rephrase the affective part of the client's statement: "It sounds as if you are frustrated by your husband's lack of concern for how busy you are and his unwillingness to help."
Clarifying	Ask a question by pairing it with a restatement of the client's statement. Client: "Yeah, he's as useful as a bike with no pedals." Therapist: "Are you saying that he could help if he wanted to or that you don't think he is capable of doing it right? What do you mean when you say, 'A bike with no pedals'?"
Summarizing	Condense two or more paraphrases or reflections into a clear and precise summary of the client's overall message: "So since your husband has stopped contributing to responsibilities such as housework, caring for the kids, and working, you have really started to feel frustrated and, as you described it, trapped."
Common mistakes	1. Parroting—simply repeating information with no productive clarification or understanding. 2. Giving inadequate attention to emotion. 3. Sending verbal and nonverbal messages that don't match. 4. Talking too much rather than listening. 5. Giving advice or making suggestions too quickly.

Behaviorism

Behaviorism, a comprehensive and well-established theory, represents a cluster of therapy modalities. These modalities, or techniques, are based on B.F. Skinner's concept of operant conditioning (Hall, 1975). Operant conditioning consists of three elements. First, a triggering event occurs. Second, a behavior takes place in response to the triggering event. Third, a consequence of the response occurs and is judged as desirable or undesirable. This consequence can be rewarding or punishing. Rewarding events reinforce the likelihood that a person's response will occur again, and punishing consequences discourage repetition of the behavior.

As a practical example, think of a time when you ran out of money. That circumstance would be a triggering event. One potential response to that event would be to ask a parent for some cash. The consequence of your response would be your parent's reaction to your request. If a parent gave you money, that action would reinforce your begging, and you would likely make the same request the next time you ran out of money. If the parent said no, that would be an undesirable consequence, and over time, you would stop asking (this result is called extinction).

In mental health settings, level systems based on these concepts are often used to encourage positive behaviors. As clients earn points for positive behaviors, they are advanced in the level system and have more freedoms. Likewise, undesirable behaviors, such as running away or ridiculing others, can be grounds for lessening privileges or freedoms. In addition, more advanced systems of reinforcement known as token economies are commonly used to encourage positive behaviors. For a description of token economies and various other techniques for behavior modification, refer to table 7.2. Note the cited sources in this table are from a series of training manuals on each technique. These brief manuals are user friendly and recommended for anyone working to master these techniques.

Attribution Theory

Attribution theory explains how people perceive their successes and failures in life and the consequences of these perceptions. To illustrate this idea, consider the story of a minor league football team that won the league championship because the other team failed to show up for the game. Interestingly, the champions had lost to the other team twice earlier in the season. After the season ended, the coach of the championship team announced that the team would return just for another chance to prove that he and his players were true champions. Attribution theory says that the factors to which we attribute our successes will affect our beliefs about ourselves. How do you think the

Table 7.2 Behavior Modification Techniques

Technique	Description	Considerations
Positive practice (Azrin & Besalel, 1999)	When error occurs, stop and practice correction successfully several times.	• Avoid scolding and punishment. • Interrupt misbehavior immediately. • Positive behavior becomes habit.
Response cost (Thibadeau, 1998)	Simply put, consequences are applied for undesirable behaviors. Examples: • Losing recess for talking • Requiring payment of a fee for a late bill • Losing points or tokens for off-task behavior	• Technique is relatively mild compared with aversive forms of punishment. • Allows immediate feedback. • Does not disrupt environment. • When possible, consequences should be logically related to the causal behavior.
Shaping (Hall, 1975)	Teach complex behavior by rewarding successful progression through increasingly complex levels of the target behavior.	• Analyze tasks to determine levels. • Ensure that progressions are attainable. • Examples: hitting a baseball and riding a bike.

(continued)

Table 7.2 *(continued)*

Technique	Description	Considerations
Chaining (Hall, 1975)	Teach complex behavior by sequentially introducing and rewarding parts of the behavior.	• Analyze tasks to determine steps or parts. • Ensure that progressions are attainable. • Can work backward or forward. • Example: In dance, teach step 1, then step 2, and finally step 3. • Each step builds on the previous one.
Fading (Esveldt-Dawson & Kazdin, 1998)	Gradually remove external reinforcers.	• Fading helps ensure that behavior is not indefinitely contingent on reward and helps shift the focus toward natural, intrinsic rewards.
Extinction (Hall & Hall, 1998a)	Ignore negative behaviors through techniques such as refusing to speak to or answer the person, looking away, turning the back toward the person, or removing self from environment.	• Pinpoint behavior to change. • Measure behavior and set goal. • Practice ignoring behavior. • Targeted behavior may first increase. • Reinforce appropriate behaviors. • Other people and staff must also ignore negative behaviors.
Modeling (Streifel, 1998)	Use prearranged models or planned models as a mechanism for learning through imitation.	• Make sure that the learner pays attention. • Ensure that the learner is physically and cognitively capable of behavior. • Model clearly and consistently. • Provide feedback and rewards.
Token economies (Ayllon, 1999)	Provide concrete reinforcers for appropriate behavior. Later, use a backup reinforcer.	• Tokens must be easy to administer. • Administer tokens immediately. • Tokens must be hard to counterfeit. • Establish and always follow rules for exchanging tokens for rewards. • Goal should be to fade out the system.
Time-out (Hall & Hall, 1998b)	Decrease behavior by removing a person from the opportunity to receive attention or rewards for undesired behavior.	• Clearly explain undesired behavior and the specific consequence. • Typically, works best with 2- to 12-year-olds. • Time-out area should be safe and free of reward. • Time-out areas should be easily monitored. • Time-outs should last 2 to 5 minutes and no longer than 1 minute for each year of age. • Add minutes for refusing to go or misbehaving in time-out, up to a maximum of 30 minutes. • Time-outs may not be appropriate for kids with a history of self-stimulation.

Note: Additional information regarding the methods presented in this table can be found in the *How to Manage Behavior* series, edited by Vance and Marilyn Hall and published by PRO-ED.

circumstances of the championship affected the coach's perceptions of himself and his team?

To illustrate the relevance of attribution theory to mental health, consider the explanation of depression presented by Abramson, Seligman, and Teasdale in their landmark 1978 publication concerning attribution theory and the concept of learned helplessness. In this work, the authors pointed out the relationship between the causal attributions that people make, the resulting development of learned helplessness, and the risk of depression.

Causal attributions are the beliefs that we hold about the causes of the events that occur in our lives. A causal attribution is our explanation as to why we succeed, fail, experience hardship, or find happiness. When we are fired from a job, we attribute it to factors such as our boss; our workmates; the fact that we didn't like the job; lack of effort; or most concerning, our lack of ability. Repeatedly attributing failures to our own inadequacies will eventually lead to learned helplessness. If a person believes that he or she is helpless and can do nothing about it, the person is more likely to become depressed.

One approach to helping people break this negative thinking pattern is to focus on the attributions that they are making. In many cases, they may be ignoring outside influences and taking blame for all their misfortune. Statements like "If I could have made my wife happy, we would still be married" ignore the fact that other factors may have led to the event. This example is an internal, as opposed to an external, attribution. The statement "I always screw up relationships; I just don't have what it takes to make it work" is not only internal but also stable, as opposed to unstable. This type of attribution means that things are viewed as unlikely to change. Finally, a comment like "I just can't have cordial relationships with women at all, even at work or with family" represents a global, as opposed to a specific, attribution. Global attributions represent a generalization of the basic belief to other settings or situations. Ultimately, internal, stable, global attributions about our failures will lead to learned helplessness and depression. The therapist's job is to bring attention to this type of negative thinking and encourage the client to think about alternative explanations for failures. The therapist must also watch out for external, unstable, and specific attributions when a person succeeds. This pattern is equally dangerous and may be reflected in comments like "I never would have won if Joe had been trying harder." For the therapeutic recreation specialist, recognizing attribution patterns is critical in understanding leisure motives and experiences. Furthermore, leisure time can serve as a laboratory for building accurate and healthy attribution patterns.

Seligman has emphasized the importance of recognizing choice about how we view the events in life. He refers to this as learned optimism, which is essentially the opposite of learned helplessness. People can learn to be optimistic by controlling thoughts that impact feelings and behavior (Anderson & Heyne, 2012b). This learned skill results in an attribution style where people attribute successes to stable, global factors and failures to unstable, specific factors (Seligman, 2002). Seligman's shift in focus from helplessness to optimism is an example of a larger paradigm shift toward positive psychology theories and philolophies. These paradigms are discussed further later in this chapter.

Self-Efficacy Theory

Related to attribution theory is self-efficacy theory. **Self-efficacy**, in simple terms, refers to the extent to which a person believes that he or she is capable of successfully performing a specific task (Bandura, 1986). As you might have guessed, self-efficacy theory can also be applied to depression.

This theory states that four factors can influence self-efficacy. The first and most powerful factor is past performance. We obviously can't change the past, but what we do in the present and future will one day become the past. Based on this logic, creating successful experiences should be a primary objective when working with clients with low self-efficacy. The second factor is vicarious experience, which can come in two forms. The therapeutic recreation specialist can model behaviors for clients (show them how to do it) or ask them to mentally rehearse success (visualize success). Doing so will bolster clients' beliefs that they can succeed at the relevant task. The third factor is arousal, so an important technique is to create an optimal level of arousal for the clients. This may mean psyching them up as a coach does a team or helping them relax when they are overwhelmed by the task at hand. Finally, verbal persuasion can be used to increase self-efficacy. Again, you might guess that focusing on internal, stable, global reasons for successes and external, unstable, specific factors contributing to failure is the best approach to bolstering self-efficacy.

The most important point to remember about attribution and self-efficacy theory is that these theories and the corresponding techniques require action on the therapeutic recreation specialist's part during therapy sessions or activities. Simply planning a day of activity and watching it take its course is not appropriate. The therapeutic recreation specialist is in the trenches interacting with clients and manipulating environments in ways that foster success. At the same time, success must be genuine, not the result of providing too much help or deceiving the client. Appropriate sequencing of activities and facilitation of experiences is critical in the process of creating real success, as is planning and anticipating situations during which these theoretical concepts can be used.

Psychoanalytic Theory

Several useful theoretical concepts come from psychoanalytic theory. One of the most significant is the acknowledgment that the unconscious mind can influence behavior. These unconscious behaviors (meaning that we are unaware of their presence and influence) often occur in the form of **defense mechanisms**. The unconscious aspect of the mind uses these mechanisms to protect our psychological well-being (Corey, 2004). In Freudian terms, a defense mechanism is a tool that the id (unconscious) uses to protect the ego (conscious awareness) from anxiety-provoking thoughts, beliefs, or situations. These mechanisms can be healthy or unhealthy depending on the circumstances and consequences of using them. For example, denial of a serious illness may lead to further health problems, but using sport to redirect aggression related to work difficulties may be an acceptable alternative to assaulting the boss (this concept is called sublimation). Whether defense mechanisms are truly unconscious or just behavior tendencies that become ingrained into daily routine is somewhat irrelevant. What is important is that clients become aware of such tendencies and the impact they may have on them. Some of the more common defense mechanisms are listed in table 7.3.

Table 7.3 Common Defense Mechanisms

Defense mechanism	Description	Example
Denial	Insisting that a source of anxiety doesn't exist	Denying that you have been diagnosed with a serious illness
Displacement	Taking out impulses on a less threatening target	Yelling at your children after a day of abuse from the boss
Intellectualization	Avoiding unacceptable emotions by focusing on intellectual aspects	Focusing on funeral arrangements to avoid facing the loss of a loved one
Projection	Attributing unacceptable aspects of yourself to another	Criticizing the work of others when you fail to complete an assigned project
Rationalization	Using faulty logical reasoning to ignore reality	Focusing on the choices that the coaches made even though you missed the winning touchdown pass in the end zone
Reaction formation	Believing or acting in a manner opposite your true feelings	Laughing hysterically and joking with friends when your girlfriend breaks up with you
Regression	Returning to a previous developmental stage	Throwing a temper tantrum in the grocery store line
Repression	Pulling information into the unconscious	Forcing yourself to forget the witnessing of a relative's suicide
Sublimation	Expressing unacceptable impulses through acceptable behavior	Using rigorous exercise as a way to express your frustration with work

Data from Fonagy and Target (2003); Corey (2004).

The psychoanalytic concepts of transference and countertransference are also relevant to the modern therapy environment. **Transference** refers to a circumstance in which the patient begins to associate the therapist with a person or situation from his or her past. This process is said to foster a productive therapy relationship. Transference may also manifest in negative ways if the client develops inappropriate expectations or feelings regarding the therapist. In contrast, **countertransference** refers to a situation in which the therapist begins to associate the client with a significant person or issue from his or her own life. This is not a good situation, but its occurrence is a real possibility. Therapeutic recreation specialists must be aware of how the client's personal situation "touches home" with them. Consider the situation of a recent therapeutic recreation intern who was also recovering from anorexia. One day, a client with anorexia was admitted to the mental health center where the intern worked, and the intern was immediately motivated to help. After a few weeks, it became apparent that the intern was so affected by the successes and setbacks of the client that her work in general, as well as her personal life, was negatively affected.

Thus, all mental health professionals should stay aware of such dynamics. Beginning psychotherapists are often encouraged to participate in counseling as a way of understanding the client's perspective and developing insight into their own psychological tendencies. For the therapeutic recreation specialist, this exercise may not be feasible, but he or she can take steps to understand how his or her personal life interacts with and influences professional performance. For the intern described earlier, the first step to coping with her countertransference was establishing open communication with her internship supervisor. Interns should be encouraged to acknowledge their internal reactions to clients and discuss these reactions with seasoned professionals. Communication between professional colleagues can be equally beneficial, and professional counseling should never be dismissed as an option. Negley (1994) described how termination of a particular long-term therapeutic relationship with a client was especially challenging for her and working through the issue with a staff psychologist was beneficial. Because therapeutic recreation services often reflect true-to-life social situations (such as community outings with friends), therapeutic recreation professionals should be especially conscious of the potential for boundaries between personal and professional relationships to fade away in the context of leisure activities. Openly discussing the nature of this relationship with clients can help remind both parties of such boundaries.

Social Contracts

Establishing social contracts, or agreed-upon norms, is a widely used concept in both therapeutic recreation programs and mental health in general. Programs that operate under this philosophy encourage clients to be accountable to one another. Issues and confrontations are brought to the group, and ownership is placed with the group to determine how to deal with such situations. Typically, a set of community principles or values is identified and used as a compass for guiding group decisions. The most practical application of this approach in therapeutic recreation is the use of value contracts in groups. These contracts are most effective when the group identifies the values by which the group will be governed, although in many cases, the values have long been established as new group members come and go. Thus, value contracts, or social norms, may need to be reestablished periodically. Social contracts ultimately empower clients to take responsibility and control of their own treatment program.

Positive Psychology and Related Paradigms

The previous section introduced a few psychological paradigms that have had a long-standing tradition within the mental health profession. One common characteristic of these perspectives is that they tend to include a deficits-based conceptualization of mental health, meaning they focus on mental illness and define mental health as the absence of illness. Deficits-based paradigms assume that clients have some sort of diagnosable mental illness and mental health workers intervene to identify and treat the condition. There are some emerging psychological paradigms that focus on an additive perspective as an alternative to a deficits perspective. Specifically, **positive psychology** is the investigation of how individuals flourish and what the social factors are that contribute to the prevention of illness, instead of focusing on the diagnosis and treatment of mental illness. Whereas previous sections of this chapter outline what happens when mental illness is developed and the methods of treatment, positive psychology and related paradigms focus on prevention of illness and the nurturing of individual

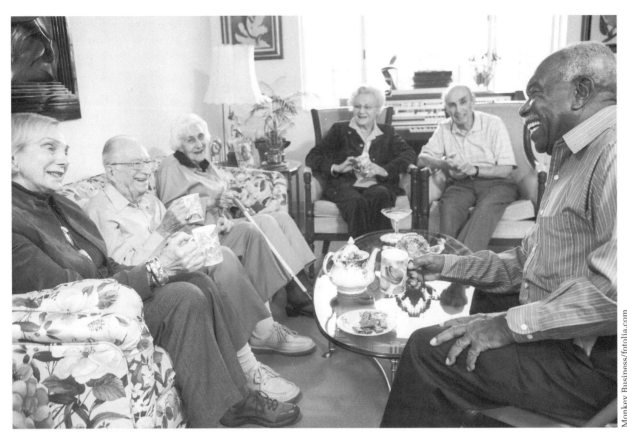

Positive psychology focuses on individual and social factors that help individuals flourish.

strengths and virtues. Seligman and Csikszent-mihalyi (2000) are largely credited for suggesting that there is a long history of positive psychology that has been ignored by theory and practice; they called for future researchers and psychologists to also focus on well-being, hope, happiness, flourishing, and the nurturing of positive individual traits, such as love, courage, interpersonal skill, perseverance, mindfulness, and wisdom. These are all concepts that are surely a good fit for the profession of therapeutic recreation, and it is no wonder that since their call in 2000, Seligman and Csikszentmihalyi's encouragement has resulted in a wider acceptance of the work of researchers focusing on the benefits of participation in recreation and leisure for all people.

Strengths-Based Perspectives

In these paradigms, mental health professionals work to identify strengths within individuals and capitalize on those strengths to assist clients in making positive changes. This means there is a focus on the identification of client strengths,

which serves to facilitate a sense of well-being. Because assessment is a large part of working with individuals and groups in mental health settings, strengths-based assessments focus on identifying and supporting an individual client's strengths, as opposed to identifying deficits in ability or mental health. Related to therapeutic recreation practice, **strengths** have been defined as "desirable personal qualities, characteristics, talents, skills, environments, interests, and aspirations" (Heyne & Anderson, 2012, p. 108). This perspective has led to the development of conceptual models of therapeutic recreation practice such as the leisure and well-being model (Carruthers & Hood, 2007; Hood & Carruthers, 2007) and an extension of that model by Anderson and Heyne (2012a) called flourishing through leisure, which added both environmental and contextual considerations that facilitate well-being (these models were presented in chapter 5).

The leisure and well-being model is a strengths-based model for guiding the practice of therapeutic recreation services and programs. The model suggests that the goal and outcomes of practice should be focused on increasing an individual's **well-being**, something the authors defined as "a state of successful, satisfying and productive engagement with one's life and the realization of one's full physical, cognitive, and social-emotional potential" (Carruthers & Hood, 2007, p. 279). This model is strengths based in that it supports the identification and development of an individual's internal and external resources (strengths) via facilitating positive leisure experiences. These experiences in turn result in the nurturing of individual strengths, which elicit positive emotions and affects, thereby increasing an individual's well-being.

The flourishing through leisure model (Anderson & Heyne, 2012a) is an additional strengths-based model of therapeutic recreation practice that expands the leisure and well-being model by extending well-being to include leisure, cognitive, physical, spiritual, social, and psychological/emotional components. In addition, the flourishing through leisure model emphasizes that therapeutic recreation services and programs should include the context and environment experienced by individuals from levels that include home and families; neighborhoods; communities; the nation; and ultimately, the world at large. This focus then extends practice beyond an individual into the community. The similarities between this model and the leisure and well-being model are the focus of therapeutic recreation practice in enhancing leisure experience and developing strengths to influence individual well-being. The major difference between these two models is that the flourishing through leisure model extends practice to include a more holistic view of well-being in addition to the careful consideration of the physical and social environments of individuals.

Solution-Focused Perspectives

Another paradigm that is related to a focus on positive psychology and strengths-based perspectives is solution-focused brief therapy (SFBT), or "solution focused." Though the development of this paradigm predates the positive psychology and strengths-based movements, it is still a relatively new paradigm for mental health settings. Steve de Shazer and Insoo Kim Berg are largely credited with the development and refinement of this therapeutic practice, based on their work at the Brief Family Therapy Center in Milwaukee, Wisconsin, in the late 1970s (Sklare, 2014;

Visser, 2013). Much like positive psychology and strengths-based perspectives, solution-focused approaches start with positive assumptions about individuals and focus on client-developed solutions instead of problems. Problem-focused approaches then are those that start with client deficits and focus on those problems, including the type and duration of the problems, factors that contribute to and enable the problems, the extent to which a client is troubled by the problems, and the long history of the problems.

It is important to differentiate the solution-focused approach from other mental health paradigms by highlighting some main philosophical assumptions of SFBT. The central philosophy of SFBT is developed on the premise that no problem can exist 100 percent of the time and there are examples in clients' lives when these problem times happen less often but go unrecognized. Additional concepts inherent in SFBT is that this approach seeks to focus on client action instead of insights to identify solutions; small change leads to large change over time; present and future focus is more important than focusing on the past (other than identifying exceptions); and the goals of therapy are positive and developed by the client, not the therapist.

SFBT attempts to assist clients in identifying "exceptions" (de Shazer, 1985) to problems and the characteristics of times when the problem is less severe or absent altogether. SFBT assumes that all clients have what it takes to improve their mental health and there are examples of when clients experience problem-free times. For example, when working with clients who report being depressed, practitioners employing an SFBT approach would focus on identifying when the client is feeling better rather than on what caused the depression. Once an exception has been identified, the therapist then helps the client identify the specific contexts, behaviors, and actions that the client did to be successful in experiencing the exception, meaning that action is more important than insight. SFBT approaches seek to determine a behaviorally specific description of the actions of clients, what they did specifically during the exceptional times to make the problem that brought them to therapy dissipate or disappear altogether. These behaviors do not have to be large, life-changing behaviors; rather, they can be small, seemingly insignificant actions that lead to large change over time. These actions are focused on the present and the future, not rooted in the past, meaning that SFBT focuses on having clients describe a preferred future and focus only on past behaviors that are helpful in creating that future. Finally, SFBT approaches assume that clients can and will make positive change, so practitioners use language that assumes positive change by assisting clients in developing their own goals for therapy; these goals are based on what clients can do, not on what clients want other people to do to solve the problems that brought them into therapy.

The process of using an SFBT approach involves a paradigm shift on behalf of the thera-pist from a problem-based model, such as those discussed in the earlier sections of this chapter, to a solution-focused model whereby clients are viewed as capable of enacting solutions they develop to reach a preferred future goal. Thera-pists use a conversational approach that mainly involves asking very specific solution-focused questions to assist clients in developing their own solutions, developing a plan to implement their solutions, and following up to measure client progress. A list of 10 common solution-focused strategies and questions is presented in table 7.4.

Table 7.4 Ten Common Solution-Focused Strategies

Strategy	Purpose	Sample questions and statements
1. Obtaining the client's description of the problem	To identify how the client currently views the reason(s) he or she is meeting with you	• What seems to be getting in the way of your being more successful during your leisure time? • What would you say is the biggest reason we are meeting today?
2. Scaling	To identify a starting point for severity of the problem according to the client To help the client be specific in describing change To track progress in resolution	• On a scale of zero to 10, where zero equals problem free and 10 is the problem at its worst, where are you today on the scale?
3. Asking the miracle question	To help the client visualize a time in his or her life when he or she was problem free—if the client can see it, he or she can achieve it.	• If the problem that brought you here disappeared, what would be the first sign? • If a miracle occurred and the problem we've been discussing were suddenly gone, what would be different?
4. Identifying positive goals	To identify a goal by asking questions using the word *instead* that involve something the client can do, not something someone else needs to do (to be used when clients report wanting someone else to change)	• If that person did change, what would you do differently? • If that person stopped _____ , how would that help you? • If that person did what you wanted him or her to do, what would that do for you? • What would you want that person to do *instead*? • If that person did change, what would you be doing *instead* of what you're doing now?
5. Identifying exceptions	To identify times when the problem is happening less or not at all	• Can you remember a time when this problem wasn't happening? • Can you remember the last time you were doing better than you are doing now? • When was the last time you noticed you were doing a little better? • When things were better, what were you doing instead?

Strategy	Purpose	Sample questions and statements
6. Cheerleading	To encourage positive success, no matter how small	• Group attendance: I noticed you were able to make it to group on time. Awesome! How did you do that? • Goal achievement: I noticed you were able to walk for 15 minutes without a break. That's really great! • Behavior issue: I noticed that today you were able to behave in group for 15 minutes. That's really great! How were you able to do that?
7. Flagging the minefield	To identify times, behaviors, and conditions that hinder positive change	• Now that you have had some success, is there anything that might get in your way of continuing to do well? If so, what might that be? • What are some things that seem to prevent you from keeping the positive change you've made from continuing? • When does the problem seem to take over?
8. Asking *what else* and *instead* questions	To elicit more ideas, thoughts, and insights from clients to generate behaviorally specific ideas, goals, and conditions	• Relationship problem: So it sounds like your parents are yelling a lot. What would you like them to do *instead*? Once they start doing that, *what else* could they do? • If the problem that brought you here were gone, what would you be doing/thinking/feeling *instead*? • If you were feeling happier, what would you be doing *instead*?
9. Asking what's *different* or *better* questions	To help the client identify exceptions	• What's *different* or *better* since the last time we met?
10. Writing a note to compliment and summarize strengths	To highlight the positive insights gained from meeting or to check in with the client if you have not had a chance to meet	• Just wanted to share with you that I noticed that your involvement in group has increased and your overall affect has improved. When you have a moment, please share with me what you are doing to make that happen.

Mental Health and Secondary Disabilities

When treating someone with a disabling condition, regardless of type, understanding the psychological challenges that the client faces is a critical step in providing comprehensive treatment. Take a moment to read the presented Client Portraits: Understanding Psychological Challenges.

Scenario 1 depicts a woman whose presenting problem is Alzheimer's disease, which is a disorder listed in the *DSM-5*, but she does not fit the stereotypical profile of mental illness. Most of her primary symptoms are oriented toward dementia (e.g., orientation) and motor functions

(e.g., gait). Still, the client's mental health is a **secondary condition** that is threatened by the primary condition (Alzheimer's). Specifically, depression is a treatable component of dementia, as are anxiety disorders. Interventions may have limited potential to restore cognitive functions, but therapeutic recreation modalities can be used to treat secondary mental disorders and significantly improve quality of life for a person with Alzheimer's disease. Review the modalities mentioned in scenario 1. Which modalities do you believe would be useful in reducing depression or anxiety? Do any of these modalities have the potential to be contraindicated?

Scenario 2 is similar to scenario 1 in that the public often does not associate the presence of

CLIENT PORTRAITS: UNDERSTANDING PSYCHOLOGICAL CHALLENGES

Scenario 1: Helen

Helen is a 92-year-old woman who resides at a long-term-care facility for people with Alzheimer's disease. The primary focus of Helen's therapy regime is to maintain cognitive and motor abilities as long as possible. Daily interventions include ongoing reality orientation, pet therapy, small reminiscence groups, and various forms of physical activity.

Scenario 2: Susan

Susan is a 16-year-old girl who has been admitted to a secured residential treatment facility specializing in the treatment of substance abuse. Susan appears well adjusted in her daily life and is involved in a variety of extracurricular activities. Her parents admitted her into the treatment program after finding methamphetamines in her bedroom for the third time. Some of the therapeutic recreation interventions that Susan participates in are values clarification and a leisure education group.

Scenario 3: Mike

Mike is a 45-year-old man who has been diagnosed with terminal cancer. He is receiving care in a rehabilitation hospital after having a large tumor removed from his spinal cord. The surgery left him paralyzed from the chest down. Doctors were not able to remove the entire tumor, and they expect it to affect vital functions within 6 months. Treatment at the rehabilitation center focuses primarily on activities of daily living and self-care.

---

substance abuse with a mental disorder (again, substance use disorders are included in the *DSM-5*). In truth, drug and alcohol disorders frequently coexist with depression, anxiety, PTSD, and other mental disorders. Addressing these mental health concerns is critical to treatment, especially in cases in which such substances are being used to cope (self-medicate).

The presenting problem in scenario 3 is not a mental disorder, but it does represent a situation in which the therapeutic recreation specialist and the rest of the treatment team should consider mental health. The immediate physical changes that the client is facing, as well as the stressors associated with the terminal nature of his condition, will no doubt affect his mental health. A therapeutic recreation specialist who works with people with physical disabilities should be knowledgeable in the area of mental health and specifically with the concepts presented in this chapter.

Common Therapeutic Recreation Modalities for Mental Health

The remainder of this chapter focuses on therapeutic recreation modalities that are commonly used in the mental health setting. Some of these modalities are also used with other client popula-

tions, but remember that any particular modality is appropriate only when it is consistent with the goals and objectives of the client. Therefore, the therapeutic recreation specialist should ensure that the content or focus of the utilized modality meets this requirement.

Leisure Education

Mental illness often has a direct effect on the same areas that leisure education is equipped to address. For example, virtually every mental illness has the potential to impair social skills both inside and outside the leisure realm. Likewise, long-term mental illness disrupts or discourages access to leisure resources that, ironically, can assist in the prevention of mental illness. Although leisure education is a broad concept in general, program content that is specific to the needs of clients with mental illness can be delivered within the framework of existing leisure education models (see chapter 5).

Values Clarification

Values clarification is a technique that can help clients examine their personal behavior, identify the values that are driving this behavior, determine whether these values are in line with their core personal values, and shift behavior to be congruent with personal core values. The values clarification process was conceptualized by Simon and Olds (1977) as consisting of three progressive categories of clarification processes (as presented in Austin, 2004). The first category involves choosing the core values by which we desire to live our lives. The second category focuses on cherishing these values. For example, this stage might involve sharing with others a decision to stop associating with known drug users. Acting is the final category, which involves behaving in a manner that is consistent with the chosen values. The power behind this technique is in the early work. As clients explore their values and how they have deviated away from what is truly important, they find it easier to share this personal desire with others and live by it.

Stress Management

Stress is a physiological reaction to the surrounding world. Our hearts pound, our muscles tighten, and our ability to function diminishes. Unfortunately, stress can have a significant effect on our mental health. Thus, helping clients relax through various means is a common aspect of therapeutic recreation services in mental health settings. Specifically, various formal techniques for relaxation are implemented, as are recreation activities that directly affect stress levels, such as yoga, tai chi, aerobics, and other fitness-based activities.

Coping Skills

One of the primary goals of therapeutic recreation is to help people develop healthy coping skills for dealing with the emotional strains and stressors of everyday life. Strong problem-solving and decision-making skills are central to developing effective coping strategies. In this treatment modality, recreation therapists work with participants to build emotional resources (e.g., confidence and self-worth); learn effective problem-solving skills; achieve acceptance; and pursue leisure-time activities that promote mindfulness, relaxation, and social connection. Participants learn that leisure is a healthy pathway to achieving relaxation as well as a powerful way to divert and distract oneself from emotional distress.

Outdoor and Adventure Programs

Outdoor recreation and nature-based experiences have been found to be a beneficial therapeutic modality. These experiences include programs that rely on experiential activities such as hiking and camping along with high-adventure activities such as rock climbing, rappelling, and white-water rafting to facilitate positive client change. Adventure programs generally are group based and

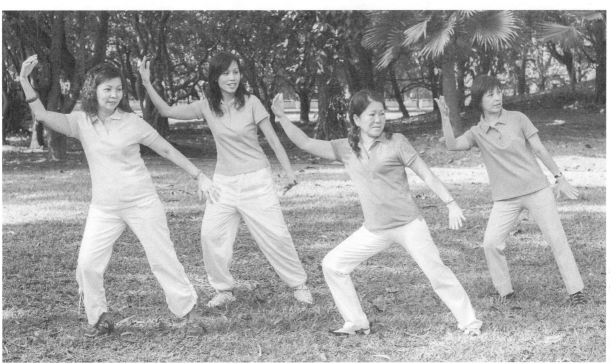

Clients can benefit from the stress-reducing effects of activities such as tai chi.

EastWest Imaging/fotolia.com

involve groups experiencing the natural challenge of wilderness activities together. As the group participates in the wilderness experience, therapists use the natural problems that arise (navigating and orienteering, setting up/breaking down campsites, cooking meals, and setting up and participating in adventure activities) to facilitate behavior change. A major component of outdoor and adventure programs is the exposure to seemingly impossible challenges, carefully facilitated by the adventure program therapists so that participants experience a sense of accomplishment and achievement. This sense of accomplishment then becomes the main mechanism for client change.

Group Initiatives

One common technique is to use group initiatives or challenge activities as opportunities to practice and master various psychosocial functions. Examples of such functions include trust, problem solving, conflict resolution, communication skills, and enhancement of self-perceptions. This strategy, grounded in **constructivism** (Fosnot, 1996; Piaget, 1970), is analogous to the concept of experiential education. Metaphors are a major therapy tool when using this modality because the therapeutic recreation specialist works toward generalizing the immediate experience to relevant real-world concepts.

Skilled facilitation is a key element of a successful group initiative. The therapeutic recreation specialist must create an environment that elicits insight and learning as a result of the experience and the associated discussion (see chapter 6 for more information on facilitation). Likewise, group initiatives, facilitation strategies, and the intended outcomes must be appropriate for the client's level of functioning. A skilled facilitator is able to create a situation that allows clients to step across the "gap" between where they are and where they are capable of going. If the gap is too small, no change will occur; if the gap is too large, clients will fail and potentially regress. This gap can be physical (e.g., a climbing wall or an elevated rope bridge), cognitive (e.g., a metaphor,

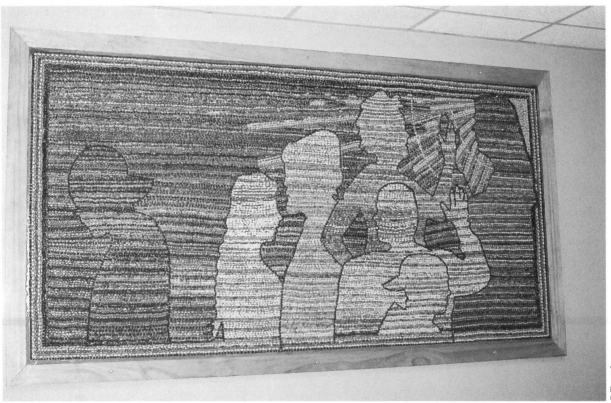

This collage made of various dried beans is on display at the Lincoln Regional Center in Lincoln, Nebraska. The collage is meant to show a silhouette of clients moving from deep depression to a celebration of life with arms raised and chins high. This moving work was the result of a therapeutic recreation intern's efforts to collaborate with the local arts council and many hours of work by clients who volunteered to take part in the project.

© Terry Long

riddle, or problem), social (e.g., cooperation, conflict resolution, or competition), or psychological (e.g., fear, anxiety, or frustration). The therapeutic recreation specialist is aware of and manipulates such factors to empower clients to cross the gap on their own or with the group.

Self-Esteem Programs

Self-esteem programs are a common therapeutic recreation modality. In some cases, these programs are activity based, focusing on building successes and a sense of accomplishment in those who participate. Other programs are more reflective, focusing on written work or journals to bolster the esteem of clients. In many cases, some combination of the two is used. A specific example of a journal-based tool for self-esteem programs is Sandra Negley's (1997) *Crossing the Bridge: A Journey in Self-Esteem, Relationships, and Life Balance.* This resource walks clients through a progression of self-reflective activities. The focus is on how people internalize messages that they receive from others and the process of challenging these messages. This workbook, as well as other worksheet-based resources, can be used with other activity-based methods, including initiatives, creative and expressive arts, and appropriately facilitated sports and games, to create a comprehensive self-esteem program.

Expressive Therapies

Expressive therapies are used regularly in therapeutic recreation programs, especially those located in mental health settings. Using drawing, painting, ceramics, clay work, writing, and a variety of other media for the expression of emotion can be a powerful therapy tool. In some cases, therapeutic recreation professionals work with art therapists to facilitate such groups. Final products that are long lasting serve as reminders and metaphors for clients even after finishing therapy.

Summary

Therapeutic recreation professionals can play a significant role in enhancing the psychological well-being of their clients. This result can occur as part of a structured treatment program for mental disorders; as a secondary goal in physical rehabilitation environments; as part of structured outreach programs for at-risk populations such as the homeless, underprivileged, and elderly; or in general community-based programs designed to enhance the well-being of people with disabilities through both inclusive and segregated recreation programs. Ultimately, every therapeutic recreation specialist must be prepared to deal with and address issues associated with psychological functioning.

DISCUSSION QUESTIONS

1. Discuss the relationship between leisure, recreation, and mental illness. Do you agree or disagree that leisure may be the most influential realm of functioning when it comes to mental well-being? Defend your answer.

2. Besides the mental disorders profiled in this chapter, what other disorders do you know of (if you don't know of any, look one up)? What are the basic characteristics of these disorders, and how could you address these characteristics through therapeutic recreation?

3. Interviewing is a major tool in assessment of clients with mental disorders. Discuss what content, issues, or questions would be important to cover in such an interview. Also, discuss other nonverbal indicators. What nonverbal behaviors may be associated with depression, PTSD, anxiety, and schizophrenia?

4. Review Carl Rogers' concept of unconditional positive regard. Can you imagine a situation in which accepting a client as a good person might be difficult? How would you deal with such a situation? Ask your instructor his or her opinion on this issue.

5. Compare and contrast a problem-based approach to mental health services to a strengths-based approach. What are the pros and cons to each of these approaches? Which approach do you think therapeutic recreation therapists should adopt? Defend you answer.

6. Review the modalities presented in this chapter as being especially useful in mental health. To what other client groups might these methods be useful? Specifically, give examples of how the behavior modification techniques listed in table 7.2 might be useful for patients with orthopedic injuries, intellectual disabilities, or cognitive deficits (such as from a traumatic brain injury).

8

Therapeutic Recreation and Developmental Disabilities

Susan Myllykangas | Alice Foose
Patricia Ardovino

LEARNING OUTCOMES

At the end of this chapter, students will be able to

- identify the difference in the terms *developmental disability*, *developmental delay*, and *learning disability*,

- identify the four types of developmental disabilities and give an example that fits each type,

- identify the main knowledge areas that a therapeutic recreation specialist should possess when working with a person with a developmental disability,

- explain the importance of age-appropriate interventions and give at least two examples,

- explain why taking a life-span approach is important when working with people with developmental disabilities,

- describe the best practices for working with people of diverse ages and different developmental disabilities, and

- explain what precautions need to be taken to address contraindications associated with at least five types of developmental disabilities.

After reading the following scenarios, try to identify what these people have in common.

- Mary is a petite, bright-eyed woman in her mid-50s who has Down syndrome. She enjoys gardening, playing rummy, and being with her cat, Sara. Mary lives with her mother, Ruth, who is 95 and whose eyesight is failing. Mary's mother worries that she will soon need to move to a nursing home.

- Jordan, diagnosed with autism, is a rambunctious 5-year-old who loves skipping stones with his older brother and is excited about starting his new school.

- Laura, born with spina bifida, is a beautiful but shy 16-year-old. She is interested in a guy in her high school class and is afraid to ask him out.

- Dominic is 12 years old, uses a wheelchair to get around, and has a diagnosis of Duchenne muscular dystrophy. He loves to hang out after school with his friends at the local park.

- Debbie is a 20-year-old woman who lives with her parents. She is searching for a job but worries that employers will focus on her cerebral palsy diagnosis and not on her skills and abilities.

What similarities did you see? Each person is dealing with life issues—illness, transitions, sexual attraction, friendship, and work—they all have unique strengths and limitations, are involved in social networks, and have a developmental disability.

What Are Developmental Disabilities?

Developmental disability is an umbrella term used to describe a group of conditions that occur because of an impairment in physical development, learning, language, or behavior (Administration on Developmental Disabilities, 2018). They are lifelong and incurable and occur before adulthood. Because they originate during early development, these disabilities often affect multiple aspects of life, including physical and mental abilities. In the United States, Public Law 106-402 describes the criteria for receiving a diagnosis of a developmental disability as having a severe, chronic disability meeting the following characteristics:

- Results from a mental or physical impairment or both
- Is manifested before age 22
- Is likely to continue indefinitely
- Results in substantial functional limitations in three or more of the following adaptive areas of major life activity:
  – Self-care
  – Receptive and expressive language
  – Learning
  – Mobility
  – Self-direction
  – Capacity for independent living
  – Economic self-sufficiency
- Reflects the person's need for a combination and sequence of special interdisciplinary or generic services, supports, or other assistance that is of lifelong or extended duration.

Common to all forms of developmental disability is an extensive delay in development of one or more adaptive areas. Although rates of development vary considerably, people with developmental disability have at least one area of delay in adaptive life that hinders their ability to live independently. With facilitation and training, many people with developmental disability are able to adapt or gain the skills needed to live independently or semi-independently.

For most of the 20th century, people with developmental disability around the world were treated like children. This view led to low expectations and minimal intervention, which in turn fostered high levels of dependence. Beginning in the 1970s, U.S. society began to view people with developmental disability from a holistic, **life-span development** approach. Simply put, society began to move away from pity for persons with developmental disabilities toward inclusion and the creation of a better sense of belonging. Legislative action in the United States was a major factor in creating this shift in perspective that supported the fair treatment and inclusion of people with disabilities (see table 8.1).

In 2001 the U.S. Surgeon General issued a national blueprint to improve the health of persons with intellectual disability (U.S. Public Health Service, 2002). Intellectual disability, one of the most prevalent types of developmental disability, is often dually diagnosed with other types of disability, such as autism and cerebral palsy. The report outlined six focuses for integrated teams of self-advocates with intellectual

Table 8.1 Significant Disability Legislation in the United States

Year	Federal code number	Law	Significance
1970	PL 91-517	Disabilities Services and Facilities Construction Amendments of 1970	Defined developmental disabilities to include people with intellectual impairment, cerebral palsy, epilepsy, and other neurological conditions closely related to intellectual impairment that originated before age 18 and constituted a substantial disability.
1973	PL 93-112	Rehabilitation Act of 1973, as Amended	Prohibits discrimination on the basis of disability in programs conducted by federal agencies, in programs receiving federal financial assistance, in federal employment, and in the employment practices of federal contractors. First law to recognize recreation as being therapeutic.
1975	PL 94-142	Education for All Handicapped Children Act	This law guaranteed a free and appropriate public education to persons with disabilities ages 6-21 years. Prior to this federal act, there were laws in place that specifically restricted students who had diagnoses of blindness, deafness, emotional disabilities, and intellectual disabilities from attending school. The law mandated that individualized education plans (IEPs) be drafted for students with special needs to provide an education in the least restrictive environment possible.
1990	PL 101-336	Americans with Disabilities Act (ADA)	The "civil rights act" for persons with disabilities. First comprehensive law to protect the civil rights of all people with disabilities across all areas of public life.
1990	PL 101-476	Individuals with Disabilities Education Act (IDEA)	This amendment to the Education for All Handicapped Children Act (PL 94-142) renamed the act and added autism and traumatic brain injury as distinct disability categories. The push to use person-first language began, and changes in terminology differentiating the terms *handicap* and *disability* played a role in the name change of this act. Focus was on the individual, not the label or condition. In addition, this law expanded the regulations to include persons with disabilities ages 3-21 years.
1994	PL 103-230	Developmental Disabilities Act of 1994	Emphasized the need to address the cultural and ethnic needs of the person served and promote dignity.

(continued)

Table 8.1 *(continued)*

Year	Federal code number	Law	Significance
1997	PL 105-17	Individuals with Disabilities Education Act (IDEA)– Amendment	This amendment to the IDEA Act of 1990 had three parts. Part A: shifted focus to the quality of teaching and learning provided to persons with disabilities. The IEP and inclusive education opportunities were emphasized; part B: provided resources related to the IEP for children with disabilities ages 3-9 years; part C: provided financial assistance to support services for infants and toddlers with disabilities up to age 3 years and their families through instructions in the individualized family service plan (IFSP)
2000	PL 106-402	Developmental Disabilities Assistance and Bill of Rights Act Amendment	Extended the definition of a developmental disability to include infants and young children from birth to age 9 years.
2010	PL 111-256	Rosa's Law	Changed the term *mental retardation* to *intellectual disability*. Named for Rosa Marcellino, a girl from Maryland who has Down syndrome.
2015	PL 114-95	Every Student Succeeds Act	Amended the IDEA through inclusion in this law. Shifted the oversight of education away from the federal government and to the individual states. Increased the percentage of government-supported funding to states for education each fiscal year until 2025, when it will reach 100%.

disability and their families, scientists, health care providers, professional training institutions, advocacy organizations, and policy makers. The six goals are as follows:

- Integrate health promotion into community environments
- Increase knowledge and understanding
- Improve quality of health care
- Train health care providers
- Ensure effective health care financing
- Increase sources of health care

Unfortunately, a 2014 article published by *Frontiers in Public Health* reported that the progress toward meeting the objectives set forth by the blueprint had been slow regarding inequities in health care for persons with developmental disabilities (Ervin, Hennen, Merrick, & Morad, 2014). A new model of integrative care was introduced and is being implemented by the Developmental Disabilities Health Center, located in Colorado Springs, Colorado. This model provides customized, integrated care for children and adults living with developmental disabilities. Care includes primary care, mental health, behavioral health, care coordination, allied health and other specialty care, health planning, and health education programs. The authors noted that evidence is clear that when access to integrated health care occurs, optimal health becomes achievable (Ervin et al., 2014). Professionals in therapeutic recreation are trained to focus on all the wellness domains of a person. Therapeutic recreation specialists are trained to offer not only purposeful interventions for rehabilitation and improvement of functioning but also habilitation and maintenance of the highest level of functioning possible of the participants served. Similar to the new model of care, integration of therapeutic recreation services and techniques within the community is an ideal way to meet the holistic needs of persons with developmental disabilities.

Understanding the Developmental Process

If interventions are going to meet the needs of the persons served and be effective at enhancing their quality of life, therapeutic recreation specialists must fully understand human development. It is important to recognize the early life effects of a particular condition but also have insight into implications that may manifest in later stages of life. This understanding must be holistic, considering all domains of functioning. Developmental delays are typically identified by examining three main developmental domains: physical, cognitive, and socioemotional (the latter is sometimes separated down into a third and fourth domain: social and emotional). Table 8.2 provides a description of typical developmental progression across these functional domains.

Table 8.2 Typical Physical, Cognitive, Socioemotional, and Leisure Development

Development	Physical	Cognitive	Socioemotional	Leisure focus
INFANCY				
0-4 months	Raises head, grasps and shakes toys, follows faces and moving objects, responds to loud noises, and pushes down with legs when placed on firm surface.	Begins to babble and imitate sounds and to respond to the word *no*.	Imitates facial movements of others and shows affection toward caregiver.	Explores the environment by responding to and imitating environmental stimuli (things that move or make noises), such as by playing peek-a-boo, shaking a rattle, or imitating simple noises; play is often solitary.
4-7 months	Supports whole weight on legs and reaches with one hand.	Finds objects that are partially hidden, tries to get objects that are out of reach, and turns head when called.	Responds to emotional expressions of others and enjoys social play, such as peek-a-boo.	
7-12 months	Uses and imitates simple gestures (waving and clapping), develops beginning walking skills, and uses crude pincer grasp (picks up objects with thumb and one finger).	Makes basic words and sounds (*ma, da-da*), responds to own name and basic commands that are accompanied by gestures (come, get, etc.).	Trusts and bonds with caregiver.	
TODDLER OR PRESCHOOLER				
2 years	Walks (heel to toe) alone, begins to run, kicks a ball, carries large toy while walking, walks up and down stairs while holding on for support, scribbles, and builds block towers of four or more blocks.	Links two to four words together to communicate ideas (*more milk, no bed*), follows simple instructions, can identify by pointing to named objects, begins to sort by color and shape, and begins make-believe play.	Begins to show independence through defiant behavior, shows separation anxiety, and imitates behaviors of others.	Play is imitative of others; still initiates little or no interaction (parallel play); play is mainly home based.

(continued)

Table 8.2 *(continued)*

Development	Physical	Cognitive	Socioemotional	Leisure focus
3 years	Climbs stairs alternating feet; kicks ball; runs easily; pedals tricycle; bends over without falling; can manipulate small objects (turns book pages one at a time, holds pencil); can make up-and-down, side-to-side, and circular marking with a pencil or crayon; turns rotating handles.	Follows a two- or three-part command, recognizes most common objects and pictures, understands placement in space (in, below, above), and uses four- or five-word sentences; speech understood by strangers.	Expresses emotions openly, separates easily from parent, and spontaneously shows affection toward familiar playmates.	Plays in presence of others with little or no interaction (egocentric–cooperative play); engages in pretend play and exploratory play; play is still mainly in the home environment.
4 years	Goes up and down stairs with no support, throws ball overhanded, catches ball, moves forward and backward, can hop on one foot for up to 5 seconds, dresses and undresses, draws a person with two to four body parts, and has better fine motor control (uses scissors and begins to copy some capital letters and square shapes).	Correctly names some colors, can count at least a few numbers, follows three-part commands, speaks in sentences of five to six words, has mastered some rules of grammar, recalls parts of a story, and works with others toward goals.	Plays and cooperates with other children, negotiates solutions to conflict, often cannot tell the difference between fantasy and reality, and imagines monsters from unfamiliar images.	Engages in pretend play; play is more independent and exploratory; plays house and other work and home roles; focuses on expression; peers and teachers begin to have influence.
5 years	Increases range of movements (hopping, somersaults, swinging, climbing, galloping); can copy triangle and other shapes, draw recognizable pictures, print some letters, and use silverware (fork and spoon); can take care of own toilet needs.	Speaks using sentences of more than five words; can count 10 or more objects; has better understanding of time; uses future tense; knows about common objects in the home (food, appliances, etc.); can recite name and address; can distinguish reality from fantasy.	Aware of gender; wants to please friends; shows more independence and can visit a nearby friend by him- or herself; can share or give and take in a group situation; peers, teachers, and the media are increasingly influential.	Play continues to mirror adult world; increasingly uses symbols and language in play; engages in expressive play that includes singing, dancing, and acting; wants to play with peers.
6-11 years	Strength increases; upper limb coordination and dexterity improve.	Can distinguish right from left; can count in multiples of 2, 5, and 10; follows rules; later, can complete tasks.	Begins forming cliques (identifying outsiders) and showing alliance to identified friends.	Enjoys collecting things, magic tricks, puzzles, and trading with others; engages in cooperative group play; starts competitive play; increase of cognitive abilities is reflected in increasing complexity of board and table games.

Development	Physical	Cognitive	Socioemotional	Leisure focus
PRETEEN				
11-12 years	Rapid growth and changes in body start to occur; must relearn or adapt coordination and gross motor skills.	Thinks ahead to make plans and set goals, uses abstract thinking, can consider several options, and has ability to take the role of others.	Becomes concerned with social image (clothes, activities, etc.); close friends are important; peers are more important than family; preteens try out roles to discover who they are; budding of sexual identity occurs; most are aware of sexual intercourse.	School is still a major focus of activity; prefers same-sex groups and team games; prefers being in groups to being alone.
TEENAGERS				
Early adolescence, 13-15 years	Rapid increase in height and weight occurs; muscle mass continues to grow; refinement of skills continues; secondary sex characteristics develop because of change in hormone levels; experiences clumsiness because of bodily changes.	Begins to set goals for the future, use abstract reasoning, and look at choosing among different ideas.	Focuses on identity; develops heightened self-consciousness.	Enjoys group activities with both genders; segregates into athletic and nonathletic groups; spends 40% of waking time in leisure; socializes informally with friends, watches TV, listens to music; begins to develop sports and hobbies; develops sexual identity; team sports become exclusive; activities are expressive and immediate; leisure is a space for peers.
Late adolescence, 16-18 years	Body and brain continue to develop; needs to sleep longer.	Can conceptualize possibilities; can plan and try out ideas; abstract reasoning continues to develop.	Focus is self and intimacy with others; begins to distinguish self from group (autonomy).	Informal and activity-specific groups provide a context for identity development; leisure provides a context for bonding, opportunities for support, and a way to demonstrate competence and meaningful activity.
YOUNG ADULT				
19-29 years	Hormonal and body-mass growth slows.	Continues to develop values and abstract reasoning.	Establishes self in context of work and family; social network often changes many times during this period because of dating, marriage, having children, divorce, change in work or school environment; continues to develop self and discover who he or she is in a changing social context.	Adapts leisure from previous interests and is influenced by the available resources, associations, time available, and family and work obligations.

(continued)

Table 8.2 *(continued)*

Development	Physical	Cognitive	Socioemotional	Leisure focus
MIDDLE-AGE ADULT				
30-44 years	Growth slows.	Development continues.	Social role provided by work, family, and need for identify from what one accomplishes; needs to balance in work, family, and leisure.	Leisure often focuses on the nurturing and development of children; reevaluates relationships and priorities; has more resources; leisure provides stability; divorce, death, and job changes can disrupt stability.
LATE MIDDLE-AGE ADULT				
45-65 years	Flexibility, strength, and muscle mass begin to decline.	Growth continues.	Focuses on dignity versus control.	Men shift values toward intimacy; women shift toward accomplishment and growth; renews activity involvement as children age.
RETIREMENT TO DISABILITY				
65 years and older	Gradual compounding of lifestyle behavior occurs; physical health varies greatly depending on whether health-promoting behaviors, such as good nutrition and exercise, were engaged in during early adulthood or whether health-risk behaviors, such as smoking, heavy drinking, and inactivity, were the norm.	Growth continues; long-term memory increases and short-term memory becomes less acute.	Reflects on accomplishments and reviews contributions made through life journey; needs to feel that he or she has lived a good life and contributed to the greater whole through children, life work, or other means (generativity).	Leisure becomes an integrating experience; quality of life is important; increases leisure involvement.
DISABILITY TO DEATH				
This phase is optional; if disability occurs, these are some possible repercussions.	Flexibility, range of motion, and muscle strength and tone decline.	Short-term memory (ability to retain new information) gradually declines.	Deals with accepting death.	With loss of physical and cognitive abilities and loss of social network members, leisure provides a context for expressing loss, continuing interests, and adapting to changes. Leisure also provides a way to pass on his or her history and gifts to the community and the next generation.

Data from DeBord (1996); Kelly and Godbey (1992); Schaie and Willis (2002); Steinberg (2002).

With development in each domain comes an increase in leisure needs, interests, and capabilities. Likewise, barriers or limitations in each domain can create difficulties or delays in a person's leisure development.

Acknowledging Strengths

Vital to working with any person with a developmental disability is the recognition that, in most cases, not all areas of functioning are delayed. For example, a teenager with a developmental disability might function intellectually around a third- or fourth-grade level. Physiologically, however, the teen's body is not developmentally delayed. The hormonal changes and urges that accompany puberty are taking place on schedule. The teen may desire to have a boyfriend or girlfriend and to kiss and be intimate, but he or she may not fully understand the ramifications of acting on those urges. The therapeutic recreation specialist may find himself or herself in the situation where a conversation with the parents or guardians might be necessary to remind them that not all developmental processes are delayed when someone is diagnosed with a developmental disability. Additionally, the therapeutic recreation specialist may choose to provide interventions that assist teens in understanding how to appropriately respond to the changes they are experiencing.

Human development varies greatly, even for people without a disability. Everyone is unique and may not fit nicely into one definition or diagnosis group. While reading the rest of this chapter, keep in mind that the information in table 8.2 is a rough overview of typical human development. Recognize that in many cases of people with developmental disability, only a few developmental areas are affected and it is common to excel in other areas, even within the same functional domain. An adult with a developmental disability still has the need for intimacy, autonomy, and generativity.

Practice Settings

Because the term *developmental disability* represents a broad range of functional domains and abilities, the nature and location of therapeutic recreation services for this population are equally broad. One major area for implementation of therapeutic recreation programs is the community public and municipal park and recreation setting. These agencies provide a variety of potential programs, including year-round recreation programs, summer camps, and after-school enrichment programs. In some cases, these programs may cater specifically to persons with developmental disabilities, although the ADA (1990) requires that services in such programs be provided in the least restrictive manner. As such, many city and county recreation agencies employ therapeutic recreation personnel to oversee inclusive recreation services. These professionals apply the therapeutic recreation process in a manner that maximizes involvement of persons with disabilities in general programs offered by the agency.

Another major provider of therapeutic recreation services to persons with developmental disabilities is in the private realm (both for profit and nonprofit). Many of these programs are community based, meaning that participants live at home and come to the agency to participate in programs. These organizations provide services such as work training and support, socialization opportunities, and various other support services. Services are similar to those offered in municipal programs. These agencies may plan camps, structured recreation, and special events, but they also may offer higher levels of support such as day programs that provide a variety of educational and therapy experiences (including therapeutic recreation).

Also in the private realm are long-term residential agencies that assist adults in living independently and semi-independently (some such agencies also operate as state or local government entities). The general focus of such therapeutic recreation programs is to support and expand the developmental needs of people with developmental disability through recreation involvement, leisure education, and promotion of **self-advocacy**.

Note that these categories represent general trends and do not reflect the fact that many private and nonprofit agencies receive funding from the government. In reality, various funding sources may support agencies that provide comprehensive services. Regardless, the role of the therapeutic recreation specialist within a particular agency will be based on the clients served.

One approach to examining the broad realm of developmental disabilities is to break them into four categories (based on the system they affect and how they manifest): nervous system, sensory

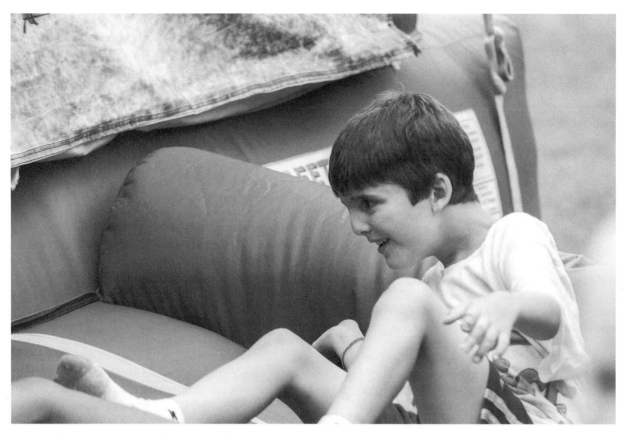

Many public park districts provide a variety of programming for people with disabilities.

related, metabolic, and degenerative (National Institutes of Health, 2018). This chapter will provide examples of each type, but the examples are not all inclusive of every disability that falls into each type. It is important to remember that the term *developmental disability* is the overall umbrella term; the types of developmental disabilities are smaller umbrellas under the larger one, and each type can have multiple disabilities falling under it.

Neurodevelopmental Disorders

Nervous system developmental disabilities affect the brain, spinal cord, and nervous system, which can affect intelligence, learning, motor control, and ultimately any aspect of functioning. Nervous system disorders can create problems with behavior, speech or language, convulsions, and movement. Examples of disabilities having an impair-

ment in neurological development are intellectual disabilities, Down syndrome, fragile X syndrome, autism, cerebral palsy, and spina bifida. Changes in the *Diagnostic and Statistical Manual of Mental Disorders, Fifth Edition* (*DSM-5*) created a category of diagnosis called neurodevelopmental disorders to refer to for diagnosing developmental disabilities of this type. This chapter will address disabilities in the neurodevelopmental disorder category and share examples of how therapeutic recreation can benefit clients with this type of developmental disability.

Intellectual Disability

With the passage of Public Law 111-256, or Rosa's Law, in 2010, the term *mental retardation* was replaced with the term *intellectual disability*. **Intellectual disability** is not a disease; it is a disability that has a variety of causes and is the largest subclass of developmental disability. In the United States, it is estimated that seven to eight million Americans, or about 1 percent of the population, have an intellectual disability (American Psychiatric Association, 2013). According to the revised criteria in the *DSM-5*, intellectual disability is characterized by

A. Deficits in intellectual functions, such as reasoning, problem-solving, planning, abstract thinking, judgment, academic learning and learning from experience, and practical understanding confirmed by both clinical assessment and individualized, standardized intelligence testing.

B. Deficits in adaptive functioning that result in failure to meet developmental and sociocultural standards for personal independence and social responsibility. Without ongoing support, the adaptive deficits limit functioning in one or more activities of daily life, such as communication, social participation, and independent living, and across multiple environments, such as home, school, work, and recreation.

C. Onset of intellectual and adaptive deficits during the developmental period. (American Psychiatric Association, 2013, p. 33)

The severity of the disability can be broken down into four diagnostic categories, mild, moderate, severe, and profound intellectual disability. The largest percentage (85 percent) of people with intellectual disabilities fall into the mild category. Persons with a diagnosis of mild intellectual disability can live independently with minimum support and have IQ scores that are between 50 and 69. The next largest percentage (10 percent) of people with intellectual disabilities fit into the moderate diagnosis level. Here, individuals can live independently with moderate levels of support, commonly reside in group homes, and have IQ scores falling between 36 and 49. Persons diagnosed with severe intellectual disabilities (3.5 percent) have more advanced needs and require constant supervision and daily assistance with care needs. IQ scores for persons diagnosed with severe intellectual disabilities fall within the 20-35 range. Lastly, persons with significant and often comorbid, profound intellectual disabilities (1.5 percent) require 24-hour care and have IQ scores below 20 (Boat & Wu, 2015).

The diagnosis of intellectual disability is used to determine eligibility for programs covered by the **Individuals with Disabilities Education Act (IDEA)**, Medicaid, and vocational rehabilitation (part B of the IDEA). Intellectual disability is often dually diagnosed with another developmental disability, such as Down syndrome or autism. An additional term that readers should be familiar with is **developmental delay**. Children reach milestones in skill development as they grow. Things like rolling over, waving goodbye, and taking a first step are all milestones. A developmental delay may be diagnosed when a child is slow to reach one of these developmental milestones. The term *developmental delay* has been used mainly in the educational system to indicate cognitive performance below the standard developmental level. This term has been applied to secure remedial or extra services to help the child develop the skills needed to function at a higher level. A developmental delay can be an early indicator of having intellectual disability or may indicate only a need for extra services. The determining factor in diagnosis of an intellectual disability is the duration of assistance needed.

It is also important to understand the difference between an intellectual disability and a learning disability. A child can be diagnosed with a **learning disability** without having a diagnosis of an intellectual disability. *Learning disability* is the general term given to a child who is having significant problems with verbal or written language or mathematical calculations, but the problems are *not* related to intellectual impairment or emotional or psychological problems. However, persons diagnosed with intellectual disabilities can also have learning disabilities. Dyslexia, dysgraphia, dyscalculia, brain injury, and developmental aphasia (loss of ability to speak) are all examples of learning disabilities. Learning disabilities are typically covered under the IDEA, but qualifying factors can vary from state to state.

Causes of intellectual disability range from genetic conditions to events or conditions occurring during pregnancy, birth, or childhood (American Psychiatric Association, 2013). Down syndrome and fragile X syndrome are examples of intellectual disabilities having genetic roots. Environmental causes of intellectual disabilities can include drug and alcohol abuse during pregnancy, illnesses such as rubella or toxoplasmosis during pregnancy, malnutrition during pregnancy, or deprivation of oxygen during birth. Some common causes of intellectual disability during childhood include diseases such as meningitis and measles, abuse or injury such as a head injury or neglect from lack of proper nutrition, and exposure to toxic environmental elements such as lead or mercury.

Program Considerations for People With Intellectual Disabilities

Program Considerations for People With Intellectual Disabilities

Therapeutic recreation for children with intellectual disabilities supplements and extends educational services and provides opportunities for socialization. Common settings are after-school and summer camp programs offered by local and state parks and recreation departments, local agencies for serving people with disabilities, and organizations such as Easterseals. The goal of the programming is to promote development of cognitive and social skills. Therapeutic recreation is specifically listed as a related service to supplement education under the IDEA. When a child is determined to be eligible for services, an interdisciplinary team develops an **individualized education program (IEP)**. Many programs, whether or not school affiliated, use the IEP to help address the specific needs of the child or teenager. As the person with intellectual disability ages, therapeutic recreation can be used to address vocational or social skills; continue cognitive development; or address transitions, such as a move or grief because of the death of a friend or close relative.

Most therapeutic recreation services for people with intellectual disabilities could be classified under the general modality known as leisure education. Leisure education has been conceptualized as a major component of therapeutic recreation, as illustrated in the leisure ability model. In addition, several scholars and practitioners have worked to develop leisure education curricula that focus on people with intellectual disabilities. Finally, specific programs or groups for this population are commonly in line with the elements of leisure education models and frameworks. Simply put, leisure education frameworks, curricula, and programs have been built on concepts that are consistent with the developmental or therapeutic goals commonly associated with people with intellectual disabilities. Social skill development, leisure awareness, appropriate use of leisure resources, and activity skill development are all potential focal points when working with such people. The following sections provide readers with a brief overview of a few intellectual disabilities.

Down Syndrome

According to the National Down Syndrome Society (NDSS), **Down syndrome** is the most common chromosomal developmental disability in the United States, affecting 1 out of every 700 babies, or approximately 6,000 babies, each year. All people with Down syndrome experience some intellectual disability, generally in the mild to moderate diagnostic categories (NDSS, 2018). A **syndrome** is a group of symptoms or abnormalities that indicate a particular trait or disease. Down syndrome results from the production of an extra chromosome during cell development. Common symptoms include poor muscle tone, hyperflexibility, lowered resistance to infection, impaired vision, slower physical and mental development, and premature aging as an adult (NDSS, 2018). The underlying genetic component predisposes people with Down syndrome to a variety of health complications, including weakness of the spine, hearing and respiratory conditions, dementia, and heart problems. Early interventions and enriched environments aid in lessening or preventing the development of poor health. Encouraging is the fact that life expectancy of a person with Down syndrome has risen from 25 in 1983 to 60 in 2012 (NDSS, 2018).

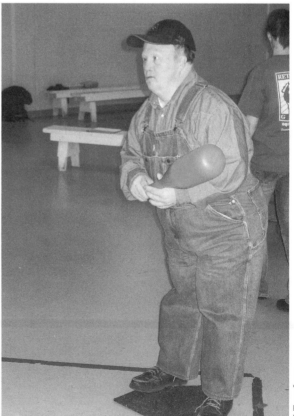

Obesity, hyperflexible joints, accelerated aging, and early-onset Alzheimer's disease are common challenges for people with Down syndrome.

© Terry Long

Fragile X Syndrome

The most common inherited form of intellectual disability is fragile X syndrome. Because the trait is carried on the X chromosome, the disability occurs more often and has more severe effects in males but can be diagnosed in females as well. Recent estimates indicated that the prevalence of those diagnosed with fragile X in the United States is 1 in 3,600 to 4,000 males and 1 in 4,000 to 6,000 females (National Fragile X Foundation, 2018). A mutation of the gene causes the body to produce insufficient protein for development. This in turn results in varying degrees of intellectual impairment; sensitivity to sensation; behavioral problems; and certain physical characteristics, including larger ears, jaw, and forehead; smaller stature; and extremely flexible joints. Other possible related physical conditions include weak connective tissue, heart murmur, and hand tremors. People with fragile X can have behaviors similar to those with autism because of their heightened sensitivity to sensations, such as loud noises and textures. This similarity extends to social behaviors and the ability to communicate in a socially appropriate manner (National Fragile X Foundation, 2018). Children diagnosed with fragile X are eligible for special education support through the IDEA (National Fragile X Foundation, 2018).

Autism Spectrum Disorders

The *DSM-5* changes resulted in a new umbrella category called autism spectrum disorder, under which now fall conditions previously classified as autistic disorder, Asperger's disorder, and **pervasive developmental disorders** not otherwise specified (PDD-NOS). **Autism** is the fastest growing developmental disability in the United States, increasing by 119.4 percent between 2000 and 2010 alone. Autism affects a person's ability to communicate, understand language, play, and relate to others. Autism occurs in approximately 1 in every 58 children and is four times more common in boys than in girls (Baio et al., 2018). Autism is related to several other developmental disorders, and three out of four people with autism are also diagnosed with an intellectual disability. About half of the people who have autism and another developmental disability are diagnosed in the moderate to severe categories. Additionally, 20 to 33 percent of people with autism also experience epileptic seizures (Spence & Schneider, 2009).

A diagnosis of autism spectrum disorder is given when the person exhibits persistent problems with social interactions and communication across multiple areas, such as deficits in social or emotional reciprocity; deficits in nonverbal communication used for social integration; and deficits in developing, maintaining, and understanding relationships. The severity of the level of diagnosis is based on social communication impairments and restricted repetitive patterns of behavior. The ultimate diagnosis also reflects the level of supportive care a person may need (American Psychiatric Association, 2013).

Characteristics commonly listed for persons diagnosed with autism spectrum disorders include inability to develop normal social relationships, delay in speech development, stereotypical play, lack of imagination, and insistence on sameness. Some or all of the following characteristics may be observed in mild to severe forms:

- Communication problems (e.g., using and understanding language)
- Difficulty relating to people, objects, and events
- Unusual play with toys and other objects
- Difficulty with changes in routine or familiar surroundings
- Repetitive body movements or behavior patterns
- A broad range of cognitive abilities and behavior—little to no language skills to highly intelligent
- Unusual responses to sensory information, such as loud noises, lights, and certain textures of food or fabrics

Program Considerations for People With Autism Spectrum Disorder

Interventions for people with autism focus on improving communication, social, academic, behavioral, and daily living skills. Use of a variety of sensory inputs, such as visual and auditory cues, is often effective in helping the person with autism learn better. Interaction with peers who do not have disabilities is important for providing models of appropriate language, social, and behavioral skills. To overcome frequent problems in generalizing skills from one setting to another, goals, experiences, and approaches should be done in a variety of settings, including, home, school, and the community. As with intellectual disabilities, therapeutic recreation specialists may encounter people with autism in a variety of settings, ranging from structured therapy or education programs to municipal recreation programs. Because autism varies widely in severity and symptomology, the therapeutic recreation specialist must adequately identify client needs and abilities through assessment and adjust the program accordingly.

As with other developmental disabilities, developing a comprehensive understanding of the client is critical to the success of intervention. Because autism usually involves restricted interests as well as substantial fixation on the interests that do exist, one major goal is to expand the client's repertoire of leisure behavior. Children who spend all their time reading the same book or playing with the same toy, often in a manner unrelated to the purpose of the toy, have limited ability to develop through typical play patterns. Stereotypic behaviors, such as rocking or bouncing (forms of self-stimulation), often reduce the possibility of broadening play interests, but by understanding the interests of a child with autism, the professional can implement effective interventions. Pairing the preferred form of play with other play behaviors can gradually lead to a more diverse play pattern, which is fuel for learning and development. This process involves hands-on work. The therapeutic recreation specialist plays with the child, integrating the preferred form of play into various activities and encouraging the child to take part. The preferred form of play can also be used to reinforce desirable behavior. In severe cases, preferred forms of play may be limited to sensory stimulation, such as use of a mirror or a vibrating toy. After the child begins to understand and enjoy using various toys in his or her intended manner, he or she is better able to socialize with other children. Early intervention is important in all cases.

Another commonly used technique is the relaxation room. Because children with autism often experience sensory overload when subjected to certain stimuli and overwhelming environments in general, they often need opportunities to recuperate. Relaxation rooms are areas that contain a variety of soothing stimuli, such as beanbags, pillows, soft-colored lights, soothing music, and even bubbles. These rooms can also provide relief for clients who crave certain types of sensory stimulation. This resource can help the child recuperate from difficult environments at school, therapy, home, or play.

Finally, community-based recreation programs for people with autism should be a regular part of the parks and recreation services provided in today's society and, when appropriate, should be inclusive. It is critical that community-based programs have staff members who understand the needs of participants with autism, set appropriate goals, and make adaptations that allow for achievement of goals.

Cerebral Palsy

Cerebral palsy (CP) is a neurological disorder caused by a nonprogressive brain injury or malformation during development (National Institute of Neurological Disorders and Stroke [NINDS], 2018). It is estimated that about 1 in 300 children have CP, which can affect body movement, muscle control, motor functioning, reflex, balance, and posture. Sometimes, but not always, a child with CP may also be diagnosed with an intellectual disability. The most common causes of CP are genetic conditions, infections (e.g., meningitis), child abuse, stroke, and head injury. CP can range from mild to severe. In the United States, about 9,500 infants and children are diagnosed with CP each year. There are four main types of CP:

- *Spastic CP* is a result of tightness of the muscles, which causes stiff movements of the arms or legs and immediate contraction of stretched muscles. People with this form of CP often have difficulty walking because of stiffness of the muscles and their legs may turn inward, causing what looks like crossed legs at the knees. This is called scissoring (March of Dimes, 2018). Spastic CP can manifest in three forms: diplegia, in which only the legs are affected; hemiplegia, in which half of the body (such as the left arm and leg) is affected; and quadriplegia, in which both the arms and the legs are affected, sometimes including the facial muscles and torso. Spastic CP is the most common form of CP, affecting about 80 percent of people diagnosed.

- *Dyskinetic CP* (also called athetoid CP or dystonic CP) is a result of too tight or loose muscle tone and manifests itself in slow, uncontrollable movements of the entire body. This disability makes it hard for the person to sit straight and walk. Some people with this form of CP will have difficulty speaking and may have problems with facial muscles, causing them to drool.

- *Ataxic CP* is rare and results in a poor sense of balance in walking and standing. People with ataxic CP may have tremors when they move, especially when control is needed, such as in writing or grasping. The person may also overshoot objects when reaching for them.
- *Mixed CP* is a combination of types. A person with mixed CP exhibits both rigid and involuntary movements. The most common type of mixed CP is spastic–dyskinetic.

CP can range from mild, in which the person has only mild stiffness in walking, to severe, in which many bodily functions are impeded. The main areas affected are locomotion (walking and other forms of movement), gross and fine motor coordination, and communication skills because of limitations in controlling muscle movement. People with CP have a higher incidence of seizure activity and may have sensation, vision, or speech problems when they overexert themselves. Lack of movement and physical activity also results in a higher probability of being overweight (March of Dimes, 2018).

Program Considerations for People With CP

People with CP experience a variety of symptoms that can make recreation activities and activities of daily living in general difficult. For example, **pathological reflexes** often accompany CP. Reflexes are usually integrated into typical motor patterns as we progress through the developmental stages, but brain injury associated with CP can cause these reflexes to persist indefinitely. These pathological reflexes disrupt normal body movements with uncontrollable movement. For example, the asymmetrical tonic neck reflex (ATNR) is triggered when the head is tilted or turned (Sherrill, 2004). Simply turning the head to track a moving ball will cause the chin-side arm to extend out and the other arm to flex. This movement is uncontrollable. Therapeutic recreation specialists can, in some cases, work to inhibit these pathological reflexes through activities that work to develop motor skills. The process of overriding uncontrolled reflex movements with controlled movement is called reflex integration and is a normal process during development. For the

individual with CP, reflex integration is inhibited, but can sometimes be fostered through repeated practice of movements that contradict the reflex. For example, ATNR intervention might include having the person creep backward and forward with the head turned to one side (creeping works to integrate the ATNR triggered by turning the head; see Sherrill, 2004, for additional techniques related to integrating pathological reflexes).

CP also involves imbalances in the inhibition or engagement of flexor and extensor muscle groups, which lead to spasticity (muscle stiffness). Spasticity causes limited flexibility and range of motion and can cause permanent joint **contractures** if untreated. Massage, stretching, and trunk rotations can be used to reduce such imbalances and maximize leisure skills. Aquatic programs

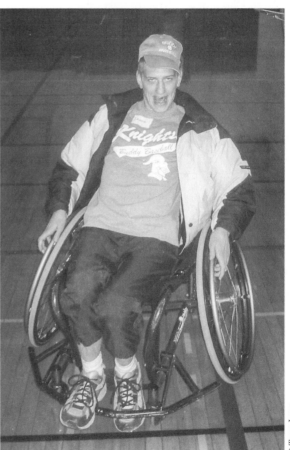

Severity of motor disturbances caused by cerebral palsy varies, with some individuals requiring the use of adaptive equipment. This young man can stand and walk but has difficulty with balance during complex activities.

are especially useful because buoyancy in the water makes movement and manipulation much easier and warm-water pools (90 to 98 degrees Fahrenheit [32.2 to 36.7 degrees Celsius]) help relieve contractures.

Two increasingly popular modalities are therapeutic horseback riding and hippotherapy. Therapeutic horseback riding can help address disturbances in postural reactions (the ability to hold the body upright) and other physical abilities and can also be used to address social and emotional issues. Hippotherapy uses the movement of the horse to relieve spasticity and hypotonia (low muscle tone). These horse-based therapies require certification and collaboration with trained professionals.

Spina Bifida

Spina bifida is a neural tube developmental condition caused by a malformation of plate cells along the spine when the embryo is forming. The term *spina bifida* means "cleft spine." This is the most common form of neural tube disability, affecting between 1,500 and 2,000 babies each year in the United States (Parker et al., 2010). The Centers for Disease Control and Prevention (CDC) and the U.S. Public Health Service have identified folic acid deficiency as a significant risk factor for spina bifida and first recommended folic acid supplements for all pregnant women in 1992 (CDC, 1992). As a result, folic acid supplements are routinely recommended to pregnant mothers. Three forms of spina bifida present problems. **Spina bifida occulta**, meaning "hidden," is the mildest form and results from one or more openings of the vertebrae, covered by skin, with no discernible damage to the spinal cord. Approximately 10 to 20 percent of spina bifida diagnoses are of this form. The second form of spina bifida, **closed neural tube defect**, occurs when the sac that protects the spinal cord, the meningocele, is pushed through an opening in the vertebrae. There are malformations of fat, bone, or meninges. This form can easily be repaired and usually does not result in injury to the spinal cord. In the third type of spina bifida, **myelomeningocele**, the spinal cord protrudes through the person's back. This is the form commonly referred to as spina bifida. This condition may result in muscle weakness or paralysis below the exposed area in the spine, loss of bladder and bowel control, and frequently (in 70 to 90 percent of cases) causes accumulation of fluid in the brain (**hydrocephalus**; NINDS, 2018). The treatment requires several operations throughout childhood and, if accompanied by hydrocephalus, placing a shunt in the child's brain to drain excess fluid. Buildup of fluid on the brain can cause further damage, resulting in blindness, seizures, or brain damage. Estimates are that 1 child in 4,000 has this third form of spina bifida (MedlinePlus, 2018). Certain medical facilities across the country that are participating in the Management of Myelomeningocele Study, or MOMS, are performing in utero surgery to repair this type of spina bifida. This highly risky surgery cannot fix neurological damage that has already occurred, but it has been shown to reduce additional losses.

With proper medical care and supplementary services, 90 percent of all children born with spinal bifida live a normal life span. Spina bifida is often classified as an orthopedic or neurological disability, but because of the early onset and possible cognitive impairments, some organizations classify spina bifida as a developmental disability. Like other orthopedic disabilities, many people with spina bifida use assistive devices, such as walkers, braces, wheelchairs, splints, or crutches. As with any lower spinal cord injury, possible loss of bowel and bladder control may require the use of a catheter (NINDS, 2018). Because of continued physical growth during childhood and adolescence, repeated operations are often needed. These procedures can result in loss of strength and low self-esteem.

Program Considerations for People With Spina Bifida

Therapeutic recreation interventions focus on increasing muscle strength and flexibility, learning how to adapt activities, and increasing a sense of self and empowerment through leisure activities. Frequent operations during childhood create a need for continual strengthening of the muscles. The same adaptations and activities used with people who have difficulty with mobility can be used with people who have spina bifida. Possible precautions relate to complications from hydrocephalus and the spinal cord lesion, which include possible seizures, cognitive impairment, apnea, swallowing difficulties, neck pain, and increased susceptibility to bladder and bowel dysfunctions and infections. Therapeutic recreation goals such as increasing upper body strength to assist in activities of daily living and building self-esteem are common.

Sensory-Related Developmental Disabilities

Sensory-related developmental disabilities interfere with a person's ability to sense the world around him or her. We use our senses to navigate our world, most of the time without even thinking about it. Children with sensory-related developmental disabilities have difficulty processing and using sensory information from sight, sound, smells, taste, and touch. Thus, vision and hearing problems can also be associated with other developmental disabilities. It is important to note that a person can have multiple challenges and fit into more than one type of developmental disability. For instance, a person with fragile X syndrome may have a neurologically caused intellectual disability but also may struggle with sensory-related issues because they are typically sensitive to loud noises. Children with autism spectrum disorders would be another example of this crossover of types of developmental disabilities.

In 1972, a University of California, Los Angeles, psychologist and occupational therapist, A. Jean Ayers, proposed that some impairments in adaptive functioning may actually be related to a neurological problem in the processing of sensory information. Ayers originally referred to this condition as sensory integration disorder. Difficulty in handling sensory information from sight, hearing, taste, smell, and touch as well as proprioceptive and vestibular senses was proposed to be the basis of the problems.

Recently, sensory integration disorder has been reconceptualized as sensory processing disorder (SPD) and is included in the *Diagnostic Classification of Mental Health and Developmental Disorders of Infancy and Early Childhood* (*DC: 0-5*). The *DC: 0-5* describes SPD as including three general types: sensory over-responsivity disorder, sensory under-responsivity disorder, and other sensory responsivity disorders (Zero to Three, 2016).

As noted earlier, sensory disturbances are frequently observed among children with autism spectrum disorder, and such disturbances are actually a diagnostic criterion for the condition.

This brings into question whether SPD is a unique condition or simply an element of autism. The *DSM-5* does not specify SPD as a formal diagnosis but does acknowledge that not all children with autism have SPD. Furthermore, it is widely accepted that some children who have sensory processing difficulties do not have autism. Thus, there is some debate on whether such sensory processing issues warrant a separate diagnosis. Many practitioners have advocated the inclusion of SPD in the upcoming 2025 release of the *DSM-6*. There is evidence to suggest that children with SPD and children with autism differ in both the severity and nature of sensory disturbances (Schoen, Miller, Brett-Green, & Nielsen, 2009), as well as in white matter abnormalities (Chang et al., 2014) and cognitive processing styles related to empathy and systematization of thought (Tavassoli et al., 2018). As of now, the debate continues regarding the need to diagnostically differentiate autism and SPD; however, it is clear that many children and adults experience sensory processing disturbances and that these disturbances warrant consideration when providing therapeutic recreation services.

Program Considerations for People With Sensory-Related Disabilities

Several sensory-based interventions have already been mentioned above regarding programs for clients with autism who may either crave or be aversive to various forms of sensory stimulation; however, it is possible that participants may experience these conditions but not have autism. Other clients may have underdeveloped sensory systems that make it difficult for them to detect sensory information and can benefit from engaging senses in a way that encourages the maturation of sensory systems. It is often necessary to assess what forms of sensory stimulation are craved, overwhelming, or underdeveloped. Therapeutic recreation specialists can then make adaptations to provide appropriate opportunities to engage in desired stimulation, modify overstimulating environments or develop a tolerance to the aversive stimuli, and engage underdeveloped sensory systems through repetition and practice. As examples, rough textures, such as a wet washcloth, are often more easily tolerated and can be used to build up to softer forms of touch, and massage or object manipulation can help develop the ability to detect tactile stimulation.

CRAIG STROHBECK, CTRS

Education: BS in Recreation and Park Administration (Therapeutic Recreation Sequence), Illinois State University
Position: Director of Residential Services
Organization St. Louis Arc, Saint Louis, Missouri

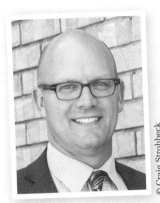

© Craig Strohbeck

My Career

During college, I had the opportunity to be employed in a variety of services that supported individuals with physical, social, and cognitive needs. As a physical therapy tech, private direct service provider, and parks and recreation team member for Special Opportunities Available in Recreation (SOAR), I gained the foundation of skills that opened doors beyond college. Following college, I was a private care coordinator for an individual with developmental disabilities (high school and transition age). After this, I was director of activities in a 180-bed skilled nursing facility (older adults). For nine years, I worked in a community parks and recreation department, where I ran facilities, coordinated senior programs, and served as the ADA liaison for individuals, families, and facilities. This gave me extensive understanding of the business side; I worked with a large and diverse staff as well as with community members of all ages with situations related to disabilities. During this time, I served as an interim director of the parks and recreation department for a period and as superintendent, reporting directly to the city manager. I then became the executive director of a community-based social skill training program for adults with more independence. This was a terrific opportunity to lead a small nonprofit and grow the organization in many ways over a period of nine years.

My current position is director of residential services with St. Louis Arc. The mission of St. Louis Arc is to empower people with intellectual and developmental disabilities to lead better lives by providing a lifetime of high-quality services, family support, and advocacy. My responsibilities include overseeing the residential needs of 13 group homes with 71 residents, inspiring a team of 125 employees, and contributing to the overall vision and direction of the agency. One of the most rewarding aspects of my work is seeing the successes of the individuals who our organization supports. We have a unique opportunity to support an aging population. Our participants are aging, but that does not mean they are not still learning. They each experience success and joy through different achievements, and it is always exciting to know how our team plays a role in that. Second, I really enjoy coaching and mentoring the team and being coached by them. I truly believe the chain of command should not be a top-down approach, but a linked continuum of people who must work together for the outcomes to be achieved.

My Advice to You

Understand that the coursework is just the beginning of the learning. You will always be learning. Understand that everyone is in a different place in their learning, and we need to respect and understand each other. Empathy is gift. Find it in yourself, use it, and work your best to support others in developing empathy. Advocacy is your job. Make it a priority. Outcomes are a reality. Dashboards are your friend. You can only achieve what you are tracking. Work is not your life. Find balance: Give everything you have while you are at work, and then give everything you have to your other interests. Relationships are important—develop them and nurture them. Give to others first. The rewards will come back tenfold.

Metabolic Disabilities

There are other ways that developmental disabilities can occur. Metabolic developmental disabilities refer to the body's metabolism, which relates to the way the body creates, uses, or breaks down materials it needs to function. Disorders that fall into this type are phenylketonuria (PKU), galactosemia, and severe combined immune deficiency (SCID), of which PKU is the most common disability.

Phenylketonuria

Phenylketonuria (PKU) is a rare, inherited metabolic disorder that if not treated can lead to brain damage that causes intellectual impairment or cerebral palsy. Because of a genetic mutation, the body is unable to break down the amino acid phenylalanine (Phe). PKU is caused by the liver's being unable to make the enzyme phenylalanine hydroxylase (PAH). The PAH enzyme normally converts the Phe to another amino acid known as tyrosine. Without PAH, an excess of Phe builds up and becomes toxic to the person's central nervous system. Treatment must begin within the first few weeks of life and consists of changing the diet to limit the intake of phenylalanine, which is found in foods high in protein, such as meats, fish, eggs, beans, nuts, and milk and dairy products, and foods containing the artificial sweetener aspartame. Since 1961, when prenatal screening began, careful diet has prevented most cases of intellectual impairment. PKU is rare, occurring in 1 out of every 10,000 to 15,000 births in the United States (Genetics Home Reference, 2018). Because a careful diet can usually prevent brain damage, the need for therapeutic recreation is limited. But people with PKU demonstrate the importance of being aware of the medical history of the client in all settings. In offering services, the therapeutic recreation specialist must understand the dietary as well as the physical needs of clients. No specific program exists for people with PKU, but when dealing with a person who has cerebral palsy or intellectual impairment, service providers should be aware of potential **contraindications**, such as the dietary restrictions indicated earlier.

Galactosemia

Galactosemia is a disorder that causes an inability to process galactose, a simple sugar found in milk. Damage to the liver, kidneys, brain, and eyes can occur in children who have this disorder and consume milk or milk products (Genetics Home Reference, 2018). If not diagnosed early, intellectual disabilities and even death can occur. Children who are not treated early may develop cataracts; unsteady gait; and delays in learning, speech, and growth. Treatment is a strict diet that eliminates this sugar, but there is still a chance that the child may develop a mild intellectual disability. This is a rare disease today because of early screenings and occurs in about 1 in every 50,000 babies in the United States.

Severe Combined Immune Deficiency

Babies born with **severe combined immune deficiency (SCID)** have an inability to fight off infections because parts of the immune system fail to operate. This disorder has also been referred to as the "bubble boy disease," in reference to a child born in 1971 with SCID who became famous for living in a sterile environment. Screening newborns for SCID is now common practice to identify the presence of this inherited metabolic disorder. If left untreated, children rarely live past the age of 2. This is an extremely rare metabolic disorder with only 40 to 100 cases being identified each year in the United States. A bone marrow transplant that replaces the immune system is the only treatment for the disorder.

Degenerative Disabilities

Infants born with degenerative disabilities may appear to be healthy but will gradually begin to lose abilities or functioning as the disorder progresses. Often, the disability is not noticed until later in the developmental stages when milestones or abnormalities in functioning abilities are noticed. Degenerative disorders, such as Duchenne muscular dystrophy, can cause physical, mental, and sensory problems, depending on the nature of the disability.

Muscular Dystrophy

Muscular dystrophy (MD) is a group of chronic, genetic diseases characterized by the progressive degeneration and weakness of voluntary muscles. MD results from a hereditary or mutated gene on the X chromosome that causes generalized weakness and deterioration of the muscles. The onset of four forms of MD occurs during childhood: Duchenne, Becker (a milder form of Duchenne), congenital, and Emery-Dreifuss. Two other forms, facioscapulohumeral MD and limb-girdle MD, occur in late childhood to adolescence.

Duchenne MD, also called pseudohypertrophic MD, is the most common type and most aggressive form of childhood MD. It accounts for over half of all forms of MD and occurs in 1 of 3,500 births. Duchenne MD is more common in males, but a few rare cases have been diagnosed in females (Muscular Dystrophy Association [MDA], 2018). The genetic defect caused by Duchenne MD results in the absence of the protein dystrophin, which helps keep the muscle walls intact. Signs of weakness, loss of reflexes, difficulty sitting up, and impaired breathing first occur when the child begins to walk (around age 2). As the disease progresses, the muscles become weaker, and breathing becomes difficult. Many children with Duchenne MD begin to need a wheelchair between ages 7 and 12. As the disease progresses, the person will experience an increase in the weakness of the heart muscle, respiratory complications, or infections (MDA, 2018). Life expectancy is increasing, with many people living into their 30s and a few into their 40s and 50s.

The other forms of MD cause varying degrees of muscle weakness that affect the ability to walk as well as the health of the heart and respiratory systems. Treatment focuses on helping the person with MD be as independent and comfortable as possible. Activities that improve movement and flexibility are recommended (MDA, 2018).

Program Considerations for Muscular Dystrophy

MD generally involves lifelong impairment that progressively worsens. Therapeutic recreation programs are, therefore, often built around providing opportunities for engagement in recreational activities that improve quality of life. Enhancing leisure is a primary goal as well as providing respite from ongoing physical and emotional challenges. In addition, therapeutic recreation programs can certainly be used to counteract some of the progressive effects of MD. A regular stretching regimen and mild to moderate physical activity can help counteract loss of mobility and maintain quality of life, but precautions should be taken with physical activity. Because needs and precautions can be highly individualized and each type of MD can warrant a different approach, consulting with the client's primary physician when developing programs involving physical activity is important. In addition, some research findings have indicated that moderate to intense forms of exercise can exacerbate the symptoms of MD, and the recovery cycle following exercise may be slower; therefore, consulting with the physician is a necessity.

Best Practices

In all stages of education and training of those with disabilities, a balance should be struck between traditional educational goals, such as learning the alphabet and how to read, and functional skills, such as learning how to cross the street safely or use the bus system. The former goals focus on skills fundamental to learning higher cognitive or physical competencies, whereas the latter goals focus on the ability to perform daily activities. Attention should ultimately be on the skills that the person needs to be as independent as possible or to live and function in the least restrictive environment.

Some additional practices to promote individual choice and independence include using adaptive equipment, offering opportunities for community integration, providing leisure education, using activity and task analyses, and providing opportunities for practice and repetition. As technology continues to expand, so too does the availability of new options for enhancing clients' skills.

One critical consideration to remember is that a person's cognitive level is not the same as his or her life-stage level. The therapeutic recreation specialist must offer and use age-appropriate activities and equipment. Although a person may have the cognitive abilities of a 5-year-old, that person should not be given only toys and activities that a 5-year-old would use. Rather than thinking of the diagnosis (such as having an IQ of 50 or not having the use of the lower extremity), the specialist should think of the person and his or her chronological age and interests. Focus should be on the person's strengths and adapting age-appropriate activities that are of interest to the client and his or her peers. Many opportunities should be provided to practice these activities, including opportunities within the larger community (i.e., community integration). Remember Mary's scenario from the beginning of the chapter? As a client who is in her mid-50s and has Down syndrome, she should not be given elementary-aged toys to work on goals. Rather, the therapeutic recreation specialist can use her interests in gardening, playing rummy, and being with her cat to achieve therapy objectives. The goal of increasing social integration could be achieved by helping her enroll in a community garden club, having her volunteer to garden at a community garden plot, or aiding her in registering to show flowers at the county fair. These activities can be accompanied by engaging her in role-playing situations before the actual events (see Client Portrait: Mary at the end of this chapter for a further explanation of this scenario).

Another technique often used to facilitate learning new skills is behavior modification. **Behavior modification**, the process of changing behavior through a combination of rewards and punishments, is frequently used with clients who have developmental disabilities. Behavior modification can be used not only to teach and reinforce a positive behavior, such as remaining focused on a task or learning a new skill, but also to reduce or stop a negative behavior, such as hitting or interrupting others. For additional information, review the comprehensive overview of behavior modification principles in chapter 7.

Another important practice is using multiple modes of communication or instructional prompts. Information can be presented verbally, visually, or even with other senses, such as smell and touch. By using multiple prompts, the likelihood that the client will remember the information is increased. Leisure activities are ideally suited for using multiple senses. For instance, in using swimming to improve a client's physical fitness and endurance, the therapeutic recreation specialist can use verbal cuing (reminders) to swim, assisted movement (a physical prompt) to develop the position of the swimming stroke, and colored markers to reinforce distance traveled. Similarly, a repeated instruction can help the client focus on the task and process information. As with any learning, the more opportunities there are for practice and repetition, the more likely it is that the client will learn the behavior or task.

As described in chapter 6, activity analysis is the process of breaking down an activity into the skills and requirements (e.g., equipment and setting) necessary for successfully doing the activity. Similarly, task analysis was described as breaking down an activity into its basic behavioral steps. Both of these procedures are especially important when working with persons who have a developmental disability. As the therapeutic recreation specialist seeks avenues for using client strengths and implementing necessary adaptations, these procedures provide a structured mechanism for finding age-appropriate activities that meet the developmental capabilities and needs of the client. Regarding intellectual impairment, task analysis can be especially useful for identifying appropriate increments or steps of learning when using techniques such as **chaining** or shaping to teach complex behaviors.

The opportunity for community integration is important for all people with developmental

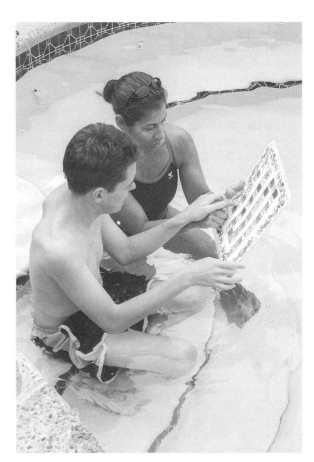

Using multiple modes of communication or instructional prompts is an effective way to reinforce learning.

disabilities. The concept developed from efforts to change the status quo from the 1970s, when the norm was to institutionalize people with developmental disabilities. The basic premise is to facilitate inclusion opportunities that offer full participation in life. Parallel to the concept of community integration is the concept of least restrictive environment. As the term indicates, every person should have the opportunity to participate in activities as he or she is able. The range of suitable opportunities will vary according to ability. Least restrictive environment often means that the person participates in community activities with some assistance. For instance, an adult with cerebral palsy might be able to snow ski after training in the use of adaptive equipment and being provided transportation to a nearby ski resort.

Leisure education is part of many of the therapeutic interventions with people with developmental disabilities. Leisure education focuses on goal areas such as expanding the range of

We briefly met Mary at the beginning of the chapter. As a refresher, she is a woman in her mid-50s who has Down syndrome. Her interests include gardening, playing rummy, and being with her cat. She has lived all her life in her family home, which now houses only herself and her 95-year-old mother, who thinks that she may need to move into assisted living. Mary says that she would love to meet other people but does not know anyone. During a recent visit from social services, the social worker determined that Mary would benefit from therapeutic recreation services. Goals would be to increase social integration and learn about community resources.

Objective

During the initial assessment interview, the therapeutic recreation specialist discovered that Mary had helped her father and some of her siblings take care of their large garden and many pets, including three horses. The animals were sold when her father died 11 years ago, so Mary now takes care of only one cat and a small flower garden. Mary spoke many times during the interview about how much she had enjoyed working in the garden and caring for the horses. At the end of the meeting, three objectives were established for the general goal of social integration.

1. Mary will attend four different activities related to gardening within the community in the next month.

2. Mary will volunteer once a week for an hour at the local stables, where she will help groom the horses in exchange for a 15-minute horse ride. Mary will talk to at least one other person (besides the therapist) for at least 3 minutes while at the stables and the gardening activities.

Activity Analysis

Before Mary attends the meetings or volunteers, she and the therapeutic recreation specialist can role-play the gardening activities and what is expected in the volunteer job. Because Mary has both gardened and helped with horses in the past, extensive activity analysis will probably not be needed with these tasks. Even so, activity analysis can be useful in teaching the social skills needed for having a conversation. By breaking down the activity of introducing oneself (such as making eye contact, taking the right hand to shake when offered, saying hello, and waiting for a response), the therapeutic recreation specialist can determine what skills need further practice and role-playing.

Behavior Modification

Positive reinforcers during role-playing and both during and after participation in the community settings can be used to help achieve the goal of increasing social integration. During role-playing, simple words of encouragement for correct actions, such as "You are a natural at this," accompanied by a smile are quite powerful. In the community, many natural reinforcers of social interaction will be present, such as getting to ride a horse and meeting people who are enthusiastic about the same activity. After being in the community, the therapeutic recreation specialist should be sure to emphasize the actions that are leading to achieving the objectives. For example, the therapeutic recreation specialist could say, "Mary, you are becoming quite the social butterfly. I noticed that you introduced yourself to almost everyone at the plant exchange and talked to three people today." Open-ended questions are an effective way to prompt Mary to give herself praise ("So what did you do at the plant exchange? What did you talk about?").

Communicating With Mary About Community Integration

The therapeutic recreation specialist can further enhance the outcome of the interventions by using multiple sensory inputs. In working with someone with a cognitive impairment, use of pictures, music, simple verbal cues, and role-playing (enacting the scenario) can help with retention of the lesson. The closer these cues come to simulating the community setting, the more likely it is that the behavior will be replicated. For example, to help Mary prepare for a plant sale sponsored by a local gardening club, a role-play could be conducted using the same items that would be present at the plant sale (potted plants, pamphlets about the plants, money, etc.). Although the objective could be to meet people by passing out flyers at the local plant sale, the props can help Mary remember the role-play. The therapeutic recreation specialist can also take advantage of many of the elements that naturally occur in the community setting to enhance the therapeutic results, such as using Mary's comfort in being around horses or plants to help her interact with others.

recreation awareness and opportunities, exploring possible adaptations of activities, improving recreation-related social skills, and mastering activity skills. Modification of activities should continue in accordance with the developmental skills and limitations of the client. As mentioned earlier, modification can be accomplished through training in the use of various forms of adaptive equipment and adapting the nature of the activity to client needs. Again, task analysis and activity analysis are important tools in identifying and developing necessary adaptations.

Summary

Development is a lifelong process. Although a person is diagnosed with a developmental disability during childhood, the delay or consequences of the disability extend throughout the person's life. This chapter has presented information about how to implement the goals required to improve the health and wellness of a person with a developmental disability. Whether the therapeutic recreation specialist works with someone with intellectual impairment or with another form of developmental disability, a fundamental understanding of how a person's life context can be enhanced by taking an integrative approach to therapy is the greatest insight that can be gained.

Therapeutic recreation can play a significant role in optimizing lifelong growth in people with developmental disabilities. Although developmental disabilities affect a wide range of abilities, the capacity to adapt activities based on needs and interests of an individual is a trademark of the therapeutic recreation specialist. Expanding this skill to include the social environment in which the person lives and works allows professionals to facilitate opportunities for enjoyment, growth, and self-advocacy. By using expertise on how leisure evolves throughout life and across development, therapeutic recreation specialists are ideally suited to create an environment to support growth, social integration, and safety in dealing with and working through life transitions.

DISCUSSION QUESTIONS

1. Describe the commonalities and differences in the diagnoses of developmental disability, intellectual disability, learning disability, autism spectrum disorders, cerebral palsy, Down syndrome, and spina bifida.

2. List the four types of developmental disabilities, and give an example of a disability for each type.

3. What are the main knowledge areas that a therapeutic recreation specialist should understand when working with a person with a developmental disability?

4. Explain the importance of age-appropriate interventions, and give at least two examples.

5. Explain why taking the life-span approach is important when working with people with a developmental disability.

6. Explain what precautions are needed to address the contraindications for each of the presented types of developmental disability.

7. Identify potential goal areas for each of the presented types of developmental disability.

9

Therapeutic Recreation and Physical Rehabilitation

Terry Robertson | Jody Cormack | Terry Long

LEARNING OUTCOMES

At the end of this chapter, students will be able to

- recognize common orthopedic and neurological conditions experienced by therapeutic recreation clients,
- explain the role that therapeutic recreation plays in providing services to people with such conditions,
- delineate modalities typically used to address orthopedic and neurological conditions in both rehabilitation and reintegration settings,
- identify appropriate application of these modalities to various orthopedic and neurological conditions, and
- describe best practice mechanisms for the delivery of such modalities, including use of protocols and critical pathways.

Physical rehabilitation services are designed to address disturbances or deterioration of physiological functions, but the nature of impairments resulting from such disturbances can go far beyond the physical realm. Physical rehabilitation services often involve programs that address impairments of social, emotional, cognitive, and physical functional skills. Likewise, causal factors and pattern of progression can vary widely even within specific diagnostic categories. As such, rehabilitation programs must provide for a broad range of client needs. As an example of the diverse needs of patients who are receiving rehabilitation services, consider that a person with a traumatic brain injury is likely to experience not only physical challenges but also a variety of other impairments related to cognitive processing, emotional stability, and social interactions. Furthermore, the need for support or additional rehabilitation does not end when patients are discharged from the hospital. A gradual community reentry with continued involvement in community-based programs is often a necessary component of recovery.

Therapeutic recreation can be a significant part of physical rehabilitation programs and is uniquely capable of addressing this broad range of client needs. Approximately 32 percent of certified therapeutic recreation specialists (CTRSs) work in rehabilitation hospitals or in the rehabilitation department of general medical hospitals (National Council for Therapeutic Recreation Certification, 2015). Many hospital-based programs offer interprofessional practice, wherein two or more health professionals collaborate in the delivery of care. Therapeutic recreation specialists work with nurses, physical and occupational therapists, **speech-language pathologists**, and other professionals to develop and implement interventions that address the social, emotional, cognitive, and physical impairments and functional limitations that lead to reduced participation in life roles. Therapeutic recreation specialists are the team members most prepared to contribute to the rehabilitation of affected functional skills, notably those necessary for successful participation in recreation and leisure activities. In addition, leisure-skill development and reintegration into the community are major goal areas that therapeutic recreation specialists commonly address during the rehabilitation process. After patients have achieved appropriate levels of function and independence, the provision of therapeutic recreation services can shift to community-based professionals who provide adapted and inclusive forms of recreation and leisure.

Common Diagnostic Groups in Rehabilitation

Patients find themselves in need of rehabilitation services for a variety of reasons. Some people may have been in an accident, and others may be experiencing deficits caused by genetic conditions or transmittable diseases. Many people need rehabilitation services because they have simply worn out part of their body (e.g., joint replacements). Other patients are receiving care for impairment that has resulted from an unhealthy lifestyle (e.g., smoking, poor diet, or drug use). This broad array of causal factors naturally results in an equally broad list of diagnostic groups representing people who potentially could receive services in a physical rehabilitation program. The following section identifies some of the more common patient categories, but practitioners will observe many other conditions in daily practice. More important than patient classification is the use of a competent assessment procedure to identify deficits in client functioning. Care plans can then be built around individual client needs.

Orthopedic Impairments

Orthopedic impairment refers to a condition caused by disruption of the musculoskeletal system. Such disturbances are common in rehabilitation, and many involve joint replacement. Typically, **osteoarthritis (OA)** leads to the progressive deterioration of joint cartilage and the formation of bone at the margins of the joint. Muscles around the joint may also be affected (Klippel, Stone, Crofford, & White, 2008). OA often requires replacement of a knee or hip with an artificial joint. OA, the most common form of arthritis, results from wear and tear on joints over a person's life span. Genetics can play a role in how quickly such deterioration occurs, but lifestyle is a major factor in determining progression. In all, there are over 100 known types of arthritis, with OA and **rheumatoid arthritis (RA)** accounting for the majority of cases (Sherrill, 2004). RA involves inflammation of the lining of joints, called the synovium, and is believed to be related to an attack on the body by the immune system. In some cases, RA is systemic, affecting vital organs and causing **pericarditis** (inflammation of the lining of the heart). The most common impairments seen with either type of arthritis are pain and inflammation in joints leading to loss of range of motion and inhibition of muscle function, which leads to weakness. Sharp, unexpected joint pain in a closed-chain activity, such as walking, may also lead to imbalance and potentially, falls. These impairments often lead to loss of function. A person with knee or hip arthritis may need assistive devices, such as a cane or walker, to reduce the compressive forces and the muscle demands on the joint when walking. Raised toilet seats are often helpful for bathroom transfers. Individuals often live with painful arthritis for many years prior to seeking joint replacement options; therefore, it is crucial that these individuals maintain functional ability and recreation and leisure options.

Other conditions, such as degenerative bone diseases or severe fractures, can lead to the need for joint replacement, but more common is the general rehabilitation of hip fractures, multiple bone fractures, or soft tissue injuries (i.e., muscle, ligaments, and tendons).

Rehabilitation following limb amputation is also common. Common goals for therapy include mastery of ambulation techniques, use of **prosthetic devices**, therapy for phantom pain, and

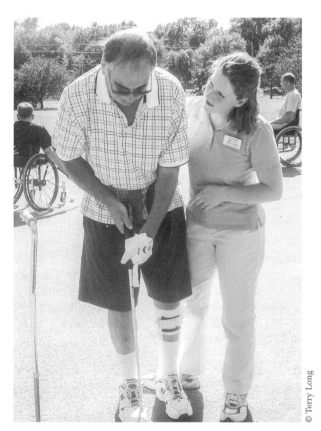

Therapeutic recreation specialists assist clients with orthopedic impairments in developing recreation and leisure skills.

© Terry Long

mastery of activities of daily living and recreation and leisure skills.

Neurological Impairments

Neurological impairments include injuries or diseases that originate in the nervous system. The two most common traumatic neurologically based injuries observed in rehabilitation are spinal cord injury and traumatic brain injury. These two classifications include a broad array of potential impairments.

Spinal Cord Injury

Spinal cord injuries (SCIs) involve trauma or other damage to the spinal cord that creates disturbance of either motor functions or sensation. The spinal cord is a bundle of nerves that carries information back and forth between the brain and the rest of the body. A series of hollow bone structures, referred to as the spinal column, protects the spinal cord. The bones that make up the spinal column are called vertebrae. The last vertebra is at the 5th lumbar level in the lower back, also called L5. The upper motor nerves, which carry information from the brain to the spinal cord to synapse, end at about the L1 or the L2 level. Therefore, all motor nerves traveling through the spinal column at the L2 level and below are lower motor neurons, or peripheral nerves. The extent of impairment from an SCI depends on the location of the injury, with injuries higher on the spinal column resulting in greater impairment. The nervous system functions much like a telephone line. When the line is damaged, service beyond the damaged area is affected, but customers who are located before the damaged line still receive service.

SCIs are classified in several ways. **Paraplegia** refers to an injury that affects only the partial trunk and lower limbs of the body, whereas **tetraplegia** (also called quadriplegia) affects the full trunk and all four limbs. A common misconception is that people with tetraplegia have no use of their arms. In truth, the nervous system is extremely complex, so certain aspects of upper limb function can be affected while others remain intact. Depending on the location of the injury, upper limb function can be disrupted to various degrees. A second classification to consider is whether an injury is complete or incomplete. Complete SCI involves loss of all functions below the location of the injury, whereas incomplete SCI involves partial loss of sensation and/or motor function. This classification depends on the severity of the injury.

A complete severing or destruction of the spine results in a complete injury. In over half of SCIs, incomplete injury occurs, leaving some functions below the injury area intact. Likewise, about half of SCIs involve paraplegia, and the other half involve tetraplegia. Damage to upper motor neurons can cause spasticity, hyperreflexia, and loss of voluntary motor control. Damage to lower motor neurons can lead to **flaccidity**, muscle atrophy and wasting, **hyporeflexia**, **fasciculations**, and weakness or loss of voluntary and reflexive motor control. Therefore, all patients with tetraplegia have upper motor neuron syndrome, and most patients with paraplegia caused by a lumbar lesion have lower motor neuron syndrome. Thus, the differences between tetraplegia and paraplegia are not just lesion level and the use of upper extremities but also other impairments that must be managed as well.

The pathology and resultant impairments for SCI result in loss of function at all levels. Following are some examples of functional loss based on a complete lesion. Patients with tetraplegia have lost trunk and lower extremity motor function in addition to some level of upper extremity motor function, depending on the level of the lesion. A key level of injury for independent function in tetraplegia is C7. Most of these individuals have full shoulder and elbow function, including triceps, but some wrist and most finger motor control is weak. The ability to extend the elbow is crucial because it allows the individual to push in a seated position to lift body weight for transferring. Most patients at the C7 level and below are, therefore, independent in functional mobility with compensation and use of a manual wheelchair and assistive devices. Patients at the C6 level may still have the ability for functional independence, but many of them require assistance for more difficult transfers and perhaps even a power wheelchair for long-distance mobility. Those at the C5 level and higher need assistance and use a power wheelchair. Any lesion at the C4 level and higher indicates that the person will begin to have difficulty with independent respiration and loss of most upper extremity movement. These individuals require a power wheelchair with mouth or chin controls and ventilation assistance. Therefore, although people with cervical SCI are classified together as tetraplegic, each person has very different rehabilitation needs based on the specific neurological level. People with paraplegia are typically independent using a manual wheelchair and may even be able to walk with orthotics and assistive devices, depending on the level of the lesion. The full use of upper extremities and some trunk control help these individuals with balance and function.

Regardless of the level of the lesion, recreation and leisure options for this population are plentiful. The typical person with traumatic SCI is male and between 15 and 25 years old. This highly active population typically wants to continue to be active after an injury. Many sports were first adapted for this population. Quad rugby and basketball are very popular. Tennis, sailing, and skiing (water and snow) for the paraplegic athlete are also very popular. The possibilities for rehabilitation and community reentry are enhanced by technology and equipment and often limited only by our imaginations.

Traumatic Brain Injury

Traumatic brain injury (TBI) is defined as an alteration in brain function or other evidence of brain pathology caused by an external force (Menon, Schwab, Wright, & Maas, 2010). Because the brain is responsible for controlling virtually every function of the human body, rehabilitation from TBI requires a comprehensive approach to recovery that is designed to address functional deficits across all domains. Unlike many other conditions being addressed through rehabilitation, TBI typically disrupts interpersonal and social functioning. Patients may be extremely self-centered, display socially inappropriate behaviors, and experience outbursts of anger or other extreme emotional states. Executive functions can also be affected, leaving the patient with difficulties in planning and carrying out self-initiated behaviors. The severity of a TBI can range from mild concussion to coma, but the TBIs relevant to this discussion typically involve a long-term rehabilitation program with significant deficits in all areas of functioning. The relatively advanced areas of functioning mentioned earlier may not even be relevant to treatment until after weeks or months of therapy.

TBI can be the result of a penetrating injury (e.g., gunshot) or a closed head injury (e.g., sporting collision or fall). Motor vehicle accidents or pedestrian versus vehicle accidents are the most common type of head injury overall, whereas falls are more common in the elderly and the very young. Closed head injuries can involve an impact from an external force or an internal shifting of the brain (a common example is a shaken baby). A blunt head trauma can not only cause brain injury at the site of the injury but also cause the brain to shift within the cranial vault and incur injury to the opposite side of the brain, depending on the force of the impact. This is called a coup–contre-coup injury and is commonly seen in the frontal and temporal poles and the anterior–inferior temporal area. Often, a hemorrhage in the brain causes a mass effect that occupies space within the cranial vault. The brain gets pushed centrally and then downward, often collapsing the lateral ventricle and then pushing down on the brain stem and ultimately the cerebellum (called a herniation syndrome). This pressure on the brain stem initially causes signs and symptoms such as the inability of the pupil to react to light (blown pupil), caused by damage to the oculomotor cranial nerve. Ultimately, pressure on the portion of the brain stem that regulates alertness can lead to coma, which is often associated with a TBI (Blumenfeld, 2010).

In contrast to focal injuries, diffuse axonal injury occurs when there is shearing of the axons as the brain moves over bony prominences within the cranial vault or there is twisting and shearing of axons with a rotational force in acceleration–deceleration injuries. This type of movement causes diffuse damage to the white matter of the axons and cranial nerves but often indicates no immediately detectable injury on a CT scan because there is no blood accumulation. Brain injuries can also occur from extended periods without oxygen (anoxia); extreme temperatures; or toxins, such as methamphetamines. A TBI is differentiated from conditions such as intellectual impairment, cerebral palsy, and Alzheimer's disease because it is neither **degenerative** nor **congenital**.

Because of the diffuse damage and potential for increased cerebellar and brain stem involvement with herniation syndromes, patients with brain injury often have a different clinical presentation than patients who have had a cerebrovascular accident (CVA). After TBI, patients often have cognitive (e.g., altered arousal and attention, memory loss, or poor motor planning), behavioral (e.g., agitation, perseveration, or socially inappropriate behavior), and motor (e.g., quadriparesis, hypertonia, spasticity, or ataxia) impairments. Patients often have secondary impairments, such as contractures, caused by spasticity, posturing, and decreased mobility.

TBIs are typically graded in the acute stage with the **Glasgow Coma Scale**. This scale evaluates patient functions in the areas of eye response,

motor response, and verbal response. The TBI is then classified as mild, moderate, or severe. The levels, often called Rancho levels, are used to assess the cognitive and behavioral status of a person as he or she progresses through TBI recovery (Hagan, Malkmus, & Durham 1979; see table 9.1). Levels I through III describe coma or near-coma states, levels IV through VI are the stages of behavioral confusion, and levels VII and VIII indicate impairment in higher-level processing. Patients often go through the stages in order, although they may move through stages quickly or revert to previous stages (caused by, for example, infection or a change in environment).

Rehabilitation in this population focuses on their cognitive, behavioral, motor, and functional needs. In addition to traumatic neurological injury, patients may experience neurological pathology that is acquired in a one-time vascular insult, such as a CVA, or progressive neurological injury is possible, as with Parkinson's disease or multiple sclerosis.

Cerebrovascular Accidents

Cerebrovascular accident (CVA) is a term used to describe conditions that involve disruption of blood flow to the brain. **Stroke**, the most common form of CVA, typically involves blood clot blockage (ischemia) or bleeding (hemorrhage) within the brain. The former cause is more commonly associated with heart disease or high cholesterol, whereas the latter is related to high **blood pressure** and the structural integrity of arteries and veins (Sherrill, 2004). Strokes typically occur as either a left-brain or right-brain stroke, with symptoms manifesting on the opposite side of the body.

Possible Consequences of Stroke—Right Brain

- Weak or paralyzed left side
- Impaired sensation on the right side
- Literal thinking style
- Lack of insight and denial of disabilities
- Distractible and inattentive
- Impaired judgment and memory
- Left-side neglect
- Quick and impulsive behavioral style
- Dysarthria—oral muscle weakness leading to difficulty in articulating speech

Possible Consequences of Stroke—Left Brain

- Weak or paralyzed right side
- Impaired sensation on the right side

- Slow and cautious behavioral style
- Broca's aphasia—impaired language structure and ability to produce speech but normal comprehension
- Wernicke's aphasia—impaired comprehension and nonsensical language production
- Dysarthria—oral muscle weakness leading to difficulty in understanding speech

Immediate provision of treatment is key to the potential extent of recovery from a stroke. For an ischemic stroke, use of tissue plasminogen activator within 6 hours of the stroke significantly increases the odds of being alive and independent at final follow-up, particularly in patients treated within 3 hours (Wardlaw et al., 2012). Most significant gains in function from neurological recovery come within the first 6 months of rehabilitation, but with intensity and repetition of practice, patients can induce brain neuroplasticity and continue to gain function for years after the stroke occurred (Nudo, 2011).

Hemiplegia, a common consequence of stroke, involves loss of sensation or movement on one side of the body. Stroke patients in rehabilitation typically face impairments related to **ambulation**, upper limb functions, and speech. Speech impairments can be associated with aphasia (left-brain CVAs) or dysarthria (left- or right-brain CVAs). **Aphasia** involves disruption of speech patterns, whereas **dysarthria** involves impaired speech motor functions (Auxter, Pyfer, & Huettig, 2005).

Aneurism, another form of CVA, involves the bursting of a blood vessel within the brain. Aneurisms are much more likely to be fatal than strokes, but when patients survive, the challenges are analogous to those associated with stroke. A subtler but equally threatening condition is the occurrence of multiple infarctions happening over an extended period. This condition results in gradual loss of function. This gradual process

Table 9.1 Glasgow Coma Scale Levels of Cognitive Functioning and Associated Response to Stimuli

Cognitive level	Level description	Response to stimuli
Level I	No response	No response.
Level II	Generalized response	Physiological response (change in heart rate, blood pressure, respiratory rate); nonpurposeful movement (general writhing).
Level III	Localized response	More specific but inconsistent response to stimuli (may push away stimuli); begins to follow simple commands.
Level IV	Confused, agitated	This is a heightened state of activity in which patients may not be able to process multiple points of stimulation, causing them to react against the person providing the stimulus. Verbalizations are frequently incoherent or inappropriate.
Level V	Confused, inappropriate	Patients can respond to some simple commands and attend to tasks for brief periods of time within a structured environment. They may begin to be oriented and follow brief conversations. Memory and new learning are still impaired.
Level VI	Confused, appropriate	Patients can follow through with simple commands and be more goal directed in their activity with external direction. Memory and new learning are still impaired but improving.
Level VII	Automatic, appropriate	Patients are oriented and can follow commands. They can complete a daily routine automatically but will have decreased ability to problem solve in new situations or if external structure is removed.
Level VIII	Purposeful, appropriate	Patients can recall and integrate past and recent events and are aware of and responsive to the environment. They show carryover of new learning and do not need external direction to complete tasks. Some executive functions may still be impaired.

EXEMPLARY PROFESSIONAL

LINDA OHNOUTKA, CTRS

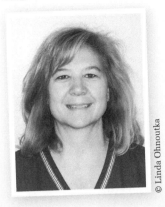

Education: BS in Therapeutic Recreation, University of Nebraska at Lincoln
Position: Recreation Therapist
Organization: Madonna Rehabilitation Hospitals, Lincoln, Nebraska
Special Awards:

- Madonna Angel Wings
- Georgann Claussen Memorial Award

My Career

My student internship was at Madonna Rehabilitation Hospitals in Lincoln, and I was able to get a recreation therapy position in 1987 after completion of the internship. Madonna Rehabilitation Hospitals provides world-class rehabilitation and physical medicine services to children and adults throughout the United States. As a specialty hospital system, Madonna's clinical expertise, innovative technologies, and cutting-edge research empower us to help people facing the most complex conditions—including brain injury, stroke, spinal cord injury, and pulmonary conditions—reach their fullest potential. We rehabilitate those who have sustained injuries or disabling conditions so they can fully participate in life, we lead research to improve outcomes, and we promote wellness through community programs.

My position as a recreation therapist at Madonna Rehabilitation Hospitals involves application of the therapeutic recreation process. I complete assessments; plan and lead individual treatment sessions and groups; and provide leisure skills training, education, and community training individually and in a group setting. I also supervise volunteers, serve as program leader for the adaptive sports and recreation program, and coordinate the student internship program. There are four certified therapeutic recreation therapists on staff who work in one or more of the following programs: acute rehabilitation, specialty hospital, extended care, skilled care, outpatient rehab, and adaptive sports. Patients and residents may participate in individual treatment sessions, leisure education, group activities, community reintegration, or any combination of these services.

I like working with clients of all age groups and teaching them ways to return to recreation when they didn't think it was possible, and using leisure activities to enhance their rehabilitation. In addition, I enjoy supervising students and watching their skills continue to develop throughout their internship. I wish the inpatients' length of stay were longer in order to have more time to work with them, but I am glad that our organization's continuum of care provides the opportunity for recreation therapy throughout the continuum. The continuum ensures maximum exposure to clients and allows us to continue to support them as they move forward with their lives.

My Advice to You

Be flexible to meet the needs of your clients and adaptable to the ongoing changes in health care. Seek out opportunities to collaborate with those from other disciplines and team with other community resources to help clients achieve their highest level of functioning in leisure activities and sports.

---

often leads to a failure to notice early symptoms. Long-term consequences include a condition referred to as **multi-infarct dementia**, which causes **dementia** because of multiple ministrokes. A similar condition is **transient ischemic attack (TIA)**, which also involves ministrokes. The differentiating factor is that TIA typically involves full recovery after several hours of impairment. TIAs can be a warning sign of impending major strokes. Stroke rehabilitation is most effective when provided by an interprofessional team (Winstein et al., 2016).

Parkinson's Disease

The loss of the neurotransmitter dopamine from the substantia nigra pars compacta of the basal ganglia causes a loss of the normal influence the basal ganglia has on voluntary movement. By 70 years of age, there is a 50 percent loss of neurons in the substantia nigra that produce dopamine (Lew & Yeung, 2014). This loss occurs in normally aging individuals and does not cause any appreciable changes in movement. Therefore, the symptoms of **Parkinson's disease (PD)** often are not observed until a significant amount (~80 percent) of these dopamine-producing cells are lost. The most common impairments associated with PD are resting tremor and a loss in the rate of force production (Morris, Morris, & Lansek, 2001). Therefore, although the patient has the potential for a full muscle contraction and normal strength, the muscle contraction cannot be accessed rapidly enough for normal function. People with PD therefore have bradykinetic (slow) and hypometric (small amplitude) movements, which result in postural and gait disturbances (Blumenfeld, 2010). Gait disturbances include a shuffling gait with slow and hypometric stepping; a festinating gait, in which the patients lean forward to start the gait cycle and then chase their center of mass, which is constantly in front of them (often, until they fall); and an akinetic gait (also known as freezing), in which the client has difficulty initiating gait, which is most typical when crossing thresholds, turning, or walking in narrow spaces. People with PD are often classified using the modified Hoehn and Yahr Scale (Goetz et al., 2004):

- Stage 0 = no signs of the disease
- Stage 1 = unilateral appendicular disease
- Stage 1.5 = unilateral plus axial involvement
- Stage 2 = bilateral disease with axial involvement
- Stage 2.5 = mild bilateral disease with recovery on the pull test
- Stage 3 = mild to moderate bilateral disease; some postural instability; physically independent
- Stage 4 = severe disability; may still be able to walk or stand unassisted
- Stage 5 = wheelchair bound or bedridden unless assisted

Maintaining strength, range of motion, and flexibility is important for continued functional independence. Large amplitude movements may be used to counteract the tendency for bradykinetic and hypokinetic movement (Farley & Koshland, 2005). Progressive aerobic high-intensity exercise can improve function while also modifying brain excitability for a neuroprotective effect (Fisher et al., 2008). Functional activity interventions in people with PD focus on techniques to improve momentum and timing of movement. Visual and auditory cues may be used for people with freezing gait disorders to augment initiation of gait (Frazzitta, Maestri, Uccellini, Bertotti, & Abelli, 2009).

Multiple Sclerosis

Multiple sclerosis (MS) is a **demyelinating disease** of the central nervous system. In 1868, Dr. Jean Charcot identified many areas of hardened plaques in the brains of individuals with this disorder, hence, the term multiple sclerosis. The cause of MS is unknown, but one of the most common theories is an immune-mediated pathogenesis causing antibodies to attack myelin sheaths. An environmental infectious agent and heredity (linked to the human leucocyte antigen [HLA] system) are also considered possible causes. There is a geographic incidence for MS that supports an environmental cause. There are higher-frequency prevalence rates in areas lying between 45 and 65 degrees north or south of the equator. If you move regions prior to the age of 15, you assume the risk of the new region (Detels et al., 1978). There is also a history of epidemic outbreaks in the Faroe Islands and Iceland (Kurtzke, Gundmunsson, & Bergmann, 1982). In addition, increased immunoglobulin and oligoclonal bands in the cerebrospinal fluid of 65 to 95 percent of MS clients point to a viral infection or antigen. The diagnosis of MS is made based on neurological exams, with evidence of damage to at least two separate areas of the central nervous system over two distinct points in time (Polman et al., 2011). As the disease progresses, MRI detects the plaques in the central nervous system, which serve as a biological marker of the severity of the disease (Rovira & Leon, 2008).

There are several clinical courses for MS, including relapsing–remitting, primary progressive, secondary progressive, and progressive relapsing. The relapsing forms of MS have clearly defined episodes of acute worsening followed by periods of improved function. The progressive forms of MS are nearly continuously worsening because of a more extensive inflammatory process that is not interrupted by a distinct relapse. The progressive forms of MS are as responsive to anti-inflammatory and immunomodulatory treatments as relapsing–remitting MS (Lassmann, van Horssen, & Mahad, 2012). Common impairments related to MS include weakness, spasticity, tremors, bowel and bladder loss of control, and visual disturbances (loss of optic nerve myelin). Fatigue and intolerance to heat that raises the core body temperature are common symptoms that can worsen impairments and function. The Kurtzke Expanded Disability Status Scale (EDSS; Kurtzke, 1983) is commonly used to classify patients according to their level of functional limitation:

- 0 = Normal neurological status
- 1-2 = Minimal objective abnormality
- 3-4 = Mild disorder, not sufficient to impede normal activities, full ambulation
- 5-6 = Ambulatory, not ordinarily house-bound, some impairment in daily activities
  - 5 = 656 feet (200 m) without aid or rest
  - 6 = cane or crutch needed for 328 feet (100 m)
- 7-9 = Severe disability, almost always in a wheelchair or bed
  - 7 = Unable to walk past 16 feet (5 m) even with aid
  - 8 = Bed patients who may be in chair or wheelchair for much of the day and retain many self-care functions
  - 9 = Helpless bed patients who can communicate and eat but not perform self-care activities
- 10 = Death due to MS

Although rehabilitation often does not improve impairments, functional activity and participation level can improve abilities (Kahn, Turner-Stokes, Ng, Kilpatrick, & Amatya, 2007). People with MS must conserve their energy and maximize their abilities (Matsuka, Mathiowetz, & Finlayson, 2007). Although they may be ambulatory with or without assistive devices or orthotics, these people may use scooters for community mobility to decrease the potential of exacerbation from fatigue. They may need to schedule activities in the early morning to maximize energy and avoid later afternoon heat. Air-conditioning, fans, and cooling vests (Nilsagard, Denison, & Gunnarsson, 2006) can assist these people in maintaining a lower core body temperature as well.

Other Notable Conditions

Cardiovascular and **pulmonary** impairments may also be observed in rehabilitation settings, and many hospitals provide specialized pulmonary or cardiac rehabilitation programs. Some rehabilitation centers have specialized programs for **thermal injuries** and treatment of open wounds, such as **decubitus ulcers** (also known as pressure sores), whereas other centers address those conditions as part of their general services. Finally, many people with cancer participate in rehabili-

tation services following surgeries associated with their treatment.

Common Therapeutic Recreation Modalities in Rehabilitation

Chapter 5 presented several of the more commonly used modalities in therapeutic recreation. This chapter points out modalities commonly used as part of rehabilitation and reintegration of persons with injuries or illnesses of a physical nature. Again, a physical cause does not ensure that impairments will be limited to the physical realm.

Functional Interventions: Recreation as Therapy

Functional intervention is typically the entry point of services for people in rehabilitation programs. Recovering functional skills is the primary concern. Other therapeutic recreation services (e.g., leisure education, community reintegration, and wellness programs) are provided simultaneously or after functional skills improve. Essentially, functional intervention involves using recreation and leisure as tools for therapy (recall the definition of therapeutic recreation in chapter 1, which specified that recreation skills could be used as a means of enhancing functioning). To illustrate this potential application, the following sections discuss how therapeutic recreation can be applied toward the improvement of cognitive, physical, and socioemotional functions.

Cognitive Rehabilitation

Cognitive rehabilitation services refer to a comprehensive therapy effort implemented by a team of professionals to restore cognitive functions in persons with TBI, stroke, or other conditions that cause deficits in cognitive functions. Therapeutic recreation specialists contribute to this effort by planning and implementing games, activities, and other cognitive tasks that exercise areas of cognitive functioning identified in the treatment plan. The therapeutic recreation specialist can present daily recreation and leisure tasks that require people to use their memory, recognize shapes and colors, place items in order, develop strategies, and perform other increasingly complex tasks.

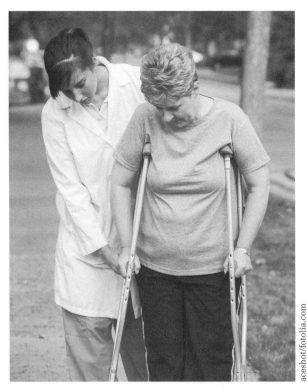

Ambulation is one of the areas of physical function that might be addressed by a therapeutic recreation specialist.

Physical Rehabilitation

The method used to address the physical deficits experienced by people is similar to the approach taken with cognitive deficits. Therapeutic recreation specialists plan and implement activities that correspond with physical deficits identified through assessment procedures. As such, the process is individualized. To illustrate how this process works, this section will discuss several physical areas of functioning, including ambulation, sensory–motor functions, strength, and endurance.

The application of the therapeutic recreation process to address ambulation is illustrated by a program that encouraged patients recovering from stroke to maintain a walking pace that corresponded with the tempo and beat of a standardized piece of music. This process was intended to encourage program adherence and maintain maximal effort. The program was a collaborative effort between music therapists and therapeutic recreation specialists working in the rehabilitation department of St. Francis Hospital in Topeka, Kansas. Sensory–motor functions are a common area of intervention and frequently involve games or puzzles that require the manipulation of objects

in space. Card games, board games, stacking games, and tossing games are all examples that require coordination of senses and motor skills (both fine and gross).

Strength and endurance are areas of significant concern for persons who have had a stroke. Many activities have been created to work on strength, endurance, and range of motion in affected limbs. One of the most simplistic but also motivating activities involves the use of clothespins and a yardstick (graduated measuring stick). The yardstick is attached to a table in a vertical position. The patient is asked to place clothespins on the yardstick, starting at the bottom and working upward. This simple activity provides immediate feedback because the number and height of the clothespins are easily determined, allowing the patient and therapeutic recreation specialist to monitor progress from day to day in a concrete way. Variations can include stacking games or the use of Velcro balls or objects instead of clothespins.

Socioemotional Considerations

As mentioned earlier, this domain is probably most relevant to those with TBI, but other conditions can also affect social skills and emotional states. For example, both stroke and multiple sclerosis can affect emotional functions. Understanding that physical impairment may cause these deficits is important in determining appropriate interventions and expectations. Likewise, therapy sessions should be planned at an appropriate social or emotional level, allowing room for improvement without overwhelming the patient with unreasonable demands. Loved ones should be educated about the nature of such social behaviors and emotional states. For many families, the loved one seems like a completely different person. As such, the effect of injury has social and emotional implications for the patient's entire family system.

Other Modalities

The modalities described in this section may also fall under the recreation-as-therapy realm, but they are mentioned separately because of their distinct purpose or function. In addition, some of these modalities, pet therapy for example, might be used in settings outside the rehabilitation setting. Because the editors of this text have attempted to avoid redundant listings of each modality in every chapter, you are encouraged to consider how each modality might be applied to other populations or situations.

Sensory Stimulation

Sensory stimulation is a technique used with people who have severe brain injury and demonstrate limited responsiveness to stimuli. Sensory stimulation is designed to engage clients who are in unconscious (coma) or subconscious states, thereby reducing the depth and length of unconsciousness (Austin, 2004). This technique can be implemented in a multimodal or unimodal fashion (Austin, 2004). Multimodal sensory stimulation involves engaging all senses during each treatment session, and unimodal sensory stimulation focuses on a single sense during each session. For both techniques, stimulation is usually applied at the lowest level that is still capable of eliciting a response (eye responses, muscle contractions).

Pain Management and Relaxation Techniques

Pain management and relaxation strategies can be useful for clients who are dealing with severe and persistent pain. Training clients to use **biofeedback**, **meditation**, **progressive relaxation**, and other pain management techniques can be a significant part of therapeutic recreation programming and can have important implications for the client's ability to control pain in the long run. Clients who may find such programs particularly beneficial include those with thermal injuries (burns); **chronic** conditions, such as RA or fibromyalgia; and **terminal** conditions, such as acquired immune deficiency syndrome (AIDS) and some forms of cancer. Massage may also be used to manage muscle pain and **spasticity**, but therapeutic recreation specialists should ensure that those providing such services are appropriately qualified. In addition, massage can be harmful for people with soft tissue injuries or recent thermal injuries.

Aquatic Therapy

Certified aquatic therapists or physical therapists typically implement aquatic therapy, but therapeutic recreation specialists can also gain certain water certifications or help facilitate such sessions. For example, the Arthritis Association offers certification programs for therapeutic aquatics instructors. These programs are often offered in community-based settings but are specifically designed for people who have conditions of **rheumatism**, or arthritis. Such people may also use aquatic-based programs for fitness and exercise because exercising in the pool reduces impact on joints and muscles. Therapy pools, that is, pools with temperatures typically ranging from 88 to 92 degrees Fahrenheit (31.1 to 33.3 degrees Celsius), can be used to reduce spasticity, increase flexibility, and encourage blood flow to injured areas. In addition, specialized strategies, such as the **Halliwick method**, have been developed for teaching people with significant disabilities to swim.

Animal-Assisted Therapy

Animal-assisted therapy, or pet therapy, is commonly used in rehabilitation, especially in facilities that involve extensive stays. True therapy animals are certified through organizations such as Pet Partners (https://petpartners.org) or Therapy Dogs International (tdi-dog.org) and have gone through an extensive process to ensure that their temperament is appropriate for the therapy environment. Because certified therapy animals require extensive time and care, they are typically brought in by outside persons who volunteer their time and services to the rehabilitation centers. Some facilities, however, have in-house animals that the therapeutic recreation staff might care for. These animals may include birds, fish, or rabbits. In some cases, uncertified dogs and cats may be present (this is more likely to be the case in long-term-care facilities). Certified service animals can be used in various ways: as motivators to encourage people with disabilities to engage in what would otherwise be unattractive or discomforting therapy activities, as a form of sensory stimulation for people with severe brain injuries, and as calming agents for patients who are experiencing substantial discomfort or anxiety. They may also be used to improve the quality of life of patients by simply being there.

Another area of animal-assisted therapy involves the use of horses. Two primary types of horse-based therapies exist. The one most likely to be tied to orthopedic or neurological conditions is **hippotherapy**. This approach uses the movement of a walking horse to relieve muscle contractures; build trunk stability; and increase strength, flexibility, and range of motion. Only certified hippotherapists should provide services, but therapeutic recreation specialists can be instrumental in arranging for and supporting such a program. The second type of horse-based therapy

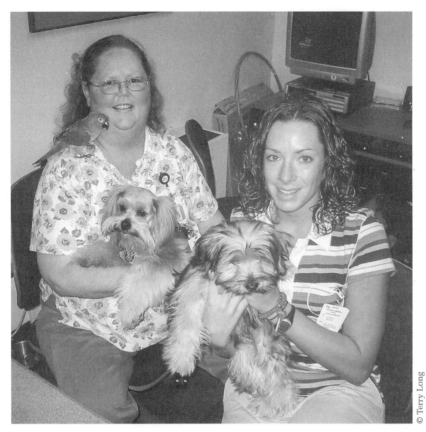

Therapeutic recreation specialists at Truman Medical Center Behavioral Health, in Lees Summit, Missouri, include pet therapy as part of their therapeutic recreation program.

is **therapeutic riding**. These programs are less directly related to physical rehabilitation but do provide an avenue for community reentry as well as cognitive and socioemotional functions. Therapeutic riding involves more than just riding the horse. The process includes caring for, grooming, and saddling the horse and forming a relationship with the horse that involves both responsibility and trust. Therapeutic riding can be used in a variety of therapeutic recreation realms, including mental health, youth development, programs for people with developmental disabilities, and aging populations. The same can be said for pet therapy in general. Such programs exist in virtually every type of therapeutic recreation setting.

Horticulture

Horticulture therapy uses plant life as a means of therapy. This technique uses the tasks associated with horticulture and metaphors related to the experience of caring for plant life. Horticulture therapy is used in a variety of therapeutic settings but is specifically relevant to physical rehabilitation for several reasons. First, planting and caring for plant life provide an opportunity for exercising a variety of cognitive, motor, and sensory–motor functions. Strength, endurance, kinesthetic awareness, hand–eye coordination, and controlled motor movements are all potential areas of functional intervention that horticulture therapy can address. Horticulture therapy can even engage social competencies through mechanisms such as the development of a community garden. Second, horticulture provides purposeful and satisfying leisure activities that can help patients cope with the psychological challenges of rehabilitation and use cognitive functions, such as memory and planning, and executive functions. Third, this modality provides the potential to develop a leisure skill that will continue after the patient returns home. Finally, horticulture therapy requires relatively limited resources and space, which are often considerations for therapeutic recreation programs.

Community Reintegration

Community reintegration programs, sometimes called community reentry, are designed to assist patients with the adjustments associated with returning home. The goal is for patients to be able to participate in activities of daily living and continue with a satisfying and healthy lifestyle. As such, therapeutic recreation specialists work with patients to identify barriers to reentry, master skills necessary for home life and community involvement, and develop strategies for involvement in recreation and leisure activities at home and in the community. In many cases, services will include field trips into the community and home visits intended to assess and address real-world functioning.

Leisure Education

Leisure education, as conceptualized in the leisure ability model (Stumbo & Peterson, 2004), addresses issues related to leisure awareness, leisure resources, social skills, and activity skills. Any of these four content areas might be relevant in the rehabilitation environment, depending on the nature of the patient's impairments. Patients with TBI are likely to experience social deficits and challenges with cognitively processing information related to leisure decisions. People who have life-changing conditions, such as SCIs, heart disease, or limb amputations, may not recognize the importance of recreation and fitness in maintaining health. Furthermore, they may be unaware of the resources available for becoming involved in such activity. These examples illustrate the importance of leisure education in making a successful transition to living with a disability. Therapeutic recreation specialists must be familiar with the content and process of delivering leisure education services to patients.

Exercise and Fitness

One potential modality that can be part of rehabilitation and is directly tied to leisure education is an exercise and fitness program. Because the dangers of sedentary living are even greater for those with a disability than for those without one, people with physical injuries can gain particular benefit from living an active lifestyle. Patients should be informed of proper exercising techniques and activity precautions associated with their particular condition. For example, high-impact activities can exacerbate symptoms of arthritis, and therapy

pool (warm-water) activities could make symptoms worse for a person with multiple sclerosis.

Some conditions require significant **precautions** during exercise. For example, SCI can affect both **maximum heart rate** and advisable levels of training intensity. The maximum heart rate for people with injuries above T7 (tetraplegia) is less than 130 and typically between 110 and 130 (Durstine, Moore, Painter, & Roberts, 2009; Swann-Guerrero & Mackey, 2008). Furthermore, training intensity should be between 50 and 70 percent of maximum heart rate. Injuries at T7 or below typically involve a regular maximum heart rate, but it is wise to consult a physician before beginning an exercise program.

Autonomic dysreflexia (AD) is a condition of extreme hypertension that is caused by an exaggerated autonomic nervous system response to a noxious stimulus. AD is experienced by 60 to 80 percent of people with an SCI of T6 or higher; it can be life threatening and requires immediate medical attention. To prevent AD, the bladder should be emptied before exercise. Other precautions include checking for regularity of bowel movements, periodically checking blood pressure, and checking for skin trauma during transfers.

Orthostatic hypotension is a decrease, or drop, in blood pressure because of the pooling of blood in the lower extremities and abdominal area. Paralysis of leg muscles compromises the body's ability to return blood to the heart. Precautions to avoid sudden drops in blood pressure include discouraging quick movements, providing sufficient time for people to move from supine to upright positions, and encouraging hydration. Having people use compression stockings and an abdominal binder can also help prevent orthostatic hypotension. These risks can be exacerbated during exercise, so it is important to monitor blood pressure.

Impaired **thermoregulation**, or regulation of body temperature, is a common difficulty experienced by people with SCIs. Overheating during exercise is much more likely to occur in someone who cannot regulate body temperature. Precautions include monitoring external temperature, providing fans and water in warm environments, and wearing appropriate clothing in cold and warm environments.

People recovering from strokes require special considerations before and during exercise. A medical examination by a physician is highly recommended to ensure that the heart is capable of exertion. The physician should approve the client's exercise program before it is implemented. **Hypertension** (high blood pressure) is a major risk factor for stroke and an important consideration when working with those who have had strokes in the past. Blood pressure should be monitored periodically throughout exercise. If blood pressure is above 200/110 mmHg, the client should stop exercising.

CLIENT PORTRAIT: EZRA

Ezra is a 17-year-old high school junior who wrecked his motorcycle into a telephone pole while street racing with a group of other riders. He received a partial SCI at the C5 vertebra, resulting in complete loss of sensation and movement in his legs and partial loss of movement in his arms. His doctors informed him that he would not regain function in his legs and would need to use a wheelchair for the rest of his life.

Ezra's Rehabilitation

A rehabilitation team, including a CTRS, began working with Ezra within days of his admission into rehabilitation. Following an assessment of Ezra's functional abilities and leisure needs and interests, the CTRS and Ezra established therapeutic recreation goals and objectives. Immediate goals focused on maximizing range of motion, strength, and endurance in Ezra's upper body and assisting the rehabilitation team in teaching Ezra about prevention of secondary health conditions, using his wheelchair, and living with an SCI. To address these goals, the CTRS encouraged Ezra to participate in a variety of activities and games that encouraged him to push his limits in the goal areas. These sessions involved activities such as gardening, cooking and nutrition, card and board games, painting and sculpture, air hockey, playing fetch with the therapy dog, aerobic and anaerobic exercise, swimming, and a variety of customized games and activities designed to work on the targeted goal areas. Many of these activities were practiced as part of a recreation/physical/occupational therapy group for clients with SCI. The physical therapist (PT) focused on mobility and gross motor functional independence, the occupational therapist (OT) focused on fine motor activities and cognitive–perceptual skills, and the CTRS focused on integrating the recreational activities as a part of the therapy. For example, in art-related activities, the PT worked on unsupported sitting balance, the OT worked on fine motor control using tools and brushes, and the CTRS worked with the clients to determine the type of art that was most meaningful for them. In bocce ball, the PT worked on mobility over uneven surfaces, the OT worked on grasping the ball and perceptual skills toward the target, and the CTRS worked on social interaction and rules for game play.

Ezra's Reintegration

Once Ezra had begun to make some of these life adjustments, the CTRS suggested that they broaden Ezra's therapy goals to include leisure education and community reintegration. At this point, Ezra began participating in a leisure education program that included leisure awareness and activity skill development. Content focused on ensuring Ezra was aware of the benefits of maintaining his previously active and satisfying leisure lifestyle and identifying barriers and resources associated with this goal. Ezra also learned about adapted sports opportunities and available equipment that could be used by a person at his ability level. As Ezra's health, knowledge, and independence increased, a plan for community reentry was developed. Ezra was fortunate that he had regained enough strength, mobility, and trunk control during his rehabilitation that he did not require an electric wheelchair. Still, he openly questioned how he could ever have a satisfying life with his injury.

Before his discharge from the rehabilitation center, the CTRS and the PT collaborated to develop a weight-training program for Ezra that could be conducted at home and at the local fitness center. The CTRS accompanied Ezra to the center on several occasions until Ezra was ready to go on his own. He also accompanied Ezra on a visit to a local Paralympic sports competition, where Ezra met several wheelchair basketball players. Finally, the rehabilitation center sponsored an adapted sport and activity clinic that introduced Ezra to several activities, including golf, rugby, scuba diving, hunting, and even dancing. After his discharge, Ezra continued to participate in sports and recreation events sponsored by the rehabilitation center as well as other organizations in the community. He was also able to return to school for his senior year, graduate with his friends, and dance with his girlfriend at senior prom.

Of course, exercise programs with a person who has a physical injury, illness, or disabling condition should always involve detailed examination of necessary risks and precautions, possible adaptations, and potential benefits. The above examples illustrate the importance of closely considering such factors when working with clients.

Community-Based Services

To this point, the described modalities have been at least partially grounded in what can be described as clinical settings. As the title of this chapter implies, the needs of people with extensive injury or permanent disability rarely end with the conclusion of an inpatient rehabilitation program. Thus, community-based services can be an inherent aspect of making the transition from the rehabilitation setting to a maximal level of independence and quality of life. The diversity noted within each disability category described earlier is even more present in community-based programs, where adapted and inclusive recreation services are provided to a broad array of participants. The task of finding the best way to engage each participant requires that therapeutic recreation specialists be competent in applying the therapeutic recreation process to a variety of participant circumstances. The general concept of community programming is not itself a specific modality, but this element is discussed here because of the importance of ensuring that the opportunity for therapeutic recreation services continues beyond formal rehabilitation services.

Best Practices

Typically, those who work with people with physically disabling injuries or illnesses will serve as part of an interprofessional treatment team. The therapeutic recreation specialist can be a critical part of this team. Team members must understand the nature of each other's work and collaborate to maximize patient benefits. As part of this team, the therapeutic recreation specialist must follow standardized procedures associated with the therapeutic recreation process.

In addition, this process must occur within the context of a larger system. Many rehabilitation facilities follow **clinical pathways**, which map out the role of each department within an agency in providing care to a particular client. Within these pathways are **treatment protocols**. These protocols outline the standard practices and procedures for care within each department. As such, treatment protocols for providing therapeutic recreation services are likely to exist within a particular rehabilitation hospital. Protocols should be developed based on evidence-based practice yet be flexible enough to consider patient preferences.

Following such structure serves multiple purposes. First, it provides a mechanism for ensuring quality care of the client. The therapeutic recreation specialist has an ethical obligation to provide quality care regardless of whether internal and external agencies are monitoring performance. This process of purposeful intervention is also necessary to maintain accreditation with the Commission on Accreditation of Rehabilitation Facilities (CARF) and the Joint Commission on Accreditation of Healthcare Organizations (JCAHO). These procedures also allow for fiscal accountability by maximizing treatment effectiveness and efficient operations.

Summary

This chapter has focused on the nature of orthopedic and neurological conditions that require rehabilitation services as well as therapeutic recreation modalities that can be implemented within the context of a rehabilitation program. These commonly observed conditions are only a sample of what the therapeutic recreation specialist may encounter. On any given day, a therapeutic recreation specialist might be exposed to a patient who broke a hip in a fall, received a TBI from a motorcycle wreck, has brain damage from oxygen deprivation, or has a condition that the specialist has never seen before. Regardless of what physical injury or illness is occurring, the responsibility of the therapeutic recreation specialist is to determine how to address cognitive, physical, or socioemotional deficits that might manifest. This task may sound intimidating, but adhering to the therapeutic recreation process and the associated standards of practice can guide the adequately trained therapeutic recreation specialist through this challenge.

DISCUSSION QUESTIONS

1. Differentiate between a neurological injury and an orthopedic injury. What commonalities and differences do you see between these two diagnostic areas?

2. Discuss the role of the therapeutic recreation specialist as the client moves through the recovery process. Do you think this role would change as the client progresses? How is this concept reflected in the therapeutic recreation models presented in chapter 5?

3. Can you think of other modalities that could be integrated into the therapeutic recreation process for any of the described conditions? State your case about why you believe that this particular modality would be useful for the chosen condition (client group).

4. Why is the use of standardized procedures outlined in protocols or critical pathways important? Do you see any drawbacks to using such a system?

5. Of the described modalities, which modality do you currently feel most comfortable with, and which modalities are most intimidating? What steps can you take to ensure that you are professionally capable of using these modalities? Do you think that any of these modalities have the potential to harm a client if used inappropriately?

10

Youth Development and Therapeutic Recreation

Sydney L. Sklar | Cari E. Autry

LEARNING OUTCOMES

At the end of this chapter, students will be able to

- describe and apply the concept of positive youth development,
- identify and describe the purpose of therapeutic recreation in positive youth development,
- identify challenges to positive youth development,
- describe the stages of the continuum of risk in youth development,
- identify and describe specific needs of youth clientele with various backgrounds,
- understand and describe influences of the environment on youth development,
- identify and describe theories related to youth development and therapeutic recreation practice,
- describe the scope of therapeutic recreation youth development services, and
- identify and describe various settings, opportunities, and modalities used for therapeutic recreation and youth development programming.

Since the earliest days of organized recreation, community programs have aimed to develop healthier youth and address social issues that challenge the positive development of young people. Indeed, the well-being of our society depends on the ability of communities to prepare well-adjusted, responsible, well-educated young people to step forward as the older generation passes. Because many of today's youth face serious challenges in their social adjustment, therapeutic recreation has had much to offer in supporting positive youth development.

In the United States, the Individuals with Disabilities Education Act (IDEA) of 2004 and the subsequent 2015 reauthorization represent significant efforts in the education system to provide adequate support and services to help young people with challenges achieve their fullest potential. Among these efforts is the increased attention given to transition services, a planning and support mechanism for helping students successfully make the transition to the community after graduation. Therapeutic recreation practitioners have played important roles in supporting such students given that IDEA includes the provision of recreation as a related service in special education.

Within both education and recreation contexts, there has been an increase in prevention- and intervention-oriented programs that have engaged youth interests and energies in prosocial activities geared toward positive development. Therapeutic recreation has played a special role in addressing concerns surrounding youth who present the most challenging behaviors.

The purpose of this chapter is to describe how therapeutic recreation principles and practices are employed to meet the developmental needs of contemporary youth. To achieve this purpose, we will (1) present terms and definitions related to youth development; (2) present theoretical frameworks to guide professional practice; (3) discuss the purpose of therapeutic recreation practice as it relates to both prevention and intervention; (4) outline the scope of therapeutic recreation practice in youth development services; and (5) describe a sample of settings, opportunities, and modalities for providing therapeutic recreation youth development programs. Additionally, we will discuss emerging issues and trends in the recreation field pertaining to youth development services.

Positive Youth Development

A philosophy that focuses on youth potential provides an optimistic context for providing therapeutic recreation services and reflects current trends in strengths-based therapeutic recreation practice (Sklar & Carter, 2016). The concept of *positive youth development* has emerged from a growing body of research concerned with the promise of youth potential. **Positive youth development** refers to a service approach that focuses on children's unique talents, strengths, interests, and potential (Damon, 2004). Partly in reaction to media and social distortions of youth, this approach to youth development connotes a more affirming and welcoming vision of young people, viewing them as resources rather than as problems for society. "The positive youth development perspective emphasizes the manifest potentialities rather than the supposed incapacities of young people—including those from the most disadvantaged backgrounds and those with the most troubled histories" (Damon, 2004, p. 15).

The approach recognizes the existence of hardships and developmental challenges that affect children in various ways but resists conceptualizing the developmental process as an effort to overcome deficits. Rather, it begins with "a vision of a fully able child eager to explore the world, gain competence, and acquire the capacity to contribute importantly to the world" (Damon, 2004, p. 15). This philosophy of practice aims to understand, educate, and engage children in productive activities rather than correct, cure, or treat them for maladaptive tendencies. The therapeutic recreation process, armed with both historic and recent developments in strengths-based practice, is uniquely situated to deliver positive youth development programs.

One model emphasizing youth potential has significantly influenced the youth-serving disciplines. The developmental assets framework (Search Institute, 2018b) provides a powerful alternative to deficit-based models for guiding youth work. According to research findings of the Search Institute, there are 40 assets (20 internal and 20 external) deemed necessary for youth to successfully navigate the journey to adulthood. Studies by the Search Institute suggest there is a relationship between the number of assets present in a young person's life and the existence of positive attitudes and behaviors. For example, the more assets a young girl has in her life, the more likely she is to exhibit thriving behaviors, such as exhibiting leadership and succeeding in school. The same girl would be less likely to exhibit negative behaviors, such as problem alcohol use and risky sexual activity (Witt & Caldwell, 2005), than her peers with a fewer number of assets.

The 40 developmental assets from the Search Institute are divided into the following categories.

- Support
- Empowerment
- Boundaries and expectations
- Constructive use of time
- Commitment to learning
- Positive values
- Social competencies
- Positive identity

Positive youth development works best when multiple resources, service providers, and institutions organize around young people. Effective youth programs put youth at the center and involve parents, school personnel, local government officials, social workers, juvenile justice personnel, youth workers, and recreation personnel. In other words, when a range of resources comes together in the interest of youth development, youth stand to reap greater benefits. The 40 developmental assets model offers a framework for therapeutic recreation specialists working with youth.

Challenges to Positive Development

With positive youth development practice as a guiding principle, therapeutic recreation specialists developing youth programs may require a context by which to understand social and environment obstacles to growing up in a well-adjusted manner. Challenges to positive youth development can be explained through a continuum of risk factors youth may face in their environments and relationships (McWhirter, McWhirter, McWhirter, & McWhirter, 2013). An examination of this continuum can help practitioners understand the variability of potential barriers to positive development (see figure 10.1).

Within this model, youth are considered to face relative degrees of challenge depending on where they fall with respect to a variety of risk factors. Youth who face few psychosocial and environmental stressors; experience favorable demographics (such as higher socioeconomic status); and have positive, caring family, school, and social interactions are generally at minimal risk for future trouble. A young person's risk factors rise, however, as stressors compound, environmental conditions degrade, and interactions with support systems become increasingly negative.

Within the next category of remote risk, a young person's demographics are less favorable; social, family, and school interactions are less positive; and more stressors exist. The child at this point in the continuum experiences certain markers of future problems that may include risky activities and behaviors more likely to appear than with a child who faces fewer and less severe risk factors. For example, although being a member of an ethnic minority does not necessarily predict future problems, minority membership is often associated with experiences of marginalization, oppression, racism, and psychosocial stressors that increase the possibility of future problems.

Within the category of high risk, stressors are numerous and compounded to the point where negative attitudes and emotions may be characterized by signs such as aggression, anxiety, conduct problems, mental illness, or hopelessness. Deficits in social skills and coping skills may further emerge from and contribute to the person's environment. Youth who fall within the high-risk category experience a number of personal characteristics that set the stage for gateway activities and behaviors.

Imminent risk implies that youth who are participating in gateway activities (e.g., mildly to moderately distressing activities that are often self-destructive) are generally on the brink of adopting deviant behaviors, such as aggression, toward other children and authority. These behaviors can lead to juvenile delinquency.

Beyond imminent risk, at-risk category activity describes the youth whose activity places him or her solidly at risk for more intense problems and maladaptive behaviors. For example, the child who is regularly truant from school is also at risk of academic failure and may ultimately lack skills

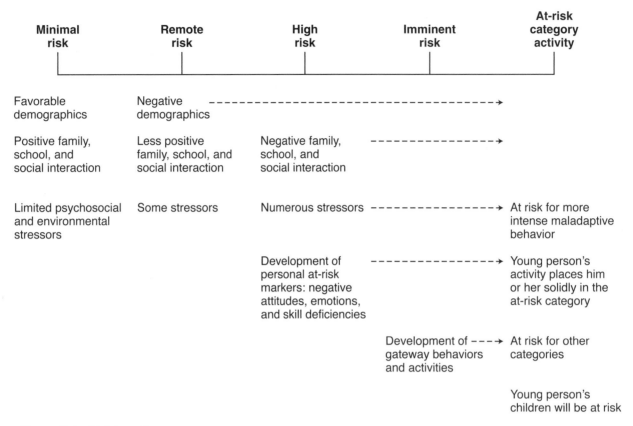

Figure 10.1 At-risk continuum.

for advancing in life. Additionally, the children of those who have reached this extreme will most likely face serious challenges to their positive development.

Internalized and Externalized Maladaptive Behaviors

When working with youth who face challenging circumstances, practitioners should also be aware of externalized and internalized maladaptive behaviors. We are typically more aware of and give more attention to externalized maladaptive behaviors, such as acting out, aggression, and anger. Internalized maladaptive behaviors, such as withdrawal, avoidance of social contact, depression, and anxiety, may pose just as much challenge to a child's development as the more easily observed externalized behaviors (Kentucky Department of Education, 2005).

The social and peer domain is the most significant area affected in the lives of children and youth with externalized and internalized maladaptive behaviors. Concerns associated with such behaviors include a lack of appropriate social behaviors and peer interactions and long-term effects of poor social skills, such as truancy, delinquency, substance abuse, and the inability to be mainstreamed into regular education classes and recreation programs.

Child Maltreatment

Also of concern to therapeutic recreation specialists working with children are those with histories of abuse or neglect. Reports of child maltreatment have risen over the years as the resources of child protective agencies have decreased (Carter & Van Andel, 2011; Jewel, 1999). Therapeutic recreation has much to offer in addressing the needs of maltreated children. Therapeutic recreation specialists may address child abuse and neglect in a variety of settings, including summer camps, schools, psychiatric settings, residential placements away from the family, and within the juvenile justice system.

The scope of therapeutic recreation services for children who have been maltreated includes assessment, education, prevention, and the promotion of well-being (Carter & Van Andel, 2011). Assessment of developmental needs can occur through observation of children in natural play environments. Leisure education can enhance motor and self-concept development and develop skills in relationship building, self-expression, coping, and resource awareness (Carter & Van Andel, 2011). Family education and skills training (e.g., time management and stress management training) may be offered to mitigate the likelihood of future maltreatment. To apply a prevention approach, the specialist should act as a positive role model, helping youth establish trusting relationships with reliable adults (Jewel, 1999).

Learning and Behavioral Disorders

Therapeutic recreation services are frequently used to address childhood problems associated with learning and behavioral disorders. Although these disorders commonly manifest during the developmental years, they may result in significant difficulties in employment or social adjustment during adulthood. Thus, interventions in the developmental years should attempt to minimize

CLIENT PORTRAIT: EDUARDO

Eduardo is a 15-year-old Latino boy who is proud of his Mexican heritage. He lives in a low-income public housing development with his mother and younger brother. Eduardo's mother is single and supports her two children by working as a night auditor at a 24-hour grocery store. Because of her work schedule, his mom is out of the home overnight and sleeps most of the day. Eduardo's father is serving prison time for a drug conviction.

Eduardo's neighborhood consists of multiple blocks of poorly maintained low-rise apartment buildings and a poorly maintained park with outdated playground equipment. Drug deals often take place on street corners. Although Eduardo is not involved in drug activity, he feels pressure from his neighborhood friends to experiment. His free time is unstructured, and he spends most of it out of the home with friends.

Academically, Eduardo is a low performer. His teachers are concerned with his disruptive classroom behavior and poor attendance. During a session with the school social worker, Eduardo said that he thought schoolwork was pointless, he was angry about his father's imprisonment, and he had nothing to do after school. Eduardo was referred to a certified therapeutic recreation specialist (CTRS) working with the local recreation department.

CTRS's Plan

The CTRS conducted an assessment with Eduardo and discovered that he enjoyed sports, being outdoors, working with his hands, and helping others. Additionally, she learned that Eduardo's lack of structured activity was putting him at risk of experimenting with drugs with his neighborhood peers.

The CTRS helped Eduardo enroll in the Latino Teen Corps, which engages members in hands-on service projects within the greater community (e.g., a peer mentoring program in which Eduardo could help teach younger children about their Latino heritage and various sports activities). Additionally, Eduardo was introduced to the after-school teen center sponsored by the recreation department, where he could receive adult assistance with homework and participate in open-gym activities. Here, Eduardo enrolled in the center's Environmental Ambassador (EA) program, in which he and other participants volunteered with agencies related to environmental conservation and preservation. The EA participants also present information and educate city officials and the community about strategies to protect the environment.

Eduardo's Achievements

The structured peer and community recreation activities helped Eduardo achieve a sense of accomplishment and belonging while being engaged in activities of his interest and background and maintaining distance from his drug-using acquaintances. With the homework assistance, Eduardo's grades stabilized and began to trend upward. The CTRS met with Eduardo and his mother to discuss common leisure interests and the importance of family-oriented leisure and to brainstorm strategies for making time for one another. Eduardo's mother was receptive and made an oral commitment to plan at least two family-oriented leisure activities per month. Finally, Eduardo was referred to the Mentoring Children of Prisoners program, where he gained an adult male mentor with whom he met once weekly. With his mentor, Eduardo engaged in active recreation activities, developed a trusting relationship, and began to share his feelings of anger toward his father.

or reduce the extension of problem behaviors into adulthood.

Intervention approaches are typically intended to (1) prevent and remediate maladaptive behaviors and inappropriate interaction; (2) assess and promote the acquisition of skills that support academic, motor, and socioemotional functioning; community involvement; and inclusion; and (3) facilitate confidence and enhance self-esteem (Carter & Van Andel, 2011). The therapeutic recreation specialist may address self-confidence and physical well-being through a variety of activities, such as aquatics, relaxation, cooperative games and sports, leisure awareness, and expressive therapies. Cognitive experiences, such as playing board games, keeping score, and reading directions, can reinforce academic skill development (Carter & Van Andel, 2011). Adventure and challenge experiences further encourage sensory integration to support cognitive functioning while also supporting development of self-confidence, self-esteem, and cooperation skills.

The Environment

Previous sections have placed youth risk factors within a continuum and identified behaviors, but one more layer needs to be added when we are considering the context for positive youth development. The trajectory of a young person's development will be influenced through an interaction of his or her personal characteristics and situational circumstances (Gordon & Yowell, 1994). This person–environment interaction may be referred to as the **ecological system**. To promote success, all parts of this system must be included within prevention and intervention measures (Kronick, 1997). Therapeutic recreation specialists need to consider the ecology of the youth with whom they are working. In a broad sense, ecology is the science of relationships between an organism and its environment. In relation to humans, the ecological perspective adopts a holistic view in seeing the person and his or her environment as a unit. In the context of working with young people, this view targets the youth (characteristics, behaviors, physiological factors) as well as the youth's relations with his or her environment. This environment encompasses the immediate settings and people (e.g., home, classroom, neighborhood, family, teacher, counselor, and peer groups) surrounding the youth as well as larger contexts in which these settings and people are embedded (e.g., cultural, political, educational,

and community institutions; Bronfenbrenner, 1989; Farmer, 1997; Germain, 1991). This relationship and interaction between the youth and environment is reciprocal and cyclical (Perkins & Caldwell, 2005). That is, the risk factors from the environment affect the youth, and the factors that make the youth at risk affect the environment (people and settings) in which he or she exists.

Theories That Guide Therapeutic Recreation Practice

Thus far we have defined how youth exist within a continuum of risk, risk factors exist as a consequence of and as an effect on the youth's environment, and positive youth development focuses on developmental needs of youth rather than on deficit-based problems. Several theories play additional and vital roles in helping us understand the relationship between therapeutic recreation and youth development. These theories tie in the social and psychological aspects of the youth who exist on the risk continuum. We begin this discussion by further exploring the ecological perspective and its implications for therapeutic recreation. We will also address another more socially based theory of social capital and then tie in more of the psychologically based theories of anomie, hope, optimism, and flow to inform more completely the practice of therapeutic recreation when working in youth development.

Ecological Perspective

What is the role of the therapeutic recreation profession in addressing the needs and strengths of youth who exist within the risk continuum? When taking on the ecological perspective described earlier in the chapter, our duty is to evaluate circumstances and environments surrounding the individual youth in addition to individual characteristics and behaviors. As we assess and target the physical, cognitive, social, emotional, and leisure needs and strengths of our clients, we have to realize that family, peers, school, law enforcement, church, and other societal factors influence their behaviors and thoughts. These people and settings can be negatively or positively influential in the strengths and needs of the youth and in the collaborative outcomes necessary within our intervention and prevention programs. Within the therapeutic process, our profession must look at the person *with* his or her environment throughout the assessment, planning, implementation, evaluation, and documentation (APIED) process. Four concepts expressed through positive person–environment interaction include human relatedness, competence, self-direction, and increased self-esteem (Germain, 1991). In therapeutic recreation, the primary goal of intervention and prevention programs is to help our youth clients attain these concepts. Ultimately, we want to help them help themselves to maximize their own quality of life (Howe-Murphy & Charboneau, 1987).

In summary, the ecological approach when working with youth provides the practitioner a guide to facilitate "a much broader range of contextual understanding" of this population (Rappaport, 1987, p. 34). A person interacts with and affects a unique combination of subsystems in his or her environment. In return, this environment (in addition to physiological and personality factors) ultimately affects the development of behaviors and beliefs of that person. Within the ecological system, one person does not "own" a disturbance, disability, or condition, and no one is blamed for it (Paul & Epanchin, 1991). In applying this approach, we can help decrease the cause–effect dynamics that place a child or adolescent in danger of future negative outcomes (i.e., **at risk**; McWhirter et al., 2013). We in therapeutic recreation can play a vital role in positive youth development by understanding and working within this perspective and the environment in which youth live, learn, and play.

Social Capital

A second theory that we are increasingly becoming aware of in therapeutic recreation and using when working in youth development is **social capital**. Essentially, social capital is the notion that human beings fair better in life when bonded together (Putnam, 2000; Putnam & Feldstein, 2003). Social capital exists when social networks have value and facilitate cooperation for a common benefit. Social capital also exists when two important ingredients are present within this network: reciprocity and trust (Cullen & Wright, 1997; Hagan & McCarthy, 1997; Putnam, 2000; Putnam & Feldstein, 2003). Reciprocity is achieved when everyone, including the youth, plays a role in giving and receiving within the relationships in the network and all contributions are respected. Trust is necessary and achieved only when members forgo a "what

can you do for me attitude" and when respect and role expectations from all within the network are clear and achievable. When boundaries of roles are less clear, dissonance and ultimately a lack of trust can occur within the relationships. This inability to trust causes greater role segmentation and isolation (Seligman, 1997).

The presence of social capital facilitates positive reinforcements for youth and offers them access to positive role models; recreational, educational, and vocational support; and mentors (Putnam, 2000). Communities that are high in social capital have the capability to realize common values, maintain higher-trusting networks, and sustain social control so that youth can become empowered members of the group (Cullen & Wright, 1997; Hagan & McCarthy, 1997; Putnam, 2000; Putnam & Feldstein, 2003; Sampson, 2001).

According to Hagan and McCarthy (1997), social capital, in general, refers to a variety of resources that originate in an ecological perspective in which social relationships connect youth to groups of other people in neighborhoods, churches, schools, recreation, and law enforcement. Social capital can connect youth to these social relationships by connections with the youths' families (traditional or nontraditional). That is, the social network of the family is important. Just as important are networks within other social groups that connect the parent–child relation to other parents, children, neighbors, teachers, police, recreation personnel, human services personnel, and church members (Hagan & McCarthy, 1997). Making such connections can only help in the transference and generalization of outcomes from the therapeutic recreation services into a youth's community and family life. If we do not work within these support networks in the community and family, the opportunities and benefits of the services that we provide could be lost after the youth go home for the day or when the youth finish our programs.

Anomie Theory and Hopelessness

Before we provide a discussion on the theory of hope and optimism, the theory of **anomie** and its relationship to hopelessness will be addressed to guide the reader to the importance of hope for youth who exist on a risk continuum. One of the challenges that youth face, particularly those in the high- and imminent-risk categories, is that of hopelessness or low hope. In general, people who are less skilled in developing attainable and realistic goals have low hope. Low hope is also exhibited when an intense negative emotional response occurs when a person's goals are blocked or he or she encounters barriers. All these reactions can create a cycle of hopelessness for the person. Furthermore, those with low hope are less likely to be able to negotiate alternative goals when faced with barriers or a blocked original goal and are less likely to view themselves as being able to adapt successfully to such situations. They are caught in a cycle of hopelessness (Rodriguez-Hanley & Snyder, 2000). In summary, people who have less success in establishing positively directed goals or in planning an appropriate means to meet goals experience low hope as a result (Snyder, 2000).

What happens when a person remains within this low-hope cycle? According to Snyder (2000), the person can follow a path to apathy through a variety of stages. Apathy is what leads a person into a state of anomie, or a state of mind in which there is a "breakdown of the individual's sense of attachment to society" (Passas, 1997, p. 80). In relation to youth, this is what we would refer to as a state of delinquency. According to Orrù (1987), anomie is a conflict of belief systems and causes conditions of alienation in which a person progresses into a dysfunctional ability to integrate within normative situations in his or her social world. Because of this alienation, people perceive themselves to be and will appear to be alienated from the economic, cultural, political, and primary socialization group systems (Orrù, 1987).

Therefore, the theory of hope plays a vital role in working with youth in therapeutic recreation settings. Facilitating and promoting hope and optimism for their futures is crucial within intervention and prevention programs.

Hope and Optimism

As many as 20 percent of youth in the United States may experience clinical depression or a related condition by the time they graduate from high school (Lewinsohn, Hops, Roberts, & Seeley, 1993; National Alliance on Mental Illness, 2016). Similar rates of youth anxiety and suicide

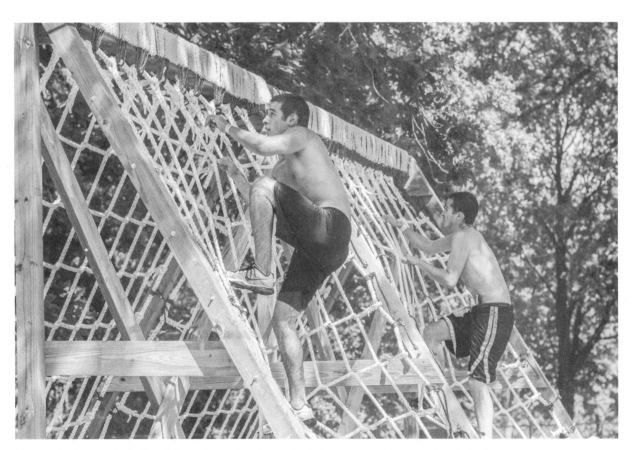

Youth optimism can be fostered through structured, meaningful engagement in recreational activity.

rates have been reported (Centers for Disease Control and Prevention, 2004; Twenge, 2000). Such marked indicators of mental illness suggest a widespread deficit in youth optimism and the need to foster hope among youth.

As a protective factor against such harms, optimism is largely an attitudinal strength. Tiger (1979) proposed a useful definition for optimism: "a mood or attitude associated with an expectation about the social or material future—one which the evaluator regards as socially desirable, to his [or her] advantage, or for his [or her] pleasure" (p. 18). Peterson (2000) suggested that optimistic attitudes are linked to "positive mood and good morale; to perseverance and effective problem solving; to academic, athletic, military, occupational, and political success; to popularity; to good health; and even to long life and freedom from trauma" (p. 44). Pessimism, on the other hand, tends to indicate passivity, failure, social estrangement, morbidity, and mortality.

Youth optimism can be fostered through structured, meaningful engagement in recreational activity. Involving young people in continual opportunities to challenge themselves, build competence and confidence, experience flow, enact self-determined choices, and take active roles in decisionmaking processes encourages future expectations for engagement and success.

Flow

Among the many problems confronting contemporary youth is the challenge of structuring time in positive developmental pursuits. Nearly 40 percent of adolescent waking hours is discretionary time (Bartko & Eccles, 2003), and youth seem to make the poorest activity choices when they are out of school (Pawelko & Magafas, 1997). Studies have shown that large portions of adolescent daily life are experienced as boredom (Csikszentmihalyi & Larson, 1984; Larson, Csikszentmihalyi, & Freeman, 1992; Larson & Richards, 1991), even among teens considered least at risk for future problems.

Developing skills for the constructive management of discretionary time is paramount to youth development (Witt & Crompton, 1996). Yet for all youth, finding constructive and interesting ways to occupy time and avoid boredom can be challenging (Witt & Crompton, 2002b). The excitement of illicit activities and the action and entertainment of video games and popular media compete with youth motivation for interesting, challenging,

and developmentally positive pursuits (Witt & Crompton, 2002b).

Research on enjoyment and optimal experience has produced the concept of flow, a term used to describe intensely absorbing, self-rewarding experiences (in which challenges match a person's skills and the person tends to lose track of time and selfawareness). Flow has been described as the experience of "concentration, absorption, deep involvement, joy, and sense of accomplishment . . . what people describe as the best moments in their lives" (Csikszentmihalyi, 1993, p. 176).

It has been suggested that the ability to engage in flow promotes overall psychosocial development of youth (Csikszentmihalyi & Larson, 1984). Young people who regularly engage in complex flowproducing activities may be less prone to boredom and anxiety and have developmental advantages over those who do not have such experiences.

Prevention, Intervention, and the Therapeutic Process: APIED

When working with youth in therapeutic recreation settings, concepts of prevention and intervention must be understood and integrated into the therapeutic process: APIED. Before reviewing how the APIED process can be applied in youth development, these two concepts will be explained in more detail.

Prevention

A major challenge that a youth-serving agency must address is targeting risk factors that may not have happened yet or that come from an environmental history. Most risk factors are known to be cumulative and synergistic. That is, they exist within a cycle and can be passed across generations (Simeonsson, 1994). The best way to target such risk factors is through prevention services because intervention and treatment services will become overwhelmed by addressing such problems alone (Simeonsson, 1994). With the growing numbers of youth and families with identified problems, human services, including therapeutic recreation, must understand and be involved with youth, families, and their communities and be able to implement prevention-based programs.

In general, prevention is defined as stopping something before it happens, but we must be aware that just as risk exists on a continuum, prevention also moves along various degrees of addressing the needs of the youth who exist on this risk continuum. The following section will discuss three areas of the prevention continuum: primary, secondary, and tertiary.

Primary prevention focuses on reducing the number of new cases of identified problems or conditions occurring within a population. Primary prevention can be defined as the primary promotion of health and development (Simeonsson, 1994). It is also seen as a logical and needed strategy to reduce physical, social, and psychological problems. Programs using such a strategy should target youth who are at increased risk based on group characteristics rather than on individual characteristics (Simeonsson, 1994). According to McWhirter et al. (2013), primary prevention would target the general population and youth who exist within the minimal and remote risk levels. Chamberlin (1994) described prevention using an analogy of a river and a drowning child. He explained that children upstream, or those youth who would benefit from primary prevention, are not being taught to swim and not being kept from falling in the river. They are still on the ground but are at risk for "jumping or falling into the river because of some family and community dysfunction" (p. 37). Examples that may relate to the involvement of therapeutic recreation include isolated and depressed single mothers who are having a difficult time dealing with stress, children who are neglected in overcrowded and unsafe childcare environments, and adolescents who are hanging around on the street corner.

Secondary prevention can be equated with early intervention or recognition (Chamberlin, 1994; McWhirter et al., 2013) and focuses on "reducing the number of existing cases and lowering the prevalence of the manifested problems or conditions in the population" (Simeonsson, 1994, p. 7). Chamberlin's river analogy explains that what occurs in this stage is evaluation of whether the children and youth who have fallen or jumped are at risk for drowning. These youth may exist on the high-risk continuum and need selective intervention to help reduce the problems that already exist (McWhirter et al., 2013; Simeonsson, 1994). Groups targeted with secondary prevention may be youth who are exposed to specific environmental stressors, such as coming from families who have low incomes, have experienced divorce, have mental health problems, or have substance abuse problems.

Tertiary prevention focuses on the reduction of harmful effects and complications that occur within an existing disorder and identified condition (Simeonsson, 1994). According to Chamberlin (1994), the child is already downstream, and the human services provider has already assessed that the child needs to be rescued from drowning from such harmful effects and complications. Tertiary prevention can also be seen as treatment and rehabilitation. The youth who need such services are within the imminent and in-crisis categories of risk (Chamberlin, 1994; McWhirter et al., 2013).

Intervention

Prevention and intervention can be difficult to distinguish from one another because the two concepts overlap. Prevention programs can often be seen as intervention and vice versa. Adam, for example, had been having trouble developing positive peer relationships in middle school and was exhibiting signs of aggression. He was referred to a wilderness therapy intervention for youth who were expected to have a difficult transition to high school. Through the program, Adam developed new friendships with peers and adult mentors and began to see himself as likeable. Adam's boosted self-esteem and developing support network in turn helped protect him from future problems associated with social isolation.

A framework (figure 10.2) presented by McWhirter et al. (2013) reconciles this ambiguity by integrating intervention approaches with the at-risk continuum presented earlier in this chapter. Universal approaches to intervention are appropriate for all young people, not just those considered at risk. For example, all children in a low-income neighborhood are provided a program, although some are at only minimal risk. Selected approaches, such as Head Start programs, offered to lower-income families (who are more likely to experience additional stressful circumstances) serve children who have increased risk of developing future problems. Booster sessions further enhance the effectiveness of interventions by adding a longer-term element. To sustain outcomes, intervention approaches must be of sufficient duration (Kirby, 2001). One-time efforts are less effective because program effects are not sustained over time (McWhirter et al., 2013). Indicated approaches target young people who are at imminent risk for problem behavior or have already adopted risk-oriented behaviors.

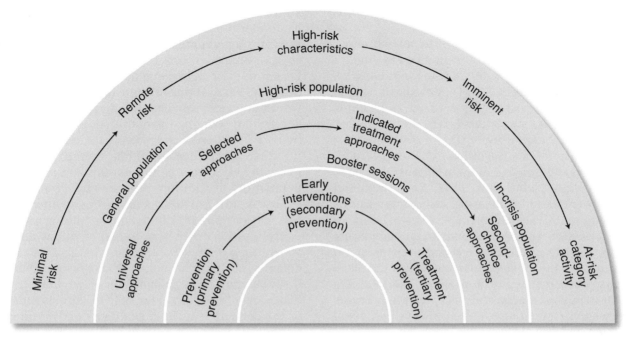

Figure 10.2 Risk, approaches, and prevention continuum.

Such approaches are developed for youth whose underlying problems, characteristics, and behaviors are directly related to an at-risk activity. For example, an anger management program may be indicated for young people who have exhibited aggressive behaviors and as prevention for future problems, such as violence or juvenile detention. Finally, second-chance interventions are needed for young people who are already engaged in at-risk behaviors, such as substance abuse or violence, or have dropped out of school or become pregnant.

Assessment

The first phase of the therapeutic process involves assessment, which helps us determine where the youth falls within the risk continuum or if he or she needs more prevention or intervention-type services and in what domains. There are several assessments that are commonly used in youth development. Although limitations can be important to assess, it is equally important to assess the youth's strengths so that later we can balance goals with appropriate programs (Anderson & Heyne, 2012b). More so, when we are at the prevention stages, it is vital that we gather and concentrate on the youth's strengths in the effort to help identify and build resilient factors.

The first assessment that is important when working in therapeutic recreation and youth development is the School Social Behavior Scale (SSBS), published by Brookes Publishing Company. The SSBS is a norm-referenced 64-item assessment that is completed by teachers or other school-related personnel on school-age children and youth (K-12). It is divided into two scales: social competence and antisocial behavior. The scale of social competence is further divided into three subscales: peer relations, self-management/ compliance, and academic behavior. The scale of antisocial behavior is divided into three subscales: hostile/irritable, antisocial/aggressive, and defiant/disruptive behaviors (Merrell, 2002). This assessment provides the opportunity to gather strengths-based data (social competence), as discussed earlier, as well as the limitations (antisocial behavior) of the youth.

In addition, several assessment instruments published by the Search Institute are important to acknowledge and discuss in relation to youth development. The Search Institute is an organization that provides resources, expertise, and research for partnering organizations, schools, and community agencies with the ultimate goal to help provide support and services to solve challenges for the youth of today (Search Institute, 2018a).

The Search Institute is founded upon the principle of positive youth development.

Currently, the Search Institute publishes four assessment/survey instruments that are vital for those working with youth in gathering strengths-based information or data. They can be purchased through the Search Institute website and include the Attitudes & Behaviors (A&B) Survey; Developmental Assets Profile (DAP); Relationships, Effort, Aspirations, Cognition, and Heart (REACH) Survey; and Youth & Program Strengths (YAPS) Survey (Search Institute, 2018a). The background and process for purchasing each survey can be found on the Search Institute website, but more information on the DAP will be provided here because of its extensive use and direct relationship with the 40 developmental assets that were discussed earlier in the chapter. The DAP is a 58-item assessment and provides a total score based on those items. It also provides individual scores for each of the external asset subscales (support, empowerment, boundaries, expectations, and constructive use of time), with a total external asset subscale score, and individual scores for each of the internal asset subscales (commitment to learning, positive values, social competencies, and positive identity), with a total internal asset subscale score (Search Institute, 2016b). In addition, the DAP measures the assets within the five contexts of personal, social, family, school, and community (Search Institute, 2016b). An important aspect about the DAP is that it targets a wide range of ages and has been used longitudinally. That is, if you have the opportunity to work with youth over a long period of time (e.g., in after-school programs), you can collect relative information on their development over the years they receive services in your agency.

Planning

Setting relevant and realistic goals with the youth and developing and choosing the most appropriate programs are important in prevention- and intervention-based services for the youth. Once the assessment data has been collected, it is important for the therapeutic recreation specialist to set goals to address specific limitations but also to target programs with the youth's strengths in mind. For example, from the DAP, the youth may score low on the item *deals with frustration in positive ways* (meaning the youth has challenges in this area) but in contrast, scores high on the item *takes responsibility for what I do* (Search Institute,

2004). Therefore, programs for that youth would be chosen to make sure that the youth takes on more responsibilities but also helps the youth cope in a positive way in frustrating situations. Programs that help develop peer leadership, trust, and empowering relationships for the youth would enhance responsibility and peer support and guidance during frustrating times. Programs that are based on such concepts include adventure therapy and team-building initiatives, and they are very common and appropriate for this population. In addition, programs based on the expressive arts provide opportunities for alternative ways to role-play and express (through art, dance, music, writing, or drama) emotions and frustrations for the youth. The youth can also demonstrate his or her ability to take responsibility by being a lead peer planner on a drama, music, dance, or art show to be presented to families and/or the community. The modalities of adventure therapy and expressive arts will be discussed later in the chapter along with leisure education, therapeutic use of sports, values clarification, and anger management.

Implementation

Within the above listed modalities, key aspects of implementation will involve technical (hard) skills and facilitation (soft) skills, as discussed in chapter 6. In youth development, providing opportunities for choice, trust, challenges, and successes, individually and socially, is important. Therefore, careful planning will be vital before it is time to implement these types of therapeutic recreation programs. Structure, organization, flexibility, openness, and guidance from the therapeutic recreation specialist will be part of this planning, and more so during the implementation phase. The more trained and prepared a therapist is within his or her technical skills for the modalities he or she implements with the youth, the more successful the programs will be in meeting client goals and outcomes. For example, in adventure therapy, the technical skills may include specialized training; client orientations; risk management paperwork; preparation of the teaching materials; physical preparation of the activities and the site; maintenance of the equipment (e.g., ropes course, white-water rafts, kayaks, campsites, rock-climbing sites, and safety gear); and continuing education for professional development, which includes accreditation and credentialing (e.g., Association for Experiential

Education [2018] and Project Adventure [2016]). Equally important in the implementation phase are the facilitation skills while running therapeutic sessions and activities. These soft skills involve the stages of briefing, leading, and debriefing/processing, which can be reviewed in chapter 6 under the section heading Implementation. Although all three stages are important, the third stage should be the most emphasized and mastered in skill when working in youth development. Processing will help youth develop connections between their experiences and the client outcomes with other aspects of their lives in other health and human services they are receiving with their families, school, and community. More so, all these skills are just as important in prevention as in intervention. The greatest advantage in processing here is to aid in transition and generalization to areas related to the ecology of youth at any point on the risk continuum (Autry, 2001; Luckner & Nadler, 1997).

Evaluation, Attaining Outcomes, and Documentation

Program evaluation and evidence-based practice have become essential in producing targeted outcomes for clients and disseminating the benefits of therapeutic recreation to many stakeholders surrounding the clients (e.g., clients themselves, families, other disciplines, administrators, insurance providers, the community, and legislators). Documentation plays a key role in the therapeutic recreation process and should be an inherent element of assessment, planning, implementation, and evaluation.

Just as prevention and intervention frequently overlap in purpose and practice, likewise do outcomes. Overall, research in the area of recreational youth program outcomes has demonstrated a multitude of benefits to youth. Evaluation of a youth recreation after-school program, for example, found that participants benefited from engagement in goal-oriented activity (which they had previously lacked), experienced feelings of acceptance among adults, and gained skills in conflict resolution and peer collaboration (Scott, Witt, & Foss, 1996).

Another study of Boys & Girls Club leaders suggested that youth who participated in the recreation prevention program developed leadership skills that increased self-esteem and perceptions of competence. The club, described by the youth members as a second home, fostered feelings of safety, belonging, and adult nurturance. The importance of supportive adult relationships and sustained program duration cannot be overemphasized because other studies have shown that outcomes are not as likely to endure post program if these elements are lacking (Autry, 2001; Boccaro & Outley, 2005; Sklar, Anderson, & Autry, 2007).

Settings and Opportunities

Youth services professionals, including traditional parks and recreation practitioners, face numerous challenges in providing adequate developmental programs because of the complex problems and behaviors that youth often present (Sprouse, Klitzing, & Parr, 2005; Witt & Crompton, 1996). Interdisciplinary collaborative approaches that include a variety of social services personnel from the community provide more powerful programs with broader influence than do single-focus attempts. Under the partnership approach to service delivery, therapeutic recreation personnel can be a strong source of support for positive youth development services (Sprouse et al., 2005), and practitioners may be found working across a range of youth development settings. Among these settings are community-based programs, schools, mental health services, residential child welfare and treatment services, outdoor programs, and services within the juvenile justice system.

Community-Based Programs

Nationwide, park and recreation departments have sought innovative ways of serving youth in their respective communities, and many of these programs represent opportunities for therapeutic recreation specialists to make significant contributions of skills and expertise. In a series of case studies on youth public recreation programs, Witt and Crompton (2002a) brought to light a number of best practices examples throughout the United States. Therapeutic recreation programs based in the community have taken strides to address the growing need for community-based services for vulnerable and challenged youth. An enduring example of a public therapeutic recreation agency that targets the needs of young people is in the mental health programs of the Northern Illinois Special Recreation Association (NISRA). NISRA collaborates with the McHenry County Mental Health Board and McHenry County Court

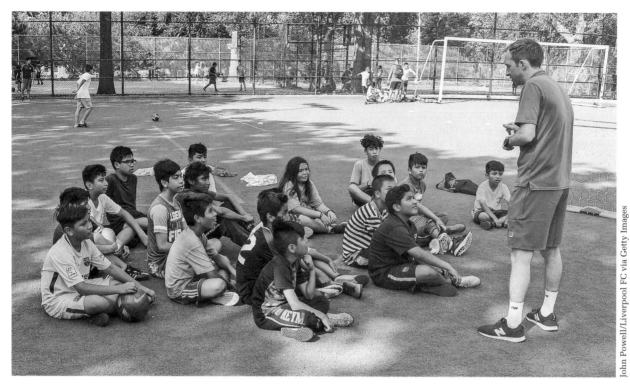

Public park and recreation departments are a common setting for delivery of positive youth development services.

Services to provide programs for youth with a range of mental health concerns. Among those served are children with severe behavioral and emotional disorders and youth who are involved in the courts, disadvantaged economically, or at risk for placement out of home or school (NISRA, 2016). These programs are designed to emphasize challenge and cooperation activities while incorporating a leisure education component. Through its youth mental health programming, NISRA focuses on both leisure education and recreational activities to provide participants with personal skill development, including self-esteem, peer interactions, positive socialization, conflict resolution, and leisure awareness (Shulewitz & Zuniga, 1999).

Not-for-profit organizations engaged in youth programming present tremendous opportunity for therapeutic recreation specialists to apply their skills in high-need settings. The YMCA of Metro Chicago uses the skills of a CTRS to employ therapeutic recreation principles to address a wide scope of youth needs in the community. For example, the YMCA supports youth with emotional and behavioral disorders as well those exposed to prolonged stress and trauma, who can have difficulty demonstrating the necessary socioemotional skills needed to be successful

in many organized sports and youth programs (Kenny Riley, personal communication, July 12, 2016). Programs emphasize intentionally building socioemotional skills, such as problem solving, initiative, empathy, teamwork, and emotion management. Tools such as the Youth Program Quality Assessment (Weikart Center for Youth Program Quality, 2016b) and the Social Emotional Learning (SEL) framework (Weikart Center for Youth Program Quality, 2016a) are used to help staff members continually improve their practice and programming. Guided by the CTRS, programs are aligned to SEL best practices, and staff members are trained to appropriately challenge, encourage, and support participants, enabling challenged youth to have increased chances for success.

YMCA of Metro Chicago offers programs on a continuum for youth needing high support to those who can participate independently. For example, youth exposed to high levels of stress and trauma are supported through the Urban Warriors program, which pairs youth with post-9/11 military veteran mentors in a 16-week curriculum. At the opposite of the spectrum, youth employment is offered, and Youth Council leadership opportunities engage young people to lead meetings and make decisions affecting teens across the association.

Schools

Schools also present opportunities for CTRSs to provide positive youth development programming. For example, a therapeutic recreation specialist position at Glenwood Academy is designated to use activity- and community-based interventions to improve the physical, cognitive, emotional, social, and leisure needs of students. The specialist position is intended to help students develop knowledge, skills, and behaviors for daily living; health and wellness; and rewarding community involvement. Located in the suburbs south of Chicago, Glenwood Academy provides "life-changing solutions for good kids from challenging circumstances impacted by poverty, violence, inadequate educational systems or lack of resources, changing the trajectory of their lives through access to increased opportunity" (Glenwood Academy, 2016).

Mental Health Services

According to the National Alliance on Mental Illness (2016), 20 percent of youth ages 13 to 18 in the United States live with a mental health condition, 11 percent of youth live with a mood disorder, 10 percent of youth have a conduct disorder, and 8 percent of youth have an anxiety disorder. Therapeutic recreation services for youth with mental disorders can be found among inpatient and outpatient clinical health care services. Treatment is normally provided under the medical direction of a psychiatrist working with an interdisciplinary team, using a variety of interventions. Therapeutic recreation professionals work with nurses, mental health counselors, social workers, and occupational therapists to provide a supportive therapeutic milieu. Among the various techniques used, therapeutic recreation interventions may emphasize experiential approaches to appropriate self-expression, anxiety and anger management, problem solving, cooperation, communication, and emotional coping skills.

Residential Child Welfare and Treatment Services

Therapeutic recreation services in residential-oriented treatment settings offer additional experiential services to support developmental success among the most challenged youth. Cunningham Children's Home, in Urbana, Illinois, for example, is a child welfare and educational services agency serving "youth who suffer from serious emotional and behavioral challenges that have been caused by abuse, neglect, mental illness, and more" (Cunningham Children's Home, 2016). The Special Therapies Department, staffed by CTRSs, provides a comprehensive recreation program, including Illinois Interagency Athletic Association teams, aquatics, music, arts and crafts, and creative writing activities.

Another residential facility, Shelterwood Academy, in Independence, Missouri, provides a therapeutic program for teens showing a variety of troubling behaviors and symptoms such as

> low self-esteem, depression or suicidal thoughts; abuse, anger, oppositional defiance or anxiety; drug use, alcohol use or other risky behaviors; loss of academic standing or school suspensions; low motivation, manipulation or poor peer choices; family or authority conflict and discord; and/or attention deficit disorder (ADD) or attention deficit hyperactivity disorder (ADHD). (Shelterwood Academy, 2016)

Staffed by a CTRS, the recreation program provides therapeutic activities and settings designed to "help each teen to take positive personal risks, engage in healthy self-expression, build self-confidence and promote greater trust among their peers" (Shelterwood Academy, 2016). In addition to use of the on-campus facilities, including a gymnasium, fitness room, and mountain bike course, the program provides a number of outdoor activities, such as camping, rock climbing, fishing, biking, and hiking.

Youth residential settings, as in the examples above, are not exclusive of educational settings. In fact, residential childcare settings are required to provide state-mandated education, though requirements may vary from state to state. Therapeutic recreation activities will typically occur outside of the hours designated for formal education.

Outdoor Programs

Therapeutic outdoor activities promoting youth development include adventure and wilderness therapy. Interventions may occur in wilderness settings or within a variety of facility-based settings, including psychiatric, educational, and correctional settings. Programs in which therapeutic recreation specialists use adventure therapy are typically treatment settings for people who have been diagnosed with mental health problems (e.g., chemical dependency or depression) or alternative programs for young offenders referred by the courts (Autry, 2001; Davis-Berman & Berman,

1999). A common approach to adventure therapy is to offer it as an ancillary treatment to traditional therapies in the psychiatric setting. This approach might involve the use of low-level teams course elements or a high-ropes course. Adventure therapy may also be delivered as a sole treatment modality (Davis-Berman & Berman, 1999) in a multiday wilderness intervention program. Whatever the delivery mode, program efficacy is well documented in the short term, but research has also demonstrated the need to conduct long-term follow-up with participants to ensure sustainable outcomes (Autry, 2001; Russell, 2002; Sklar, Anderson, & Autry, 2007).

Juvenile Justice System

People under age 18 who engage in patterns of behavior that deviate from cultural norms and threaten the welfare of others are labeled as delinquent (Carter & Van Andel, 2011) by the juvenile justice system. In the United States, the juvenile justice system includes approximately 4,000 juvenile courts that specialize in the problems of youth. Most of these courts operate with a philosophy that even the worst delinquent is not a criminal but instead an erring, vulnerable child who needs help. Police arrest about 2.8 million young people for crimes annually, but the courts

EXEMPLARY PROFESSIONAL

GAYLE RESH, CTRS, CPRP, CDP, LNHA

Education: BS in Education (Emphasis in Health, Education, and Recreation), University of Nebraska at Lincoln
MA (Emphasis in Therapeutic Recreation), University of Nebraska at Omaha
Position: Life Enrichment Coordinator
Organization: Southlake Village Rehabilitation & Care Center
Special Awards:

* Exemplary Therapeutic Recreation Professional, Nebraska Recreation and Park Association (1993-1994)

* Fellow Award, Nebraska Recreation and Park Association (2002)

* Distinguished Service Award, Nebraska Recreation and Park Association (2005)

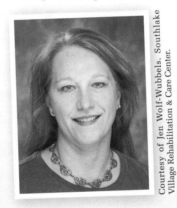

Courtesy of Jen Wolf-Wubbels. Southlake Village Rehabilitation & Care Center.

My Career

My career really started when I volunteered at Lincoln Regional Center as part of an undergraduate therapeutic recreation class. This experience led to a position with Lincoln Regional Center, where I worked as a recreation therapist for more than two decades. My responsibilities involved developing and implementing therapeutic recreation programs for a variety of patient groups receiving mental health services. After 26 years, three months, and two days, my career shifted in 2011, and I began working for Vetter Health Services as the life enrichment coordinator at Southlake Village Rehabilitation & Care Center. This facility provides living options in the areas of short-term rehabilitation, care for patients with Alzheimer's or other dementia, and skilled nursing. My responsibilities include evaluation and documentation of life enrichment programming, including cognitive, social, emotional, and physical programming. I play a lead role in development of care plans, particularly in the realm of nonpharmacological approaches.

In addition, I have always been involved in professional associations related to therapeutic recreation. This is a critical part of advocating for clients and the profession, but it is also very important to professional development. Associations that I have been a member of and worked with in the past include the Nebraska Therapeutic Recreation Association, the Nebraska Recreation and Park Association, and the American Therapeutic Recreation Association. I have also worked as an adjunct instructor for the University of Nebraska. Being involved in these activities has not only been rewarding, but has significantly enhanced my professional abilities and my overall career.

My Advice to You

Be flexible, be varied, and always be willing to learn.

process about only 1.8 million as delinquents (O'Connor, 2004).

Therapeutic recreation work with young offenders occurs in both residential settings and community-based programs. Residential programs include juvenile prisons, youth detention centers, and youth camps. The therapeutic recreation specialist in the residential program functions as a member of a treatment team that serves incarcerated youth, who may also be substance abusers or have intellectual impairments or psychological disorders. Therapeutic recreation specialists in these settings lead skill development classes; supervise recreation areas, such as the library and exercise and game rooms (Carter & Van Andel, 2011); and conduct leisure education classes, including leisure awareness and social skill development. Community-based services involve day treatment services, diversionary programs, and public parks and recreation department programs (Carter & Van Andel, 2011).

In community settings, therapeutic recreation specialists collaborate with law enforcement, education, and nonprofit and government agencies to provide direct services to youth considered at risk of involvement with the courts (Carter & Van Andel, 2011). A primary focus within the community is prevention of future problems (Shultz, Crompton, & Witt, 1995). Therapeutic recreation plays a valuable role in preventing youth from engaging in risky behaviors, such as substance abuse, that contribute to criminal acts (Witt & Crompton, 1996). Resiliency factors (skills and attitudes needed to adapt and cope with everyday life; Carter & Van Andel, 2011) become the focus of many community programs that emphasize tolerance, a sense of acceptance, resource awareness, and collaborative relationships and services that address both nonrecreative needs and positive leisure experiences (Allen, Paisley, Stevens, & Harwell, 1998).

Modalities for Youth Development

Several modalities exist that are relevant for working with youth and promoting positive youth development. They include adventure therapy, leisure education, the expressive arts, sports, exercise, values clarification, anger management, and assertiveness training (Austin, 2013; Dattilo & McKenney, 2011). The first three modalities will

be discussed in more detail, including possible outcomes settings and assessments to use within each of these modalities.

Adventure Therapy

Adventure therapy is an intervention approach widely used with young people in which outdoor experiential activities are employed to accomplish treatment-related goals (Groff & Dattilo, 2011). Adventure experiences, characterized by perceptions of risk and challenge by choice, equip therapeutic recreation specialists with useful techniques to facilitate behavioral and attitudinal change within their clients (Groff & Dattilo, 2011). Through purposive facilitation, adventure therapy can provide empowering outcomes for youth who experience low self-perceptions and engage in self-destructive behaviors (Autry, 2001). Specialized training is necessary to deliver adventure therapy programming safely and appropriately. Training opportunities are available through college curricula, professional workshops, or certification programs offered through individual programs and facilities (Association for Experiential Education, 2016; Carter & Van Andel, 2011; Project Adventure, 2016). Therapeutic recreation specialists who deliver adventure therapy may work in a number of settings, including clinical mental health facilities, community-based diversional programs, backcountry wilderness programs, and residential wilderness camps for juvenile offenders. An assessment tool directly related to measuring outcomes of coping and stress of adolescents in therapeutic recreation and adventure therapy is the Response to Stress Questionnaire Outdoor Adventure Version (RSQ-OAV; Russell, Widmer, Lunberg, & Ward, 2015).

Leisure Education

Leisure education is a modality that is based on the philosophy that everyone, regardless of race/ethnicity, gender, socioeconomic status, religion, ability, age, sexual orientation, or any other characteristic, has the right to experience leisure (Dattilo, 2015). Leisure is a human right and is included in three (numbers 13, 24, and 27) of the 30 articles of the United Nation's Universal Declaration of Human Rights (United Nations, 1948; Veal, 2016; Wise, 2016). It is also based on the assumption that leisure will not improve quality of life unless people know *how* to use it (Csikszentmihalyi, 1997). This is why the term *education* is relevant.

Therefore, it is important to offer such programs in youth development to help establish a foundation and a long-term goal into adulthood of a healthy leisure lifestyle. In the contribution of leisure education to positive development, children and youth will benefit from learning the background and application of strategies for leisure awareness, leisure skills, social interaction skills, decision making, planning, and leisure resources in the community (Dattilo, 2015; Stumbo & Peterson, 2009). Leisure education in youth development may be provided in therapeutic recreation settings, such as schools/alternative schools, after-school programs, juvenile justice, mental health, and substance abuse treatment agencies. Several assessment tools related to measuring outcomes for the various components of leisure education with youth include Free Time Boredom Measure, Teen Leisurescope Plus, Measurement of Social Empowerment and Trust, and Idyll Arbor Leisure Battery (Burlingame & Blaschko, 2010).

Expressive Arts

The expressive arts, as introduced earlier in the chapter, include the following media for physical, emotional, cognitive, and social expression: dance, movement, drama/theater, music, art, storytelling, poetry, and writing (Atkins & Appalachian Expressive Arts Collective, 2003; Austin, 2013; Dattilo & McKenney, 2011). All these media are effective, meaningful, and powerful when working in therapeutic recreation and youth development; however, the following articles from *Therapeutic Recreation Journal* provide an overview of relevant outcomes for youth from creative writing and drama interventions. In the journal's article on recreational therapy evidence-based practice on creative writing and substance abuse treatment, Snead, Pakstis, Evans, and Nelson (2015) reported several outcomes: increases in self-disclosure, therapeutic alliance and trust, self-confidence, self-awareness, physical health, coping skills, social skills, self-expression, and goal attainment. The authors also reported a decrease in trauma symptoms, stress, depression, and anxiety. In their article on recreational therapy evidence-based practice on using theater and drama interventions to reduce bullying in school-age children, Ross and Nelson (2014) reported the following outcomes for Drama in Education: a decrease in bullying incidents, an increased

understanding of the issues, empowerment of students to realize their roles in stopping bullying, an increase in empathy, a transferability of skills to real life, and the recognition from parents and the students that the program was helpful. Expressive arts in youth development may be provided in therapeutic recreation settings, such as substance abuse treatment agencies, mental health, schools/alternative schools, after-school programs, and juvenile justice. Assessment tools related to measuring outcomes for the various media within expressive arts include the Cooperation and Trust Scale (Witman, 1992) and various assessments as outlined and reviewed in the special issue on assessment in the creative arts therapies (Johnson, 1988).

Additional Modalities

Additional modalities relevant to working in youth development and therapeutic recreation include the therapeutic use of sports, exercise, values clarification, anger management, and assertiveness training (Austin, 2013; Dattilo & McKenney, 2011). These modalities engage the youth to develop individual assets (e.g., coping skills, values, decision making, empowerment, self-determination, and physical fitness) and successful social relationships with friends, family, and the community members surrounding them. The ultimate goal of all the modalities discussed in this chapter is to "encourage youth to think about who they are becoming and how they can be intentional in working toward a positive future" (Search Institute, 2016a).

Summary

Grounded in a philosophy of strengths-based service delivery, therapeutic recreation is well suited to provide positive youth development programming. As a profession, therapeutic recreation is well established in designing outcomes-based programming with the most vulnerable populations. The therapeutic recreation process of APIED can be readily applied to youth development service settings. Whether treatment goals lie in prevention, diversion, or primary treatment, therapeutic recreation offers a universal process, established service models, and standards of practice to the broad field of youth development.

DISCUSSION QUESTIONS

1. Compare and contrast the concept of positive youth development to the at-risk continuum. What are the pros and cons of either approach, and how might they be used to guide therapeutic recreation practice?

2. Examine the 40 developmental assets at www.search-institute.org/our -research/development-assets/developmental-assets-framework/. Which assets were present in your life while you were growing up? How did these assets contribute to your development?

3. Describe the importance of taking an ecological perspective when working in therapeutic recreation with at-risk youth. What are some factors within the youth's environment that a therapeutic recreation specialist would need to consider when providing intervention services? When providing prevention services?

4. Briefly describe the theories that guide the therapeutic recreation profession when working with at-risk youth. Provide examples of therapeutic recreation programs that would put each theory into practice for a youth such as Eduardo (see Client Portrait: Eduardo).

5. Compare and contrast the concepts of prevention and intervention in youth development services.

6. Describe the importance of applying the APIED process in youth development. Discuss key aspects within each stage of the APIED process that specifically need to be addressed in therapeutic recreation and positive youth development. Make sure to tie in the concepts of prevention and intervention in your answers.

7. Several modalities were discussed in the chapter that are important in therapeutic recreation and youth development. Choose two of these modalities you are most interested in, and compare and contrast the outcomes each modality will have in contributing toward positive youth development.

11

Therapeutic Recreation and Senior Populations

Laura Covert-Miller | Cameo Rogers

LEARNING OUTCOMES

At the end of this chapter, students will be able to

- describe key characteristics of the aging community that have implications for therapeutic recreation practice,
- identify common employment opportunities in therapeutic recreation that involve working with the senior population,
- explain the role that therapeutic recreation plays in providing services to the senior population,
- delineate modalities typically used to address the needs of senior therapeutic recreation clients, and
- use these theories and modalities in various client scenarios involving the development of therapeutic recreation programs for seniors.

Therapeutic recreation specialists working with older adult clients take on a coaching role, using therapeutic interventions designed to minimize excess disability; transition to an internal locus of control; develop greater perceptions of choice and freedom; and overcome perceived and actual barriers to functional recreation, leisure, and social pursuits. Leisure-based interventions are used to promote motor abilities (e.g., balance, coordination, strength, and endurance), cognitive skills (e.g., attention span, problem solving, and decision making), social skills (e.g., initiating conversation and developing and maintaining friendships), mental health, and opportunities to flourish through leisure experiences.

Therapeutic recreation specialists serving older adults should understand their health concerns and how deficits associated with aging may contribute to excess disability. **Excess disability** is a term that was coined to describe a phenomenon where individuals with disabilities were observed with levels of disability that were greater than their actual level of impairment (Brody, Kleban, Lawton, & Silverman, 1971; Sabat, 1994). Sometimes, after an older adult requires assistance with care, the caregiver begins to do things for the older adult and, over time, may minimize the older adult's role in choice, conversation, and tasks. Therapeutic recreation can provide the older adult with techniques and skills to cope with and adapt to functional losses. Therapeutic recreation specialists are key players in minimizing excess disability, drawing from techniques such as modeling, demonstration, and hand-over-hand assistance and use of available adaptive equipment to empower ability in older adults.

Throughout this chapter, the coaching roles therapeutic recreation specialists play in an older adult's life will be reviewed. These roles range from understanding factors that can negatively or positively influence excess disability to utilizing theories related to minimizing excess disability and maximizing individuals' roles in activities and socialization. In addition, this chapter explores evidence-based interventions and techniques used with older adults to improve functional, social, and cognitive functioning.

The Aging Population

In the field of aging, there is debate regarding the specific age at which a person should be classified as part of the aging population. For this chapter, an older adult is considered to be any person age 65 or older, which is a commonly used threshold in current aging literature.

As of 2015, there were 47.8 million adults over the age of 65 living in the United States. This age group represented 14.9 percent of the U.S. population, equaling one in every seven Americans (Administration on Aging [AoA]), 2016). By the year 2030, there will be 72 million adults over the age of 65, equaling one in five Americans (Centers for Disease Control and Prevention [CDC], 2013). Not only will therapeutic recreation specialists have ample opportunities to work with older adults, but they will also be working with an increasingly diverse population. In 2015, 22 percent of older adults identified as being in a racial minority group (AoA, 2016). Between the years 2014 and 2030, the Hispanic population is expected to increase by 110 percent; African American population, 90 percent; American Indian and Native Alaskan population, 93 percent; and Asian population, 104 percent (AoA, 2016).

Although the older adult community is growing and diversifying, older adults may experience decreases in social support as they age. Nearly 56 percent of community-dwelling individuals 65 and older live with their spouses. Of all women who reach the age of 75, 32 percent are living alone. There are 13.6 million adults over the age of 65 who are living alone, 68 percent of those being women (AoA, 2016).

Opportunities for social interaction are certainly a concern for the senior population. The frequency of family and friend visits sharply declines approximately 6 months after an older adult moves into a long-term-care residential community, with as many as one-third of residents receiving no visitors (Choi, Ransom, & Wyllie, 2008). As many as 22 percent of nursing home residents may be "**elder orphans,**" with no surviving family to visit (Fujiwara, Emmert, & Carney, 2015). By being aware of the decline in social networks, therapeutic recreation specialists can examine social resources and identify needs for development of friendships among peers in care settings and/or the community.

Social support is not the only decrease older adults could experience. Income levels can decline. According to the AoA, approximately 4.5 million adults over 65 were living below the poverty level in 2014. The median income for adults 65 and older in 2014 was $22,248. Social Security is the main income for 84 percent of older adults.

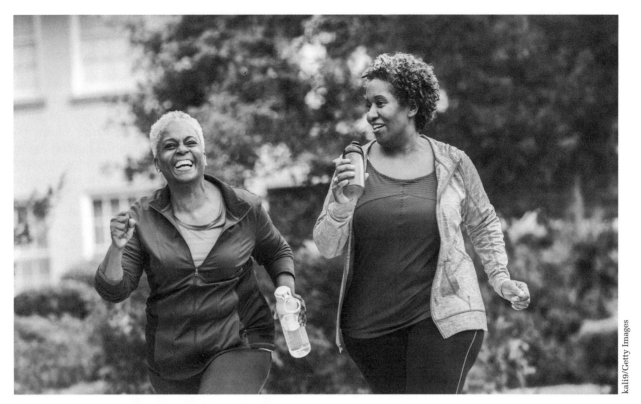

Physical activity—especially with a friend—can help to minimize age-related declines in wellness measures such as health and social support.

The remaining income consists of earnings, assets, and pensions (AoA, 2016).

Being aware of these demographics provides a better understanding of the common characteristics of the aging population. Another key area to be mindful of is the changes in health of the aging adult. A majority of older adults report having one or more chronic conditions. The most frequently reported conditions include diagnosed arthritis (49 percent), all types of heart disease (30 percent), any type of cancer (24 percent), diagnosed diabetes (21.7 percent), and hypertension (high blood pressure or taking high blood pressure medicine, 71 percent; AoA, 2016). Older adults may not only be diagnosed with a chronic condition but may also be living with some type of disability that affects self-care, ambulation, cognition, vision, and hearing (AoA, 2016).

Having chronic illness and disability may increase the likelihood of needing residential care. As of 2014, there were 1.5 million adults 65 and over living in a residential-care setting. For the age group of 85 and older, 10 percent lived in residential care (AoA, 2016). Seventy percent of adults age 70 and over can expect to have a need for some level of residential care services in their lifetime (Harris-Kojetin, Sengupta, & Park-Lee, 2016). The rates of dementia and depression are higher in long-term residential care settings than in other care settings, including home health, hospice, and adult day services (Harris-Kojetin et al., 2016). Residential care services are provided when there is a need for daily assistance in completing activities of daily living, including toileting, dressing, ambulation, eating, bathing, and transferring in and out of bed (Harris-Kojetin et al., 2016). The onset of chronic conditions can lead to excess disability in older adults. If older adults become accustomed to others completing tasks for them, they may stop accomplishing tasks they could ordinarily complete on their own.

Career Opportunities With Seniors

The 2014 CTRS Job Analysis results identified the growing population of therapeutic recreation specialists serving older adults: 30.4 percent of respondents identified the primary client population as geriatric. Of the total respondents, 17.1 percent identified their primary service setting as a skilled-nursing facility, one of the many environments where residential care is provided (National Council for Therapeutic Recreation Certification [NCTRC], 2015).

Although long-term care is where a majority of therapeutic recreation specialists work with older adults, this is not the only option. Therapeutic recreation specialists can also work within hospitals, outpatient services, parks and recreation departments, adult day care settings, private practice, fitness/wellness centers, and Program of All-Inclusive Care for the Elderly (PACE). PACE is a Center for Medicare & Medicaid Services (2018). Therapeutic recreation specialists working with a PACE program would be responsible for conducting assessments to gauge independence and developing individualized care plans in order to maintain and improve each individual's physical, social, emotional, and cognitive functioning. Examples include fitness groups, expressive arts groups, social outings, and educational workshops.

This list is not exhaustive of all the opportunities in the aging field. Going forward, there will be much growth and numerous opportunities for therapeutic recreation specialists to pursue a career in the aging field.

When looking for jobs in the aging field, job titles will vary. Traditionally, therapeutic recreation specialists start by identifying position titles around therapeutic recreation or recreational therapy, or that are associated with their credential, certified therapeutic recreation specialist (CTRS). It is often the case that job titles assigned by employers do not align with these terms, so it is important to review the entire job description when searching for a position. A job descripton may not have the title of therapeutic recreation specialist, but the requirements for that job may be consistent with the therapeutic recreation training and credentials. Examples of such titles include life enrichment coordinator; wellness coordinator; older adult programmer; rehabilitation technician; resident program coordinator; expressive therapist; activity therapist; rehabilitation specialist; and in some cases, activity director, with the understanding that the organization will allow the therapeutic recreation specialist to move the program toward a therapeutic approach instead of only diversional activities.

Theories of Successful Aging

Throughout the years, various ideas about how people age have been proposed. Some theories may still hold true, and other theories have been dismissed as a result of continued research regarding transitions in aging. The following section presents several early and contemporary theories on aging that are relevant to therapeutic recreation.

One early framework for understanding aging is the **activity theory**, which emphasizes the importance of maintaining valued life roles as one ages (e.g., father, grandmother, friend, or coach). Proponents of the activity theory have asserted that successful aging is dependent upon the maintenance of life activities associated with such roles. This perspective directly challenged the **disengagement theory**, which was an early theory based on the assumption that it is natural, and even beneficial, for aging individuals and society to socially disengage from one another. (see Cumming & Henry, 1961). Activity theory presents the alternative perspective that, to age well, individuals must retain and adapt activities as they age (McGuire, Boyd, Janke, & Aybar-Demali, 2013). As such, recreation patterns throughout one's life can have a significant effect on how a person ages. Under this theory, a CTRS would orient therapy goals around enabling participation in activities of interest, particularly those associated with the life roles that contribute to the individual's identity and self-worth. By focusing on these two elements, a CTRS can help decrease a concern for excess disability through providing activities to improve one's self-worth.

Continuity theory, another early framework, asserts that neither disengagement nor continuation of activity interests guarantees successful aging. Instead, the theory emphasizes the importance of personality and environment in aging successfully, noting that the extent to which an individual can successfully maintain life roles and activities is a function of personality-related aging patterns and the circumstances that the individual must navigate (see McGuire et al., 2013, for a more detailed explanation of specific aging patterns). One valuable contribution of the continuity theory is that it acknowledges that not all individuals will react to life circumstances in the same manner and that understanding a person's personality style is an important aspect of assisting him or her in navigating life events and the aging process.

Two additional early frameworks that are relevant to therapeutic recreation are the **selective optimization with compensation (SOC) theory** and the **socioemotional selectivity (SES) theory**. The SOC theory is based upon the belief that individuals decrease personal goals and activities as they age because they want to maximize the abilities they do have (Freund & Baltes, 2002). This theory can be applied to therapeutic recreation interventions in that the therapeutic recreation specialist can provide leisure education to assist older adults in adapting their selected activities to continue participating, especially when chronic medical conditions may be present.

SES theory postulates that, as individuals become older, they begin to decrease their social networks and keep only those relationships that have strong emotional ties (McGuire et al., 2013). Per the theory, older adults will decrease both the number of activities they engage in and the extensiveness of their social networks; however, current research has indicated increased activity and socialization positively affects an older adult's health-related quality of life and positive health behaviors (CDC, 2005). Therapeutic recreation specialists who recognize early the patterns discussed in the SOC and SES theories have the opportunity to intervene and increase socialization and activities among older adults and decrease the possibility of excess disability through activities and the creation of individual goals.

Several contemporary frameworks for aging have been presented in recent years. The **convoy model of social relationships** focuses on the importance of social networks as people age. An individual's convoy, or entourage, is made up of a personal network of family, friends, and other social ties. These social networks can increase an individual's well-being as he or she ages. The social support the convoy provides can help individuals cope with life stresses, including those related to aging. This model also emphasizes the importance of social support to assist the development of an individual's **self-efficacy** (Antonucci, Birditt, & Akiyama, 2009). This theory can be reflected by social opportunities that are provided within residential-care settings and social groups within communities.

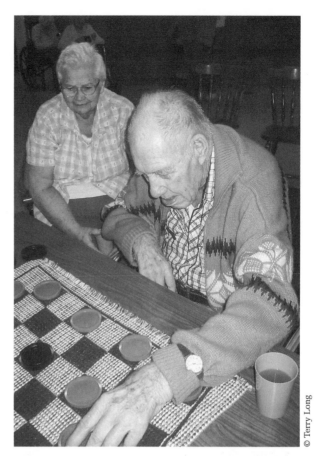

Social networks can increase people's well-being as they age.

Another contemporary theoretical perspective relevant to therapeutic recreation with older adults is the theory of **cognitive plasticity**. Cognitive plasticity is the underlying cognitive potential of an individual (Willis, Schai, & Martin, 2009). Per this theory, plasticity may occur at the behavioral, sociocultural, or neural level (Willis et al., 2009). Behavioral plasticity may be enhanced through cognitive training, which includes repetition of cognitive tasks to accomplish a specific therapeutic goal (Willis et al., 2009). Therapeutic recreation specialists working with older adults may use cognitive training methods to enhance leisure-skill mastery.

The **cumulative inequality theory** provides another contemporary theoretical perspective relevant to therapeutic recreation; this theory illustrates the level of either advantage or disadvantage experienced by individuals or groups of people within society (Ferraro, Shippee, & Schafer, 2009). The level of inequality may be affected by various demographic or developmental factors; once disadvantage or advantage occurs, it may affect other areas of life (Ferraro et al., 2009). The level of disadvantage may create barriers to accessing resources and opportunities for recreation, leisure, and social pursuits. As noted earlier, older adults may be susceptible to disadvantage in regard to social support, income, disability, and accessibility.

Self-determination theory, another contemporary framework, may help therapeutic recreation specialists improve their understanding of what motivates people as well as how to understand specific personality traits (Ryan & Deci, 2000). An example of how to apply this theory to recreation and leisure is related to the characteristic of self-motivation. When self-motivation is present, likely, there is internal locus of control, meaning that individuals feel a strong sense of choice and control in their environments and personal experiences (McGuire et al., 2013; Ryan & Deci, 2000). For self-motivation to be present for leisure participation, three variables need to be present: competence, relatedness, and autonomy (McGuire et al., 2013; Ryan & Deci, 2000). Therapeutic recreation specialists can support achievement of competence through leisure education and modalities that promote skill development (e.g., teaching someone how to use Skype to connect with friends and family). To engage the relatedness variable, therapeutic recreation specialists should seek to understand the personal and social resources of clients; they can attempt to identify where clients' goals match their goals for social networks. Therapeutic recreation specialists can support growth of autonomy by engaging clients throughout the therapeutic process, offering choices, ensuring appropriate levels of risk and challenge, and identifying personal goals.

Person-centered care provides a framework that helps care providers remain focused on the individuality and well-being of clients (Mitchell & Agnelli, 2015). Person-centered care creates a model of care where the person receiving the care is at the center of the decision making regarding treatment and services that will be provided. Traditional care models have a medical model that is adopted from acute care, where physicians, nurses, and other health care professionals make many of the decisions for the person receiving care and may or may not consult the client for feedback. Person-centered care promotes giving the person receiving care a greater sense of control and autonomy in care decisions; this framework

is the current leading model for contemporary residential-care settings.

Like the concept of person-centered care, therapeutic recreation is beginning to embrace more person-centered frameworks to service delivery, including the **strengths-based approach**. Anderson and Heyne (2012a; 2012b) described historical methods of therapeutic recreation service delivery as a deficits approach where problems, barriers, disease, and disability were the main focuses of assessment and treatment planning. These authors also advocate for an alternative strengths-based approach that focuses on identifying interests, strengths, aspirations, talents, and possibilities for growth.

Common Modalities

Theories provide a framework for understanding clients' needs and how therapeutic recreation specialists might help them meet those needs. Modalities are specific methods or techniques that are used within the context of a relevant theory. For example, classic learning theory suggests that rewarded behaviors will reoccur, so a therapeutic recreation specialist would use modalities such as a token economy to teach and maintain desirable behaviors. The modalities described in this chapter can be used in the context of relevant theories to help clients meet therapeutic recreation goals.

Physical Activity

Regular physical activity has been found to have many benefits, but research focused on aging and physical activity is just starting to be recognized. Some of the benefits of physical activity include improved muscle mass, strength, bone mass, flexibility, and aerobic endurance (Chodzko-Zajko et al., 2009; Garber et al., 2011; Haskell et al., 2007; Thompson et al., 2003) as well as improving and maintaining physical function and preventing or reducing falls (Chodzko-Zajko et al., 2009; Kerr, Rosenberg, & Frank, 2012; Nelson et al., 2007). Physical activity can decrease the risk of and help manage stroke, type 2 diabetes, some forms of cancer, high blood pressure and cholesterol, cardiovascular disease, osteoporosis, and chronic obstructive pulmonary disease (Chodzko-Zajko et al., 2009; Garber et al., 2011; Nelson et al., 2007; Physical Activity Guidelines Advisory Committee, 2008; Thompson et al., 2003). Physical activity can also help in areas of cognition. Research has found physical activity can enhance cognitive functioning (Bolandzadeh et al., 2015; Steves, Mehta, Jackson, & Spector, 2016; Vidoni et al., 2015), lower the risk of cognitive decline and dementia (Chodzko-Zajko et al., 2009; Garber et al., 2011; Weuve et al., 2004), and decrease the chance of developing neurodegenerative disorders (Bielak, Antsey, Christensen, & Windsor, 2012). Physical activity also provides mental health benefits such as a decreased risk of depression (Chodzko-Zajko et al., 2009; Physical Activity Guidelines Advisory Committee, 2008), improved quality of life and well-being (Chodzko-Zajko et al., 2009; Physical Activity Guidelines Advisory Committee, 2008), and reduced stress and anxiety

EXEMPLARY PROFESSIONAL

KENNY RILEY, CTRS

Education: BS in Therapeutic Recreation, Grand Valley State University
MA in Community Development, North Park University
Position: Teen Advisor in the Office of Learning and Evaluation
Organization: YMCA of Metropolitan Chicago, Chicago, Illinois

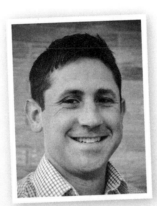

My Career

I started my career at the Kentwood parks and recreation department as a field work student in what will probably always be the best summer job—providing assistance to the athletes in their adapted water-ski program. The following summer I interned at what is now Lurie Children's Hospital in Chicago. When there was an opening, I was hired as a lead recreation therapist in the department of child and adolescent psychiatry in the Partial Hospitalization Unit at Lurie Children's Hospital. While at Lurie Children's, I worked with a social worker to start and research an outpatient social skills therapy group for adolescents with clinical depression and anxiety. After six years of acute treatment, I started to focus more on preventative care and worked in a low-resource Chicago public school with Umoja Student Development Corporation. Through this position, I was able to leverage my social-emotional and behavioral health experience to support students and teachers coping with challenges and build relationships using restorative justice philosophy.

In 2014, I moved to my current role at the YMCA of Metropolitan Chicago, where I have the opportunity to work with youth development professionals in both the suburbs and city to ensure high-quality experiences for all youth.

The YMCA of Metropolitan Chicago has 22 centers and dozens of program sites serving more than 500,000 people annually. The YMCA provides educational programming and health and wellness opportunities for individuals of all ages and socioeconomic statuses. Developmental programs are provided for young people from preschool through the teenage years. My role is to promote integration, coordination, and collaboration in support of the YMCA mission and strategic goals to ensure school readiness and academic achievement for all program participants. I serve as a subject matter expert in the design of training modules, workshops, and strategic partnerships.

My favorite thing about my various positions is the opportunity to meet wonderful people and hear about their passions and, every once in a while, help them to find new ones. I enjoy working with staff members as they try new techniques to help participants gain the skills they need to move toward recreation independence.

My Advice to You

A degree in therapeutic recreation leads you to so many worthwhile endeavors. Don't be afraid to take on a new position or create a new one that previously did not exist. Take time to attend conferences, meet others in the field, and get involved in your state and national organizations. I have found therapeutic recreation professionals to be some of the most caring people, not only in regard to their clients but also to their colleagues. We all want to see the next generation of therapeutic recreation professionals be successful, and you will find that many of us are more than willing to provide mentorship, job opportunities, or job search advice if you only ask.

levels (Chodzko-Zajko et al., 2009; Garber et al, 2011; Stephan, Sutin, & Terracciano, 2014).

Common goals associated with physical activity include maintenance and/or improvement in aerobic endurance, muscular endurance and strength, balance, and flexibility (Chodzko-Zajko et al., 2009). Other goals that can be addressed through physical activity include improved cognition, reaction time, coordination, bone density, mobility, and gait patterns and reduced falls (McGuire et al., 2013); improved socialization (Chang et al., 2014); reduced stress; and coping with depression (Chodzko-Zajko et al., 2009; Garber et al., 2011). There are many specific techniques that can be used to address physical activity among older adults, such as walking/hiking, jogging, water aerobics, dancing, and sports. Following are examples of effective applications of physical activity.

Physical Activity Classes

A physical activity program for older adults should contain aerobic, strength, balance, and flexibility activities (Chodzko-Zajko et al., 2009), and program goals should include social engagement, boosting confidence and feelings of self-worth, and creating feelings of adequacy. Traditional physical activity classes are not always successful when programming for older adults, but the following strategies can help ensure success. Practitioners need to create a welcoming and positive social environment. Whenever possible, it is important to include cognitive and social elements in classes, such as focusing on coordination drills when performing aerobic movements. Leaders need to create environments that promote self-efficacy among participants. For instance, clearly describing, modeling, and adapting each movement is vital to building a sense of confidence and ensuring success for all participants, whether novices or experienced.

An example of an evidence-based physical activity program is EnhanceFitness, developed by the University of Washington Health Promotion Research Center. The program consists of stretching, flexibility and balance exercises, low-impact aerobics, and strength training. The focus is to maintain or improve functional abilities and independence. The EnhanceFitness program provides training workshops for professionals, which include program protocols, leading classes, performing fitness assessments, and how to collect data during the program (Belza & PRC-HAN Physical Activity Conference Planning Workshop, 2007).

Yoga and Tai Chi

Yoga is an example of a specific technique within the physical activity category that has been found to be beneficial for older adults. Research has indicated yoga not only provides improvements in balance, strength, and flexibility, but also has shown cognitive benefits as well. A study conducted by Eyre and colleagues (2016) found individuals who completed weekly 60-minute yoga sessions with meditation for 12 weeks demonstrated improvements in depression and memory recall. Yoga can be taught in the traditional floor format or adapted for sitting on a chair. The yoga format for older adults follows the traditional yoga format, but some modifications may be necessary for individuals who have health concerns in performing all the moves as intended.

Tai chi consists of various postures that are taught in sequential order. The movements are slow and rhythmic. Attention to body movement, breathing, relaxation, and weight shifting and inattention to negative thoughts are all elements of

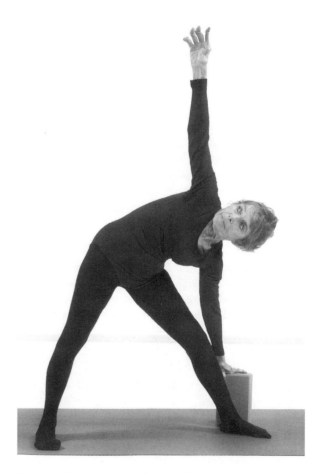

Yoga provides many benefits for older adults.

tai chi practice. Tai chi has been shown to improve physical and cognitive function (Taylor-Piliae et al., 2010) and assist in the management of arthritis and other chronic diseases. Tai chi exercises can be implemented into various physical activities, with the goal of reducing falls (Tousignant et al., 2013).

Sports

As adults age, one should not assume the desire to participate in various sports declines. Research has indicated involvement in senior sports is affiliated with increases in physical and social activities and engagement (Cardenas, Henderson, & Wilson, 2009). One example of an organization promoting senior sports is the National Senior Games Association. The games are held every other year in a different location in the United States for participants ages 50 and up. Examples of the 19 sports offered are archery, cycling, pickleball, swimming, triathlon, horseshoes, and bowling (National Senior Games Association, 2016). Another example of sport competition for older adults is the National Veterans Golden Age Games. This competition is for U.S. veterans who are 55 and older and receiving care from the U.S. Department of Veterans Affairs. Examples of sports include air rifle, boccia ball, shuffleboard, and track and field. A core responsibility of the therapeutic recreation specialist is to provide leisure education to older adults about the opportunities to participate in such athletic games. Another role the therapeutic recreation specialist would fill is to help each athlete improve or maintain his or her overall fitness, teach the specific sport skill sets, enhance self-efficacy, and provide social and emotional support.

Wheelchair Biking

Although cycling for older adults has been popular, wheelchair biking is an option for individuals who may not be able to bike because of health concerns or disabilities. The wheelchair bike consists of the back half of a bicycle attached to a wheelchair, allowing the chair to serve as the front wheel. The wheelchair has adjustable padding and footrests and headrests, and can be tilted back for the rider. Research conducted by Buettner and Fitzsimmons (2003) examined the effects of a daily 2-week wheelchair riding intervention on dementia and depressive symptoms among older adults living in residential care. Outcomes indicated a decrease in mild to moderate depressive symptoms among the participants.

Boxing

Using boxing as a form of physical activity for older adults may seem untraditional and intimidating, but research is indicating that boxing can have many positive effects, specifically for older adults with Parkinson's disease. Benefits of boxing include improved gait, balance, activities of daily living, and quality of life (Combs et al., 2011). An example of a boxing program specifically for Parkinson's disease is Rock Steady Boxing. The gym originated in Indianapolis, Indiana, and currently has over 600 gym affiliates worldwide. There are various levels of classes designed to accommodate various Parkinson's symptoms and individuals' overall levels of fitness. Within the class, participants do not box with each other, but perform drills and workouts similar to a traditional boxing training program. Class structure consists of a warm-up, an exercise portion, and a cool-down. The exercises completed will vary, but the structure of the class remains consistent throughout the program. Cardiovascular, strength, flexibility, and balance exercises are all included. The gym's structure not only includes addressing the physical aspects of Parkinson's, but also focuses on other areas the disease can affect, such as voice activation and socialization.

Lifelong Learning

Providing education to older adults is an additional modality that therapeutic recreation specialists may use when working with this population. Continuing education workshops provide many benefits for older adults. Some reasons older adults attend workshops include to enhance general knowledge, invest in personal development, increase social interaction, learn more to help others, and make productive use of their free time (Cachioni et al., 2014). Workshops can provide comprehensive programming to meet various goals related to social, cognitive, physical, and emotional domains. Various techniques used include hands-on activities, group discussions, and lectures (Zijlstra et al., 2009). Educational workshops can be found in both community and residential-care settings. For example, fall prevention workshops focus on education and prevention of falls. Educators provide information on fall risks and exercises to improve balance and strength. Through the education, self-efficacy is developed to help decrease the risk of falls (Smith, Jiang, & Ory, 2012; Zijlstra et al., 2009).

Educational workshops do not need to be limited to only fall prevention. The topics are endless, but other general areas include healthy living, creative arts, technology, advances in fields of interest, brain health, support groups, chronic diseases, and disability. One evidence-based practice example of lifelong learning was created by the Stanford Patient Education Research Center. The name of the program is Chronic Disease Self-Management. It is a 2 1/2-hour, 6-week-long workshop held in various community settings, such as libraries, churches, senior centers, and hospitals. Content covered in the workshop includes techniques to help deal with problems associated with chronic diseases; appropriate exercises for maintaining and improving strength; appropriate use of medications; communicating with friends, family, and health professionals; nutrition; decision making; and how to evaluate new treatment methods. The basis of the workshop is to help build self-efficacy by creating confidence that participants can master new skills. Research results indicated those who participated in the program showed improvements in exercise, cognitive symptom management, communication with health professionals, self-reported general health, health distress, fatigue, disability, and social/role activities limitations (Lorig, Sobel, Ritter, Laurent, & Hobbs, 2001).

Creative Arts

Creative arts programs are known to be effective treatment modalities in working with older adults (Fritsch et al., 2009). These types of programs promote decision making and expression of individuality and life experiences and beliefs; therefore, creative expression interventions promote a person-centered model of working with older adults (Fritsch et al., 2009). Therapeutic recreation specialists facilitating creative expressions should use strengths-based approaches. The goals of creative expressions groups should not solely be completion of a painting, craft, or project; there should be specific therapeutic goals in mind that enhance recreation, leisure, and social functioning of the participants.

TimeSlips, a facilitated creative writing and storytelling method, has been shown to increase client engagement and improve staff-to-resident interactions throughout residential-care communities (Fritsch et al., 2009). Facilitators use a variety of thought-provoking photos that may be funny or strange to get the group to look at details of the photos and share what they see and think may happen next. Facilitators are trained how to use a variety of questions throughout the group to promote individual participation; every comment or sound offered by participants is validated and folded into the creation of a story.

Music

Music may be used as a tool in group sessions to achieve therapeutic goals, including a reduction in anxiety (Sung, Lee, Li, & Watson, 2012) and agitated behavior (Lin et al., 2011) and an activation of the entire limbic system in the brain responsible for processing emotions and working memory (Jäncke, 2008). Music & Memory is a program where staff members in residential-care communities use iPods to create personalized music playlists for older adults with dementia. The effect of the Music & Memory program has been widely shown in the movie Alive Inside (2014).

The Java Music Club is a structured program that provides a framework for a mutual support group for older adults, co-led by both the therapeutic recreation specialist and an older adult participant; the group incorporates music, art, and spirituality and provides the opportunity to voice feelings about a variety of topics chosen by the group. The goals of the Java Music Club include offering choices and opportunities for decision making along with providing opportunities to engage residents in peer support or focusing their energies on developing meaningful and authentic, supportive relationships (Cunningham, n.d.; Theurer et al., 2015).

Memories in the Making is a group art program for individuals in early to midstage dementia designed to enhance socialization through creative expression and the use of sensory stimulation techniques. The individual with dementia engages with a variety of art media and is paired with a care partner and trained volunteer (Alzheimer's Association, 2017). Participants in the program demonstrated higher engagement, positive feelings of self-worth, and greater attention span than participants in other group activities (Kinney & Rentz, 2005).

Additional modalities within the realm of creative expressions that may address treatment goals for older adults include scrapbooking or creation of memory books, photography, journaling, art journaling, poetry writing, and legacy writing. Goals the therapeutic recreation specialist may consider for the treatment plan include improved feelings of self-worth and leisure competence, sensory stimulation, or stress management and coping skill development.

Animal-Assisted Therapy

Animal-assisted therapy is an evidence-based practice for older adults. Animal-assisted therapy can positively affect behavioral symptoms and socialization of older adults with dementia, reduce depression in older adults living in institutionalized settings, improve physical function of older adults, and decrease levels of agitation for older adults in residential-care communities (Cherniack & Cherniack, 2014). Therapeutic recreation specialists should identify active treatment goals for older adult clients related to the animal-assisted interventions; there are physical, cognitive, and social goals that may be achieved through interaction with the therapy animal.

Technology-Based Modalities

The use of technology as a therapeutic modality to improve social connections for older adults has rapidly increased in recent years. Technology applications provide a means for overcoming barriers of limited access to beneficial resources and services as seen in studies on the use of teleconferencing for family caregivers (Czaja, Loewenstein, Schulz, Nair, & Perdomo, 2013; Meyer, Marx, & Ball-Seiter, 2011). The generation of **Baby Boomers** is more likely than previous generations of older adults to have been previously exposed to technology, which will lead to less likelihood of perceived lack of technological competence than with previous generations (Fox, 2004, as cited in McGuire et al., 2013).

An example of a technology intervention includes the use of interactive touch screen technology, such as the It's Never 2 Late (iN2L) computer system. The iN2L system combines a touch-screen computer system with a simplified icon-based software design. In a case study completed with Westminster-Canterbury on Chesapeake Bay, a nonprofit life-care community, the therapeutic recreational coordinator managed therapeutic recreation interns in working one-on-one with elders with dementia to engage them with the touch-screen systems; an outcome that was unanticipated was that some residents self-initiated engagement outside of intervention times with an intern (Powell, 2016).

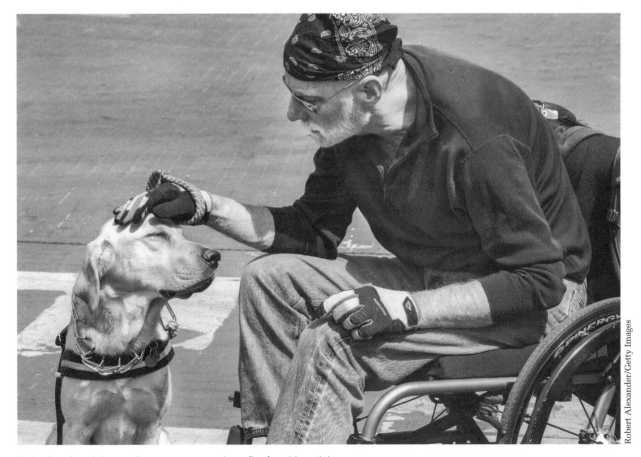

Animal-assisted therapy has many proven benefits for older adults.

Robert Alexander/Getty Images

Julio, an older adult with advanced dementia, lives in a long-term-care community. Through a comprehensive assessment, the CTRS determined Julio's historical occupation and leisure history included living in Rome, being a sought-after artist, restoring artwork in cathedrals, and speaking three languages. The CTRS, by using touch-screen computer technology via the iN2L system, engaged Julio in using a computerized paint program to practice the fine motor skills of gripping and moving the touch screen–sensitive paintbrush on the screen. The CTRS started a playlist of Julio's preferred music, and nonverbal prompts were used to regain attention to the painting task as needed. Julio engaged in using various grips of the paintbrush to achieve different strokes; maintained eye contact; nodded his head in response to questions from the CTRS; remained engaged by painting on the touch screen; and then, with prompts, transitioned work to a traditional canvas with paint and paintbrush. Julio maintained attention in the painting session for more than 30 minutes without rest breaks or diversion from the task. Julio's affect brightened; he smiled and sang and hummed to the music playing in the background.

Therapeutic recreation specialists may use a variety of technology-based tools for treatment interventions, including multiple cognitive training tools and multiple interactive touch-screen target games, word games, and trivia. Therapeutic recreation specialists may use sensory and relaxation tools, including experiential sensory videos of fishing, gardening, crocheting, and farming, to promote reminiscence. Outside of the iN2L and other similar tools, therapeutic recreation specialists can use any hardware with Web access to connect to online cognitive training programs, such as Dakim or Lumosity; entertainment sites, such as Netflix and YouTube; and social networking sites, such as Facebook, Twitter, and Instagram.

Technology not only provides the benefits noted above, but can also improve socialization for older adults with friends and family. Skype has been shown to decrease loneliness assessment scores for older adults after only 1 week of intervention; depression scores have been shown to be reduced after 3 months of routine Skype intervention (Tsai & Tsai, 2011).

Dementia Frameworks

The dementia practice guideline for recreational therapy (DPG) and the N.E.S.T. approach (needs, environment, stimulation, techniques) provide evidence-based frameworks for treatment of disturbing behaviors observed in dementia care.

The DPG and N.E.S.T. programs outline a comprehensive description of dementia, provide guidelines for assessment, offer an illustration of the need-driven dementia-compromised behavior (NDB) model, which specifies that behaviors observed in dementia may be a result of unmet needs or goals of the person with dementia (Algase et al., 1996). The DPG and N.E.S.T. approaches promote greater problem solving for why behaviors occur and recommend implementation of evidence-based therapeutic recreation interventions to improve various skills in the physical, cognitive, and psychosocial domains (Fitzsimmons, Sardina, & Buettner, 2008).

When they are familiar with the evidence-based protocols offered in these programs, therapeutic recreation specialists become powerful assets to residential-care community interdisciplinary teams that are trying to find strengths-based engagement options to use as a means of preventing apathy, agitation, or anxiety. These evidence-based protocols also equip therapeutic recreation specialists to become vital to discussions involving nonpharmacological treatment of behaviors that may occur for residents with dementia.

Therapeutic recreation specialists serving older adults in long-term-care communities must understand and follow regulatory standards provided by the Centers for Medicare & Medicaid Services (CMS) regarding the activity program. Long-term-care communities are expected to promote the "highest practicable level of well-being," defined as provision of care and services to prevent any avoidable declines and/or minimize lack of improvement in functioning (CMS, 2016).

In long-term care, therapeutic recreation specialists will use therapeutic modalities designed to enhance well-being in the mental, physical, social/emotional, and spiritual domains. Many long-term-care communities expect that a therapeutic recreation specialist will be able to build the therapeutic recreation program, so an understanding of evidence-based practice and frameworks for therapeutic recreation program development is essential.

Therapeutic recreation specialists working with older adults with dementia may consider use of simplified tasks and activities based on Montessori techniques proven to increase engagement and attention (Van der Ploeg & O'Connor, 2010). Another potentially useful approach is an adaptation of validation therapy, called integrative validation therapy, which provides guidance for caregivers who promote positive perceptions of older adults with dementia and therapeutic tools for communication (Erdmann & Schnepp, 2014).

All of the above modalities and frameworks can help to address excess disability. Through providing engaging roles and goals for older adults, the discussed modalities and frameworks can assist in providing a person a sense of purpose, self, and accomplishment, a common goal in therapeutic recreation.

Summary

Older adults encounter many life changes as they age, from health and financial concerns to social well-being. By having a basic understanding of aging theories and frameworks, such as activity theory and person-centered care, therapeutic recreation specialists possess skills and knowledge that can positively assist older adults in life changes through evidenced-based interventions, such as physical activity, creative arts, and technology-based modalities.

DISCUSSION QUESTIONS

1. Explain how basing interventions on the activity theory can play a role in decreasing excess disability for an older adult.

2. Describe how the self-determination theory can influence a therapeutic recreation specialist's approach to encouraging physical activity for an older adult.

3. Discuss at least two challenges (found in this chapter) that an older adult may experience as he or she ages. Choose one of those challenges and a modality discussed in this chapter. Explain how the chosen modality can help to positively address the chosen challenge.

4. Explain how the techniques associated with the discussed dementia-based frameworks can help decrease disturbing behaviors observed among those diagnosed with dementia.

5. Interview a person over the age of 65. Discuss with him or her any health, financial, or social challenges he or she may have encountered and the techniques he or she used to cope with those challenges.

6. Complete an online search for therapeutic recreation specialist positions. Search for the titles of life enrichment coordinator, wellness coordinator, older adult programmer, resident program coordinator, activity therapist, expressive therapist, and activity director. Compare the job descriptions. What are the commonalities and differences between the job descriptions? Describe how the skills of a therapeutic recreation specialist fit the associated job descriptions and titles.

12

A Global Perspective of Therapeutic Recreation

Rodney Dieser | Heewon Yang
Shane Pegg | Shinichi Nagata

LEARNING OUTCOMES

At the end of this chapter, students will be able to

- describe similarities and differences between the historical development of therapeutic recreation in the United States and in other countries,
- identify political, socioeconomic, and cultural factors that might affect the nature of therapeutic recreation services in various regions of the world,
- describe current trends and issues in the therapeutic recreation profession as they exist in several countries, and
- discuss alternative possibilities regarding the conceptualization, development, and delivery of therapeutic recreation services in the United States as well as other countries.

This chapter comprises several short narratives that describe various issues and examples of therapeutic recreation from a global perspective. Rod Dieser begins with a discussion of Canada. Next, Heewon Yang describes how therapeutic recreation has developed in South Korea. Shinichi Nagata summarizes the influence of therapeutic recreation on recreation-based services for people with disabilities in Japan, and last, Shane Pegg describes therapeutic recreation from an Australian perspective. Through this exploration of how therapeutic recreation services and other related concepts manifest around the globe, students can expand their understanding of possibilities within other frameworks and cultures.

Therapeutic Recreation in Canada

As in the United States, intolerance for people with special needs was widespread in Canada throughout the 1800s. Most people with special needs were hidden in Canadian society through institutionalization. According to Hutchison and McGill (1998), not until the late 1920s did Canada move away from an institutional–custodial model of care to people with special needs living in the community (see Hutchison & McGill for a listing of Canadian legislation and critical events related to deinstitutionalization). Before the 1980s, most provinces and territories in Canada had informal therapeutic recreation programs usually associated with broader health and human services professional organizations, such as the Adapted Programs Committee of the Canadian Association for Health, Physical Education, and Recreation (Velde & Murphy, 1994). A brief overview of **Canadian federalism** (political ideology of Canada) will be useful in explaining therapeutic recreation in Canada because the issue of Canadian federalism is at the core of contemporary therapeutic recreation practice and professional development in Canada (Dieser, 2002b; Dieser, 2005/2006; Ostiguy & Dieser, 2004).

Canadian Federalism

Canada is a bilingual country: English and French. The country consists of 10 provinces (similar to states in the United States) and 3 large northern territories. Furthermore, the provinces and territories exhibit strong cultural differences. For example, Quebec has a large French culture,

Alberta has a large English culture, and Nunavut has a large Inuit culture. Furthermore, within these broad provincial and territorial regions are within- and between-group differences. For example, a small French-speaking population (4 to 6 percent) resides on Baffin Island in Nunavut, and among Canadian provinces, Saskatchewan has a higher population of First Nation people (Canadian American Indians) than other provinces (Statistics Canada, 2004).

Multiculturalism (the political ideology of the mosaic) is at the core of Canadian federalism. Canadian federalism is a political system in which the constitutional authority to make laws and public policy is divided between a national government and regional governments (Brooks, 2000). The result is that throughout Canada, provinces and territories have a paramount role as guardians of regional and cultural identities and differences (Vipond, 1991). Canadian federalism is an "expression of both diversity and unity" (Gagnon, 1995, p. 23). As such, Canadian provinces and territories have jurisdiction over health and human services, such as programs to help people with disabilities (Cameron & Valentine, 2001). In short, this means that provinces and territories in Canada can have distinctive health and human services legislation, public policies, and human services programs (unlike, for example, in the United States, where the Americans with Disabilities Act allows the federal government to override the states on a variety of issues). Hence, Canadian federalism, which allows diversity in provincial and territorial health and human services programs, is different from American federalism, which is based on homogeneity, standardization, and melting-pot cultural practices (Laselva, 1996).

A Brief History of Therapeutic Recreation in Canada

Both knowingly and unknowingly, the political ideology of Canadian federalism has been at the root of professional therapeutic recreation development in Canada. Until 1996, when the Canadian Therapeutic Recreation Association (CTRA) was incorporated, Canada had no national therapeutic recreation professional organization such as the American Therapeutic Recreation Association in the United States. Instead, provincial and territorial therapeutic recreation organizations (e.g., British Columbia Therapeutic Recreation Association, Therapeutic Recreation Association of Quebec, or

L'association de loisir thérapeutique du Québec) had strong professional leadership roles in their respective provinces and territories.

Today, the mission of the CTRA (see www.canadian-tr.org/about) is to advocate and develop the profession of therapeutic recreation by

- promoting and facilitating communication between and among members in therapeutic recreation,
- developing and implementing a plan that will lead to national certification of therapeutic recreation practitioners,
- promoting and advancing public awareness and understanding of therapeutic recreation,
- developing and promoting the adoption and implementation of professional standards for the delivery of therapeutic recreation services, and
- supporting excellence and advancement in education and research in therapeutic recreation.

In May 2009, the Canadian Therapeutic Recreation Association and the American-based National Council for Therapeutic Recreation Certification (NCTRC) agreed to a partnership whereby the NCTRC credential (certified therapeutic recreation specialist, or CTRS) would be the recognized certification credential in Canada. Prior to this, there was a professional debate regarding whether the CTRA should adopt a Canadian-based (Canadian federalism) framework, titled the Mosaic Certification Framework (MCF), or align with the U.S. NCTRC model (or hold off on developing a credentialing certification framework for the short term; Diane Bowtell, personal communication, October 14, 2005). Dieser's scholarship (2002a, 2004b, 2005a) argued that MCF was a better route for Canadian therapeutic recreation to go because (1) it allowed different provinces/territories of Canada to serve their diverse populations (e.g., Francophone culture of Quebec or the Inuit culture of Nunavut) and (2) it rejected the American individualistic melting-pot political ideology that served as NCTRC's foundation (see Dieser, 2002a; Dieser, 2004b; Dieser, 2005b). In addition, Dieser (2002a, 2004a, 2005a, 2005b) outlined how the MCF is based on three important axioms. The first axiom is to follow the political ideology of Canadian federalism, which would develop a national therapeutic recreation credentialing and certification framework in which the CTRA would work in partnership with the 10 therapeutic recreation provincial organizations and the 3 therapeutic recreation territorial professional organizations. This action would support Canadian federalism because it would allow provincial and territorial therapeutic recreation professional organizations to protect regional and cultural differences. Table 12.1, adapted from Dieser (2005b), underscores the relationship between Canadian federalism and the MCF.

Table 12.1 Relationship Between Canadian Federalism and the Mosaic Certification Framework

Canadian federalism	Policies of the CTRA
Divides public policy between a national government and regional government organizations (provincial or territorial therapeutic recreation [TR] organizations) and universities and colleges	Divides TR policy (e.g., education) between a national organization (CTRA) and regional organizations
Recognizes the paramount role of provincial or territorial governments as guardians of regional identities and differences	Recognizes the paramount role of provincial and territorial TR organizations as guardians of regional identities and differences
Establishes practical and flexible institutional arrangements and relationships that allow intercommunity cooperation	Establishes practical and flexible TR institutional and provincial or territorial arrangements and relationships that allow intercommunity cooperation
Celebrates cross-cultural diversity in educational structure in different regions of Canada	Celebrates cross-cultural diversity in curriculum

Adapted by permission from R.B. Dieser, "Outlining a Canadian Framework for Therapeutic Recreation Professionalism: A Mosaic Certification Framework Part II (Planting seeds)," *Tribune* (2005): 7-9.

The second axiom of the MCF is to follow collaboration and unity within a paradigm of diversity among the CTRA, provincial and territorial therapeutic recreation organizations, and universities and colleges. Unity can occur by having the CTRA identify the entry-level core competencies through genuine dialogue with university and college administrators and provincial and territorial therapeutic recreation organizations. For example, Dieser (2005/2006) suggested four standardized courses oriented toward (a) foundational aspects of therapeutic recreation (e.g., history, concepts, theories, therapeutic recreation practice models, and professional organizations), (b) therapeutic recreation program design, (c) therapeutic recreation intervention and facilitation techniques (e.g., animal-assisted therapy, bibliotherapy, and community integration), and (d) leisure theory (e.g., Neulinger's leisure paradigm, postmodern leisure, flow, and serious leisure).

The third axiom of the MCF is to have a strong multicultural commitment. Provincial and territorial therapeutic recreation organizations and universities and colleges can collaborate to develop a list of specialty multicultural courses and fieldwork experiences that are relevant to their regions.

Table 12.2, adapted from Dieser (2005/2006), underscores the similarities and differences of the MCF and the NCTRC. The result is that beyond taking the four standardized classes, students who graduate from one university in Canada would have competencies and skills different from students who graduate from another university. For example, the University of Regina (Saskatchewan) could require that all therapeutic recreation students take course work and a fieldwork experience related to First Nation culture, whereas the University of Waterloo (Ontario) could require students to take multiple course work in assessment and evaluative procedures. The MCF, like Canadian federalism, relies on the concept of tolerance, harmony, and unity within a paradigm of diversity. Although CTRA agreed to a partnership where the NCTRC certification credential is recognized, the MCF still offers an alternative credentialing or organizational framework, one that values embracing diverse cultures, for other countries to adopt.

Concerns and Conflict in the Profession

One of the unique aspects of the therapeutic recreation profession in Canada is that there is a large group of therapeutic recreation specialists who hold a 2-year college diploma (what is known as an associate's degree in the United States). In the province of Alberta, for example, 44 percent of those in the therapeutic recreation profession have a 2-year degree (Alberta Therapeutic Recreation Association, 2010). Because of NCTRC credentialing, these professionals, the people who built the profession of therapeutic recreation, are being abandoned or forced to go to university to earn a bachelor's degree to gain NCTRC credentialing. Past president of the Alberta Therapeutic Recreation Association, Lorraine Grover (personal communication, November 12, 2010) stated the following as she reflected on how the CTRA-NCTRC partnership is dividing and hurting the profession of therapeutic recreation in Alberta and across Canada: "Rather than using CTRS as a potential examination to provide the general public with an assurance of a baseline of competency, a rather large group of [2-year diploma] recreation therapists have been excluded." Further, as Dieser (2012) noted, there is concern that this will divide the broader therapeutic recreation profession in Alberta and across Canada (similar to how therapeutic recreation is a divided profession in the United States; see chapter 2). Although other Canadian Provinces are grappling with the bachelor's degree versus two-year diploma debate, in January 2017, the Alberta Therapeutic Recreation Association membership voted that a bachelor's degree will serve as the entry to practice. This will commence April of 2021 (see http://www.alberta-tr.org/for-the-public/qualifications-of-a-recreation-therapist.aspx).

Connected to seeing therapeutic recreation differently in Canada (and around the world), in 2015, *Leisure/Loisor*, the *Journal of the Canadian Association for Leisure Studies*, dedicated an entire journal (volume 32, issue 2) to reimagining therapeutic recreation and transforming practice. Collectively, the seven articles reaffirmed how therapeutic recreation needs to return to its roots of leisure and use leisure (not therapy) to help people, such as confronting ageism (Genoe & Whyte, 2015), inclusion for women leaving prison (Fortune & Yuen, 2015), and care sharing as a form of social justice through dance (Eales & Goodwin, 2015). This issue was bookended by Sylvester (2015) advocating for critical reflection to challenge and reimagine dominant therapeutic recreation views (i.e., deficit-based medical model approaches) and Arai, Berbary, and Dupuis (2015) encouraging more playfulness and social justice

Table 12.2 Similarities and Differences Between the NCTRC and the MCF Credentialing Processes

NCTRC	MCF
1. A baccalaureate degree or higher from an accredited college or university with a major in therapeutic recreation or recreation or leisure with an option in therapeutic recreation.	1. CTRA would develop a national credentialing structure in which (a) a therapeutic recreation technician holds a 1- or 2-year diploma from a college, (b) a therapeutic recreation specialist holds a bachelor's degree from a university, and (c) a recreational therapist holds a master's or doctorate degree from a university. The diploma or degree must be from a college or university with a major in recreation, leisure, or therapeutic recreation studies.
2. A minimum of 18 semester hours or 27 quarter hours of therapeutic recreation and general recreation content course work with no less than 12 semester hours or 18 quarter hours in therapeutic recreation content.	2. For national consistency, CTRA maintains that the TR technician, TR specialist, or recreational therapist must have entry-level competencies in
3. Supportive courses to include a total of 18 semester hours or 27 quarter hours of support course work with a minimum of (a) 3 semester hours or 3 quarter hours of course work in the content area of anatomy and physiology; (b) 3 semester hours or 3 quarter hours of course work in the content area of abnormal psychology; and (c) 3 semester hours or 3 quarter hours of course work in the content area of human growth and development across the life span. The remaining semester hours or quarter hours of course work must be fulfilled in the content area of human services as defined by NCTRC (e.g., adapted physical education or psychology).	a. leisure theory (e.g., serious leisure, flow, classic leisure, postmodern leisure, and Neulinger's leisure paradigm); b. foundational aspects of therapeutic recreation (e.g., history, concepts, theories, TR practice models, and professional organizations); c. therapeutic recreation program design; and d. therapeutic recreation intervention and facilitation techniques (e.g., animal-assisted therapy, bibliotherapy, and community integration). 3. Specialty courses and field placement developed by university and college departments in partnership with provincial or territorial therapeutic recreation professional organizations will be different in different provinces or territories and universities or colleges. Examples: critical thinking, community development, clinical TR practice, community TR practice, women in politics, leisure education, medical terminology, leadership, qualitative evaluation, marketing and promotion, tourism, disabling conditions, recreation programming, issues and trends in health care, ethics in human services, counseling psychology, health promotion, human anatomy, park design, film studies, adapted physical education, outdoor education, computer technology, research and evaluation, abnormal psychology, sociology of mental disorders, history of human services, environmental philosophy, family ecology, statistics, theories of sex and gender, management and administration, disaster relief, crime and public policy, or sign language.
4. A field placement experience of at least 480 hours over 12 consecutive weeks in therapeutic recreation services that uses the therapeutic recreation process as defined by the current NCTRC Job Analysis Study under the supervision of an on-site field placement supervisor who is NCTRC CTRS certified.	4. Specialty course and field placement focused on multiculturalism will be different in different provinces or territories and universities or colleges. Examples: cross-cultural therapeutic recreation, cross-cultural counseling, cross-cultural communication, cross-cultural perspectives on mental health, critical pedagogy in indigenous education, First Nation perspectives on nature, fieldwork placement into a diverse culture, indigenous feminism, cross-cultural policy reform, French language, classic Chinese poetry, Korean art, Spanish language, Japanese music, history of Ukrainian Canadians, Hungarian dance, foods from East Asia, international relations, history of Canadian multicultural policy, Francophone culture, ritual and symbolism, cultural museum studies, cross-cultural conflict resolution, cross-cultural substance dependency, gender in cross-cultural perspective, cross-cultural gerontology, social inequality, world religions, cultural perspective of death and dying, or cross-cultural leisure theory.

Adapted by permission from R.B. Dieser, "Outlining a Canadian Framework for Therapeutic Recreation Professionalism: A Mosaic Certification Framework Part 1," *Tribune* (2005): 6-9.

in therapeutic recreation (as opposed to rigid and standardized protocols).

Therapeutic Recreation in South Korea

The historical origins of therapeutic recreation in South Korea may be found in the leisure and recreation movement of the 1960s. O-Joong Kim, a pioneer in the field of leisure and recreation in South Korea, established the Leisure and Recreation Association in Korea (LRAK) in 1960 (Kim, 2000). South Korea was in an adverse economic, political, and social situation in the 1960s because the country had gone through national tragedies, such as the colonization by Japan (1910-1945) and the Korean War (1950-1953). Thus, during the 1960s, the primary purposes of recreation programs were to provide Korean people with pleasurable experiences and help increase economic productivity through enjoyable recreational activities (Noh & Lee, 2004).

In 1963, Ewha Women's University offered recreation as an academic course for the first time in South Korea, and in the late 1980s, several universities created recreation-related majors in their graduate programs. These academic efforts introduced the concept of therapeutic recreation to South Korea (Noh & Lee, 2004).

It was not until the late 1980s that the public began to view recreation as an essential component of people's lives. People regarded recreation as simple games, and recreation leaders were considered game leaders. But since 1988, when South Korea hosted the Seoul Paralympics, opportunities for sports and recreational services for people with disabilities and interest in recreation and therapeutic recreation have steadily increased in South Korea. The following sections address therapeutic recreation professional organizations, the therapeutic recreation certification system, therapeutic recreation education and training programs, and the challenges of growth faced by therapeutic recreation professionals in South Korea.

Emergence of Professional Organizations

In the 1990s, people with social work backgrounds ignited the development of therapeutic recreation in South Korea. For instance, in 1990, Jun-Ahn Chae established the Center for Recreational Services for People with Disabilities, and in 1992, Chae started several experimental therapeutic recreation programs for people with intellectual disabilities. In the following year (1993), Chae established the Korean Therapeutic Recreation Association (KTRA), which is regarded as the first therapeutic recreation professional organization in South Korea. KTRA contributed to the development of therapeutic recreation in South Korea in many ways. For instance, the organization introduced the concept of therapeutic recreation to the Korean general public; initiated therapeutic recreation services in health care settings, including hospitals and rehabilitation centers; established a clinical center; and started education and training programs for potential therapeutic recreation specialists.

Until recently, KTRA had been working primarily on three service areas: (a) development and provision of therapeutic recreation programs to clients in several areas, (b) research on the effectiveness of therapeutic recreation intervention programs, and (c) education and training programs for future therapeutic recreation specialists. Although the initial efforts, in both research and practice, have been directed primarily to older adult populations, KTRA has been trying to expand its target populations to include people with developmental disabilities, psychiatric disorders, and mental illnesses as well as children and adolescents (KTRA, 2006).

Since 1995, several books about therapeutic recreation have been published, and academic publications, such as theses and dissertations, have been available. But during the 1990s, most of the material and resources regarding therapeutic recreation introduced only the leisure ability model (Peterson & Gunn, 1984, Stumbo & Peterson, 2004), focusing on recreation participation and appropriate leisure lifestyles.

Several professional organizations and institutes were established after the emergence of KTRA. For example, Daehan Therapeutic Recreation Association (DTRA) was founded by Jaesub Yoon in 1995. Yoon and his colleagues decided that therapeutic recreation needed a more focused organizational advocate. That is, they were more concerned with the clinical practice of therapeutic recreation and viewed therapeutic recreation as a specific tool of treatment or rehabilitation effective in combating difficulties associated with primary disabilities. Examples of their primary practice and research areas included (a) natural and ecological therapeutic recreation programs

KAYLA HAAS AND LILLY BRODERICK

Education: BA in Therapeutic Recreation (Cooperative Program), University of Waterloo
Position: Community Coordinator
Organization: Sadie's Place for Innovative Inclusion

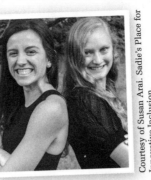

Courtesy of Susan Arai. Sadie's Place for Innovative Inclusion.

Our Career

At Sadie's Place (http://sadiesplace.com), our mission is to bring into being new ways to experience dialogue, create relationships, and engage in practices of inclusion among members of community. We focus on how our practices of inclusion help to build relationships and create reconnections in community. We shift the idea of *place* from *having a place* to *making or creating places that are inclusive* so persons with disabilities are richly woven into the fabric of community.

At Sadie's Place for Innovative Inclusion, we put into motion our three pillars of practice: Bridging to Community (building relationships between members of Sadie's Place and people and organizations in the Kitchener-Waterloo region of Ontario), Inclusion by Press (our button-making social enterprise), and Living Inclusion (our education and knowledge-sharing platform). We engage in relational reflective practice to deepen our understanding of disabling practices and to ensure people, relationships of inclusion, and community flourish within our organization.

Kayla: My introduction to therapeutic recreation was through volunteer work in a clinical setting. Initially I was convinced that clinical practice was where my passions would thrive. My love of community practice grew through coursework and therapeutic recreation experiences in community. Sadie's Place was my last co-op job, and it taught me so much about developmental services, disability studies, meaningful engagement in community, and my own passions. Experiences in clinical practice honed my program facilitation and interpersonal skills, and helped me to realize my work in that field would not be sustainable: I needed an environment that valued recreation experiences as a vehicle for relationship building, rather than skill development, and supported my passions instead of pushing me to fit into a prescribed box.

My role at Sadie's Place was what I dreamed of as an undergraduate student. I love connecting with people in small groups or one on one and having time to develop meaningful therapeutic relationships. My passion for community practice is reignited every day by the incredible team I work alongside. I look forward to the opportunity for growth and new learning that is always available. Working at a nonprofit means we need to be creative with our resources (because these can be limited). I dislike the devaluing of community practice and the perception that it is less legitimate than clinical practice.

Lilly: After my co-op placement as a community inclusion and leisure collaborator at Sadie's Place, I knew I wanted to continue to be a part of a community-informed organization. Upon graduation, I was humbled by the opportunity to continue to work at Sadie's Place as a co-coordinator. My heart will always have a piece of Sadie's Place in it.

Working for Sadie's Place, I love being able to learn every day through experiences, create collaboratively, work in an organization with mindful practices, and explore passions each day (including my own). I like being able to come to work with the thought that "today is going to be a great day." At times, working in a small nonprofit organization means you have a lot of great projects you are passionate about but only so many hours in the day to complete them—finding work–life balance can be difficult, and emotional and physical burnout can happen.

My Advice to You

Kayla: Take risks! Answer questions in class, try out for teams, reach out to new people, and study abroad. Some of my best and deepest learning came from moments when I was out of my comfort zone but took the risk anyway.
Lilly: Ask questions. Be curious about everything in life. Collaborate with those around you. Don't be afraid to learn from your experiences every day. Enjoy what you are doing in your work, and be sure to surround yourself with people who are just as passionate as you are. Finally, always make time for self-care—you can't pour from an empty cup.

for people with mental illness and psychiatric disorders, (b) therapeutic recreation intervention programs for sexually abused adolescents and victims, and (c) therapeutic recreation intervention programs for older adults with dementia. During the first decade of their practice, DTRA published 8 books and 11 academic journal articles and hosted more than 200 sessions of educational seminars and workshops. However, since 2008, their eagerness to promote the field of therapeutic recreation in Korea has almost ceased, and no further academic or practical efforts were initiated after 2008.

Focused more on the purposes of academic and educational opportunities for both the public and future therapeutic recreation specialists, Yongkoo Noh established the Korean Therapeutic Recreation Research Center (KTRRC) in 2001. Again, the primary focus was to promote academic growth of therapeutic recreation through research and scholarly activities. KTRRC has provided several academic seminars, workshops, professional conferences, and educational and training sessions. For instance, KTRRC published the *Korean Therapeutic Recreation Journal* (*KTRJ*), a scholarly journal in therapeutic recreation in South Korea. Although the academic and scholarly activities initiated by KTRRC served as a springboard for the development of therapeutic recreation in South Korea, KTRRC did not have a long life span because of the lack of research activities in the field. Simply, there were not enough scholars and researchers in the field who could share their knowledge in the therapeutic recreation-related areas. The absence of academic programs in higher education settings in Korea is the primary reason that *KRTJ* was discontinued in 2007.

Therapeutic Recreation Certification and Education Systems

The Korean Council for Therapeutic Recreation Certification (KCTRC), established in 2001, administers the certification exam. KCTRC is an independent, nonprofit credentialing body for the profession. Although KCTRC was initiated primarily by leaders from the KTRA, leaders from other entities have recently joined. Collaboration among members maintains the power balance among organizations.

KCTRC has an organizational structure similar to that of the NCTRC in the United States. For instance, KCTRC has three committees: the Standards Review Committee (SRC), Standards

Hearing Committee (SHC), and Exam Management Committee (EMC). Since 2002, the organization has offered the certification exam twice a year. Although KCTRC has an organizational system similar to that of the NCTRC, the minimum standards and qualification requirements for potential therapeutic recreation specialists in Korea are nowhere near the level of the requirements of the NCTRC. Moreover, the number of applications for the certification has dramatically decreased in recent years.

Currently (as of 2017), KCTRC offers two levels of therapeutic recreation certifications. The first level requires a total of 45 hours in training (3 hours per week for 15 weeks) and 15 hours of fieldwork experiences; the second level requires a total of 30 hours in training (2 hours per week for 15 weeks). For both levels, the candidates must pass the certification exam to be certified. Interestingly and unfortunately, the difficulty level of the current standards and requirements was significantly lowered compared to the initial standards and requirements set in 2006. It is speculated that they intentionally lowered the standards and requirements of the certification because of the recent decrease in the number of applicants.

In terms of educational training opportunities for therapeutic recreation in South Korea, because therapeutic recreation is still in its exploratory stage, no academic institutions offer degrees in the field. But more than 30 universities and colleges in South Korea offer courses related to therapeutic recreation, and several universities offer leisure and recreation management programs or have related departments. Most of the instructors who teach therapeutic recreation courses have academic backgrounds in either physical education or sport management. Other instructors have academic backgrounds in social work, special education, or rehabilitation (KTRA, 2006).

Challenges to Growth of the Profession

The growth of therapeutic recreation in South Korea during the first 15 years was remarkable. In particular, the development of professional organizations and research centers, publication of an academic journal, and development of an autonomous credentialing body were remarkable achievements in such a short period. However, it appears that, since the year 2008, the field of therapeutic recreation in South Korea has not been growing and, in fact, has been gradually declining.

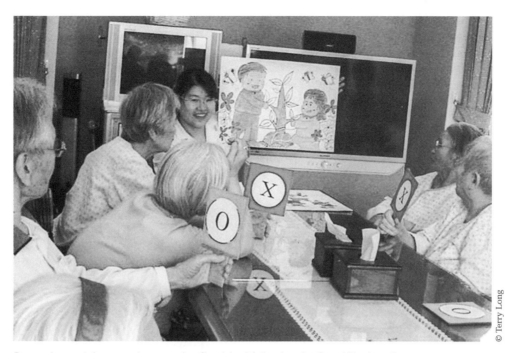

Recreation and therapeutic recreation flourished following the Seoul Paralympic games.

Several interpretations and considerations can be made regarding the decline of the field of therapeutic recreation in South Korea. First, the rapid growth of therapeutic recreation in South Korea in the early days engendered some important concerns. For example, one of the serious concerns is whether the standards and requirements of the current certification system in South Korea warrant the provision of qualified therapeutic recreation professionals. This question raises a concern about establishing a healthy identity and sound image of therapeutic recreation in South Korea. Without a scientific, reliable, outcome-oriented knowledge base and without producing qualified health care professionals, the long-term success of this new profession is problematic. In particular, producing certified therapeutic recreation specialists who are not fully equipped with the necessary academic background and practical skills in the field may even possibly cause harm to potential clients. Thus, the development of appropriate education and training systems, such as academic programs at colleges and universities that produce quality therapeutic recreation specialists, may be a prerequisite for therapeutic recreation in Korea to reestablish its identity as a profession.

Related to the need for the development of academic programs in higher education in Korea, advocating therapeutic recreation to third parties and the public with evidence-based practice would be an important but a very challenging task to pursue. Although it must be very challenging to accomplish this task as evidenced by the absence of academic programs in higher education settings in Korea, there must be some other approaches that therapeutic recreation practitioners in South Korea can take.

The strategies may include communicating with professors in related fields and health care providers in their communities about the field of therapeutic recreation and its effects on the primary human domains. Providing therapeutic recreation programs/services in collaboration with other kindred professions and inviting these professions to collaborate on research projects can be another way to produce evidence-based research and enhance the awareness of the therapeutic recreation profession among the public. That is, collaborative efforts through interdisciplinary approaches for the provision of therapeutic recreation services and evidence-based research projects could possibly promote the growth of therapeutic recreation and might be an effective way to gain the general public's attention.

Second, therapeutic recreation organizations and practitioners in South Korea could communicate with faculty who are in the field of therapeutic recreation in the United States to pursue the same tasks or to request evidence-based research outcomes. To avoid the difficulties associated with the language barrier, it would be a good idea to communicate with Korean faculty who work in the United States. There are four Korean faculty members who are employed in the field of therapeutic recreation in the United States, and a large number of Korean students are currently pursuing graduate degrees in the United States.

Finally, attending professional therapeutic recreation conferences in the United States might be another very effective way to communicate with therapeutic recreation professionals in the United States to establish a network for future communication, collaboration, and consultation.

In summary, during the first 15 years (1993-2008) of therapeutic recreation, the field grew rapidly in both quality and quantity of education and training programs. However, as described above, a premature administration of a certification system before the establishment of proper academic and educational systems may have put therapeutic recreation in South Korea in a perilous situation. Producing certified but not fully prepared therapeutic recreation specialists in today's competitive health care market might have made the general public in Korea question the validity of the profession. Therefore, strategic and long-term plans for the future growth of therapeutic recreation in South Korea must be considered. The therapeutic recreation profession in South Korea is encountering a very challenging time, making it important for therapeutic recreation professionals in South Korea to communicate with each other and work on the challenging tasks that lie ahead.

Therapeutic Recreation in Japan

Japan's unique historical and cultural background has created circumstances that require an examination of therapeutic recreation from a nontraditional perspective. First, the traditional "recreation therapist" job title does not exist in Japan. Therapeutic recreation is not a publicly recognized word or concept, but there are fragmented specialists (e.g., physical therapists, occupational therapists, social workers, care workers, nurses, and adapted physical education teachers) working within the region to deliver services that reflect the inherent characteristics of therapeutic recreation. Second, there is a certification program for what might be considered therapeutic recreation (i.e., fukushi recreation; *fukushi* means welfare and

well-being in Japanese [Takeuchi, 2014]), which helps those fragmented specialists to facilitate recreation with therapeutic purposes. Literature to date that has explored or advocated for therapeutic recreation in Japan has predominantly focused on fukushi recreation (e.g., Nishino, Chino, Yoshioka, & Gabriella, 2007; Takeuchi, 2014; Yoshioka, 2016). For the most part, *fukushi recreation* is a term that is used only for services in long-term-care settings. Another area that Japanese health care specialists have begun to promote is adapted physical activity. This section explores the application of therapeutic recreation in Japan from both the fukushi recreation and adapted physical activity perspectives as well as a few other specific examples of how therapeutic recreation services have manifested in Japan. Challenges regarding the development of therapeutic recreation services in Japan are also explored.

Fukushi Recreation Tradition

Japan has experienced amazing growth among the aged population in the past few decades, and the practice of fukushi recreation was its response. The origin of long-term-care therapeutic recreation services in Japan was in the Social Welfare Worker and Certified Care Worker Act of 1987, which included "theory and methodology of recreation" in the training of long-term-care workers (Takeuchi, 2014). The partial requirement of a training course became an independent certification when the fukushi recreation worker certification was established in 1993. There was a direct Western influence in the development of the certification system because advocates for certification were trained in therapeutic recreation at U.S. educational institutions. The increase in fukushi recreation workers has addressed the needs of quality recreation at long-term-care institutions. The Long-Term Care Insurance Law of 2000, which required long-term-care institutions to provide recreation, has assisted the growth of therapeutic recreation. In accordance with the most recent change in the Long-Term Care Insurance Law in 2015, which is focused on prevention and community services, the field had to expand its paradigm from institutional care to disease prevention care, which fukushi recreation has been used to address. As such, the changing needs of aging trends led to an increase in what might be considered therapeutic recreation services in long-term-care settings (Miyoshi, Ueno, & Shimoyama, 1999; Murray, 2011).

Adapted Physical Activity Tradition

Adapted physical activity is relatively popular in Japan. Initially, programs and services for individuals with physical disabilities were developed and significantly influenced by neurologist Ludwig Guttman, who introduced Stoke Mandeville Games in the United Kingdom. In 1960, orthopedist Yutaka Nakamura traveled abroad to study Guttman's advanced rehabilitation methods based in physical activity. After returning to Japan, Nakamura promoted sports for people with spinal cord injury, and his efforts brought the Paralympics to Tokyo in 1964. The annual National Sports Festival for People with Physical Disability began in 1965. Since then, the Japanese adapted sports movement has continued to grow at a rapid pace. In addition, each prefecture (a Japanese administrative district area similar to a state in the United States) has an organization that promotes sports and recreation for people with disabilities. Equally important are the sports centers that are built exclusively for people with disabilities. Twenty-three sports centers have been opened since 1974 to ensure accessibility to facilities and the programs (Japan Para-Sports Association [JPSA], 2012).

Unlike the situation for people with physical disabilities, sports and recreation for people with developmental disabilities was politically untouched until 1992, when the Ministry of Health (predecessor of the current Ministry of Health, Labor, and Welfare) began the National Sports Festival for People with Intellectual Disabilities. This sports festival had been held independently from the one for people with physical disabilities; however, the two National Sports Festivals were integrated in 2001, following the domestic and international trends on integration of fragmented services for different disabilities. At the grassroots level, recreation activities for people with developmental disabilities have been promoted by Ikuseikai, a family advocacy group, as well as the Special Olympics (Watanabe, 2006). Ikuseikai had a special committee on sports and recreation, which later became the Japan Federation of Intellectual Disabilities (JFID) in 2000. The JFID promotes elite sports programs and sends delegations to international competitions. In contrast, the Special Olympics focuses more on sports participation than performance and has had a significant presence in Japan since 1994.

Services for people with mental illness have been even slower to develop. In fact, the Mental Patient Custody Act was established in 1900 on the assumption that individuals with mental illness were a threat to society. The Mental Health Custody Act legitimated confinement of people with mental illness to their homes, and police officers supervised whether confinement was done appropriately. Shuzo Kure, a psychiatrist, initiated the ending of this law. Kure claimed the humanistic treatment for individuals with mental illness and led his colleagues in the movement in the late 1910s. Imperialism slowed progress, but the movement finally came into bloom when the Mental Patient Custody Act was abolished and the more humanistic Mental Health Act was passed in 1950 (Akiyama, 2000). Kure is regarded as the father of therapeutic recreation in psychiatry in Japan because he used recreational activities to treat patients with mental illness (Ishikawa & Harada, 2012). The movement in recreation increased in strength in the 1980s, and currently, recreational activities are a common element of psychiatric practice. According to the Japanese Federation for Mental Health and Welfare (JFMHW, n.d.), community sports and recreation, such as volleyball and futsal, have become increasingly popular. The JFMHW continues to advocate for sports and recreation programs for people with mental illness. Starting in 2008, volleyball programs for persons with mental illness are now included in the National Sports Festival (JPSA, 2012).

Training and Certification

Fukushi recreation worker is the certification that most closely reflects traditional therapeutic recreation service delivery models. The certification is overseen by the National Recreation Association Japan (NRAJ) and was established in 1993. As of 2013, there were 5,789 individuals holding fukushi recreation worker certification (NRAJ, cited in Takeuchi, 2014). For the development of this certification, returnees who had studied therapeutic recreation in the United States had significant influence. Thus, the training contents include the therapeutic recreation process and related practice models (Nishino et al., 2007).

Many returning therapeutic recreation specialists became professors at universities and colleges, resulting in published works interpreting therapeutic recreation in the Japanese context. For example, Suzuki (1995) wrote a book, *Therapeutic Recreation: Recreation to Reduce Disability and Maintain Health*, for Japanese audiences. Suzuki interpreted the principles and philosophy of therapeutic recreation in the Japanese way so that the related skill sets can be applied in the Japanese context.

Adapted sports instructor is a certification for minimal levels of adapted sports facilitation. The JPSA established this certification in 1985, and it currently has three levels (i.e., elementary, intermediate, and advanced) as well as specialty certifications in specific sports and sports medicine. There were 19,804 instructors registered throughout Japan in 2016, many of whom teach special physical education, care work, and social work and are volunteers working with nonprofit agencies (JPSA, 2016).

Examples of Therapeutic Recreation Practice Settings

Culture has significantly influenced the development of therapeutic recreation in Japan. As noted above, the role of recreation and leisure in Japan has followed a unique evolution that directly mirrors its economic, political, and cultural history. As such, cultural context is a critical consideration when studying therapeutic recreation in Japan. In particular, it is important to understand how applications of therapeutic recreation are empowered, but also restricted, by cultural norms and traditions. This understanding provides insight into the dangers of ethnocentric conceptualizations and applications of therapeutic recreation but also provides enlightenment regarding alternative frameworks for practice.

Services for Older Adults

Recreation activities are popular in long-term-care facilities, day-care centers, and geriatric health services facilities. The programs often involve generic group recreation, with only half of the facilities implementing individualized plans for recreation (Moriyama & Doi, 2009). Still, the development of fukushi recreation has led to widespread implementation of formalized services throughout Japan.

There are also some unique therapeutic recreation modalities that have developed in Japan. In recent years, the use of socially assisted robots (SARs; Tapus, Mataric, & Scasselati, 2007) has become popular in long-term-care facilities. A humanoid recreation leader, PALRO, and a therapeutic seal robot, Paro, are widely used as part of programming, and research shows their effectiveness (e.g., Wada & Shibata, 2007). The robots

have been used in a variety of ways. For example, PALRO has been used to physically demonstrate and audibly explain to clients physical rehabilitation movements, and both robots have been used as sources of companionship and social interaction.

Therapeutic Summer Camp

One innovative example of how therapeutic recreation has surfaced in Japan is the Solapti Kids Camp. A Japanese CTRS, Takashi Wakano, directs the therapeutic summer camp, which serves children with serious health conditions, such as pediatric cancer and heart disease. Solapti Kids Camp provides summer and winter camps with typical camp activities, such as horseback riding, archery, zip-lining, tie-dying, cooking out, snowball fighting, and sledding. The programs are typically 4 days long because of the participants' stamina. To ensure the safety and appropriateness of the programs, the APIE (assessment, planning, implementation, and evaluation) process is utilized in Solapti Kids Camp. The interview with the clients often includes a doctor and a nurse as well as a family member of the participant. In this way, the programs ensure the least restrictive environment for the participants to challenge themselves. They also value challenge by choice. Through Solapti Kids Camp, the participants not only enjoy nature but also make friends who have similar experiences and improve their self-esteem.

Hospital Therapeutic Recreation

Typical hospitals do not have therapeutic recreation programs or staff. One exception is Ishikawa Hospital, where a CTRS works as a rehabilitation specialist and provides therapeutic recreation programs (Mori, 2014). Another hospital, Tsurumaki Onsen, hires non-CTRSs as recreation staff. Recreation staff provides not only in-house activities, such as calligraphy and gardening, but also community reintegration trips. The hospital charges a "leisure fee" for all the patients because therapeutic recreation is not a reimbursable service in Japan. In addition, the recreation staff often co-treat their patients with a reimbursable service, such as occupational therapy.

Challenges for Therapeutic Recreation in Japan

Therapeutic recreation services are increasingly popular in Japan (although it is not labeled as ther-

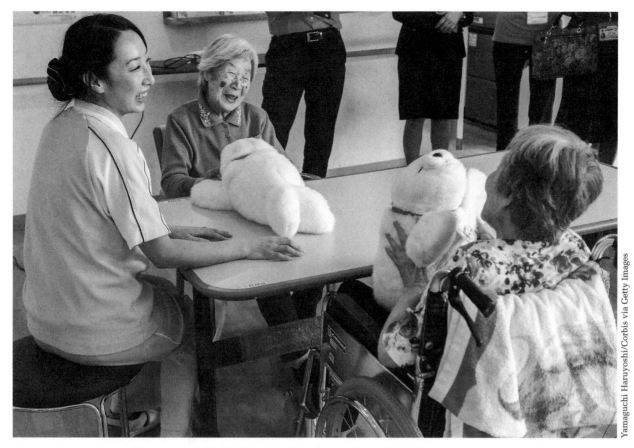

Nursing home residents interact with the Paro therapeutic seal robot in Yokohama city, Kanagawa prefecture.

apeutic recreation), and there are major opportunities to promote and develop services. However, the country's traditional attitude toward leisure in general is a challenge. Japan experienced remarkable economic growth after World War II as the country worked hard to rebuild and recover from the damages of war. The Japanese people have historically valued hard work and productivity; thus, nonproductive time and activities, such as leisure and recreation, are traditionally interpreted as laziness. As a result, a therapy grounded in leisure sometimes conflicts with the norms of Japanese society.

There is, however, a growing leisure element within Japanese society, which has created an openness to leisure and related services that were once seen as having little value. In addition, the lack of "leisure knowledge" within Japanese society has created a need for leisure education. For example, retired workers often experience difficulty transitioning back into their communities because they feel undervalued, guilty, and disconnected from people outside of their work. These individuals would benefit from therapeu-

tic recreation interventions. In fact, Tsukamoto (2013) found that the leisure-based activities helped retired individuals transition back to their communities.

Another challenge to the development of therapeutic recreation services in Japan is the fact that the fukushi recreation worker certification is not a mandatory requirement for facilitating recreation for special populations. Thus, many people run recreation programs without prior training. The lack of fukushi recreation workers compromises the quality of services (Murray, 2011; Nishino et al., 2007).

Physical and social barriers are also problematic in Japan and make community reintegration and inclusion difficult to achieve. For example, because there are segregated sports centers for people with disabilities, there is an expectation that persons with disabilities do not need to use public facilities for recreation. Public sports centers often refuse access to those with disabilities because of a lack of understanding. Continual advocacy regarding the importance of inclusion is needed to improve this situation.

Therapeutic Recreation in Australia

Although therapeutic recreation has been firmly embraced in many developed countries as a useful form of intervention in helping people live a healthier and more satisfying life, in Australia the concept (and indeed the practice) has yet to be fully accepted in the health care setting. The historical development of therapeutic recreation and leisure services and even the terminology used in this country (i.e., diversional or leisure therapy instead of therapeutic recreation) have led to a fractured notion of what the term means today and what that service entails in many parts of Australia. Such services being referred to are those that help people develop, make choices about, and participate in a leisure lifestyle that may ultimately lead to a higher quality of life through increased physical health, emotional well-being, and social connections (Martin, Cox, Kendall, & Price, 2017; Stumbo & Peterson, 2004).

Indeed, the range of therapeutic recreation staff titles used across the country is diverse. The more commonly used titles are leisure therapist, recreation therapist, diversional therapist, activities or recreation officer, and activity therapist. Although the title for staff engaged in therapeutic recreation provision may vary significantly based on locality, the industrial award under which the person is employed and whether the person is in the public or private health care system, the day-to-day tasks and core service values are generally consistent with those espoused as appropriate by the primary professional body in this country for therapeutic recreation staff, the Diversional & Recreation Therapy Australia (DRTA). DRTA has a current membership in excess of 2,000 individuals spread across the full gamut of operations in the health and aged care sectors, including rehabilitation and hospital units, community centers, residential aged care, palliative care units, and mental health services (DRTA, 2017). Its philosophy and vision are similar to those outlined by similar overseas organizations, such as the U.S.-based NCTRC (2016). For instance, the DRTA (2017) considers diversional therapy to be "a client centred practice and recognises that leisure and recreational experiences are the rights of all individuals. Activities are designed to support, challenge and enhance the psychological, spiritual, social, emotional and physical well-being of individuals" (p. 1).

Historical Development of Therapeutic Recreation Services

Although most researchers acknowledge that therapeutic recreation had its formal origins in the health care industry in Australia in the early 1940s, its history can be traced back to World War I, when nursing staff used forms of recreation to assist in the rehabilitation of injured servicemen who had returned home after fighting in the European sector. Such services were also geared to assisting those with permanent disabilities to assimilate back into community life. After World War II and in recognition of gaps in the range of health services offered to those seeking assistance, the Australian Red Cross initiated training courses in basic crafts to health care staff. Although the 3-month-long courses were offered to the public until 1976, they were significantly modified from their original form in the late 1960s to accommodate the growing recognition that the diversional activities required in the health care sector were far broader than just handcrafts alone and staff members therefore needed to be suitably skilled to adapt a range of services to suit the needs of their clientele (Diversional Therapy Association of Australia [DTAA], 2005). Concurrent with this shift, the commencement of the deinstitutionalization process in Australia in the late 1960s and early 1970s, perhaps best exemplified by significant reforms in the psychiatric and disability sectors, saw therapeutic recreation become a formally accepted area of study and a vocational outcome in the late 1970s. This was achieved by the progressive establishment of recreation courses at colleges of advanced education throughout Australia from 1976 onward. The DTAA was formed at this time as an outcome of a meeting of seven graduates of the Red Cross course who had a common interest in improving service to their primarily older adult clientele (DTAA, 2003).

These early and somewhat limited training offerings, usually offered at the undergraduate associate diploma or diploma level, have evolved to the point that a limited number of universities throughout Australia now offer programs with a specific therapeutic recreation focus, primarily at the undergraduate bachelor's degree and postgraduate master's levels. Consistent with the early development of these programs, empirical research in the Australian setting began to emerge in the early 1980s regarding the benefits of therapeutic recreation. The focus was to evaluate the principles and practices that guide interventions

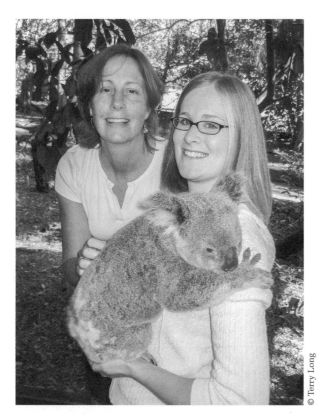

Options for therapeutic recreation are endless in Australia, where even some zoo creatures can help provide a little "pet therapy."

© Terry Long

with consumers of therapeutic services (Trowbridge, 1988). Unfortunately, many therapeutic recreation practitioners have not aligned with the shift in the Australian health care sector toward services driven by evidence-based outcomes and workplace preparation grounded in an appropriate range of training and education opportunities (Pegg, Stumbo, & Bennett, 2017).

Ongoing Australian National Reform

The provision of therapeutic recreation services in Australia over the past two decades has been greatly influenced by a sweeping array of reforms, most of them at the federal level, with respect to the health and community services sectors. Nationwide reforms to community-based public health services, particularly those services targeted toward people with mental illness and older adults, have significantly impacted the professional landscape. Each of these reform agendas has brought forth greater consideration of quality of life issues and has recognized for perhaps the first time that legislation, policies, and funding at the national and state levels must be properly aligned to achieve successful implementation of the proposed reforms across the nation. For example, the National Health Strategy, a key nationwide initiative announced by the Commonwealth government in 1994, noted for the first time at the federal level that health services need to be holistic. Since then, government policies and community actions have increasingly reflected the relationship between leisure and health. For instance, efforts made in recent years with respect to the Active Australia and Get Activated campaigns within the health care field have focused on the importance of community-based living and the need for physical activity to be incorporated into a more holistic and healthier lifestyle (Australian Institute of Health and Welfare, 2016; Australian Sports Commission, 2016).

Similarly, the National Mental Health Plan, first released in 1992 and updated in 1998, has focused on promotion, prevention, and early intervention; development of partnerships in service reform; and the quality and effectiveness of service delivery. These core reforms were reinforced further in 2006 with the tabling of the Parliament of Australia Senate (2006) report, titled *A National Approach to Mental Health—From Crisis to Community*, which recommended, among other things, that greater attention (and resources) be given to the issues of social reintegration of consumers and the level and quality of rehabilitation services, inclusive of therapeutic recreation–based programs, available to them. This was followed in 2013 with the endorsement by the Australian Health Ministers' Advisory Council (AHMAC) of the national framework for recovery-oriented mental health services, which in acknowledging the lived experience of the individual, provided "guidance on tailoring recovery-oriented serves to respond to the diversity of people with mental health issues" (Department of Health, 2014, p. 1).

In more recent years, each state and territory government has enacted new legislation or substantially revised past legislation to better align regional systems and program offerings with the Commonwealth's focus on recovery-oriented practice and service considerations such that individuals with mental health issues are better able to reside in communities without the need for forced or involuntary treatment and care. Critically underpinning this reform agenda has been the notion that recovery is considered a process and not just an end point.

In terms of aged care, the Home and Community Care Act 1985 and the Aged Care Act 1997 were the initial platforms used to reform the systems and processes in place to "support healthy ageing for older Australians and the provision of quality, cost effective care for frail older people as well as their careers" (Department of Health and Ageing, 2003, p. 3). Such support included at the time what was then considered to be alternative or other therapies. Under this banner, therapeutic recreation and other leisure-based services have continued to be funded in residential-care facilities across Australia. In fact, the more recent aged care legislative review that led to the enactment of the Aged Care (Living Longer Living Better) Act of 2013 has served to reinforce the critical importance of maintaining individual choice over service and setting options as people age.

Although most of the significant reforms have been initiated at the national level, each reform has in turn been affected at the state and regional levels by the ideology and policies of the state or territory government in power and even more at the local level by the service provider and health care practitioner overseeing program delivery. In terms of therapeutic recreation services in Australia, such practitioners have been traditionally either occupational therapists or diversional therapists, with many offering services that reflected their past education and training and were flavored by their professional philosophy of service provision. Occupational therapists, for example, continue to align strongly with the medical model of health service provision. They are key members of case management teams, in which they are being required to undertake large caseloads encompassing mainly the evaluation of client competencies (activities of daily living) and the associated administration of services. Case management in Australia today is an integral component of the overall services offered by health service providers. With its implementation, however, has come the progressive withdrawal of many occupational therapists from the face-to-face delivery of programs.

As a consequence, the shift in duties for occupational therapists has been a boon for many therapeutic recreation–based staff members because they have been required to step in to fill the void. As such, diversional therapists have remained hands-on because their services are now in demand more than ever. They too have been asked in recent times to be more accountable for what they offer and how they perform.

In the past, a significant number of diversional therapists had expressed the view through their professional links that they were uncomfortable with the notion of being required to undertake any form of critical evaluation to demonstrate client outcomes or even to justify service offerings. This was an unfortunate stance to take because greater accountability for health care expenditures in the Australian setting was a critical pressure point of the ongoing reform process. In recent years, younger and, it must be said, better-educated graduates are more accommodating of this work expectation, so a change in mindset is occurring but perhaps not at the rate some might hope.

Therapeutic recreation professionals in Australia, through their everyday interactions with consumers, play a major role in supporting people with a wide variety of care and health needs by facilitating improved leisure functioning that results in a better quality of life. Despite this fact and the increasing amount of evidence to support their involvement in allied health services, many professionals and paraprofessionals in the health and community care fields continue to dismiss therapeutic recreation services in the Australian setting as little more than time fillers and diversionary activities. Whatever the current challenges to the profession in North America, they are multiplied in the Australian setting.

Although issues of professional training and accreditation, social change, national health care reform, and the level of government funding at both the federal and state levels have all affected how therapeutic recreation is perceived and used in Australia, the harsh reality is that it remains generally a concept (and service) not well understood by the Australian public. Moreover, therapeutic recreation remains a form of service that appears to be under constant threat.

Although recent action nationally by the DRTA, and even regionally by the leisure therapists aligned with the Leisure Therapy Support Network in the State of Queensland, to establish and then enforce minimum standards for the professional preparation and in-service education of therapeutic recreation practitioners can be seen as a purposeful step in the right direction, numerous issues remain to be addressed. As has been noted by a range of authors (e.g., Pegg & Darcy, 2007; Stumbo, Martin, & Ogborne, 2004) in the not-so-distant past, until therapeutic recreation professionals in Australia take action to articulate and document a clear purpose to service provision, develop more standardized services to clients, demonstrate an ability to target and achieve valued client outcomes, improve the credibility of service provision and service providers to other providers and payers, and achieve greater equity with other health care and human services professionals, such employees and the services they offer will continue to sail on troubled waters.

Summary

Students have much to learn from these international descriptions. The presented information provides a historical context for understanding the meaning and nature of therapeutic recreation as it exists within these countries. The chapter also illustrates the importance of multicultural competence and the potential dangers of applying models and methods from one culture to another without considering cultural appropriateness. Another important lesson is that therapeutic recreation is indeed an international profession and opportunities for growth and collaboration exist at this level. To explore these and other issues related to this chapter, students should review the discussion questions and share their thoughts with classmates. These questions are designed specifically to help students recognize the limitations and opportunities associated with each of the described systems. Furthermore, exploring the value of alternative perspectives and approaches to therapeutic recreation can be a useful tool in envisioning future possibilities at both the national and international levels.

DISCUSSION QUESTIONS

1. Identify the similarities and differences between the NCTRC and the MCF credentialing processes.

2. Explain the role of multiculturalism in Canada, Canadian identity, and the MCF credentialing processes. In addition, how does NCTRC address the issue of multiculturalism, or cross-cultural, competencies?

3. What similarities and differences exist between the U.S. history and perspective of therapeutic recreation and those of other countries?

4. Recreation and leisure are inherent parts of culture. What implications does this present regarding the purpose and nature of therapeutic recreation? How might traditional American or Western perspectives be irrelevant or unhealthy when applied to other cultures?

5. What steps can you take to ensure that you are competent in your work with people from other cultures?

13

Envisioning the Future: Therapeutic Recreation as a Profession

Terry Robertson | Erick Kong

LEARNING OUTCOMES

At the end of this chapter, students will be able to

- identify primary elements of the model of personal and professional development,
- apply the proposed model to develop a long-term plan for personal and professional development,
- identify at least three social, economic, or cultural trends that may affect the therapeutic recreation profession in the future, and
- recognize and use six paradigms for understanding and addressing future trends, challenges, and opportunities in therapeutic recreation.

No one knows the future, nor does any nation, professional organization, political party, or corporation. The future is yet to be determined. What we do know is that unexpected events, political influences, global or local economics, and social and physical needs are always changing. Everything, from natural disasters and technological advancements to new expectations of consumer groups, has the potential to create change, and that includes you! Amid all this change, and as you will see later in this chapter, our profession is predicted to continue to grow, and we need to make sure we are ready to grow to meet the need. To do this successfully, we also need to commit to our own learning and sharing what we learn with others. We need to become a learning community full of professionals who can and will adapt to changes in our profession, the changing needs of our clients (e.g., patients and consumers), and changes in our world. We need to continue to build our evidence-based practice and share this evidence with others.

As we write this chapter, communication, economic, and social systems are all changing, as are professional opportunities, practice techniques, and formats of service delivery. As a profession, we (and you as an individual) must continue to grow and change to be current, competent, relevant, available, and beneficial to others. We need to think beyond our initial practice standards and current approach to the profession. We need to consider how we promote what we do and the benefits (outcomes) of our profession to others so that we become better integrated into broader service delivery systems as well as within the lives and minds of consumers (i.e., clients, patients, participants, and communities) and other professionals. To be clear, this continuous state of change offers both opportunity and risk, which requires that we have a growth mindset to be successful. According to research (Harvard Business Review, 2018), individuals who believe their talents can be developed (through hard work, good strategies, and input from others) have a growth mindset. They tend to achieve more than those with a fixed mindset (those who believe their talents are innate gifts or their place in a community or system is never changing). They achieve more because they worry less about looking smart and put more energy into learning. If this approach is adopted by a profession or an organization, it can become a learning organization or profession. If we are not careful stewards of our profession, we run the risk of losing our useful place within society. Just look around your own campus or community. Cultural change agents are all around us, and the potential for an increased pace of change is growing as a result of technology (increased access to communication and information) and our global society. So the profession is open to you—the future leaders, providers, administrators, and educators. You have the responsibility to make the profession the best it can be for you, those you serve, and society. Finally, you should note that you will be able to influence these changes during your career. If you can harness the opportunities while navigating the risks, you have a tremendous opportunity to lead the profession into the future.

Embracing Our History

In chapter 2, you read about the history of this profession. Using this book and through your class, you have studied some specific details about how to work with individuals and/or groups of individuals with disabilities or other risk factors. You may have searched the Internet, gone on site visits, or volunteered, but they too are all now history. They are part of your learning and eventual practice. However, if it is not clear yet, we believe that the practice of our profession will be very different in 5 years, much less 10, 20, or even 50 years from now. Part of why it will be different is because of you and the work you will do. Part of it is because the world is changing as a result of technology (new inventions and the speed of access to real-time global information). The impending changes all around us do represent a continuation of what has occurred in the past. However, as you will see, change is both perceptual and incremental. Just remember that change is a process, not an event. Imagine, if in your own life, you took pictures (or 1-minute videos), one a day; saved them to your phone or the cloud (sound familiar?); and then looked at them a year later. Get the picture? You would see how you and those around you have changed. It is important to know that your history helps shape who you are today. So in this profession, you too will be contributing to this change. It is true that you, just like a community, an organization, or a profession, need a plan and, of course, the desire to grow and change to be both purposeful and successful. As a snapshot of some of our history, the following milestones will shed light on how this growth and change have occurred over time and how quickly the future can arrive.

EXEMPLARY PROFESSIONALS

KERI FAGER, MS, CTRS, CADC

Education: BS in Therapeutic Recreation, East Carolina University
MS in Therapeutic Recreation, Northwest Missouri State University
Position: Therapeutic Recreation Coordinator
Organization: Rosecrance Health Network, Rockford, Illinois

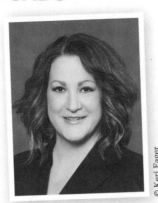

© Keri Fager

My Career

In determining a career, I always knew I wanted to help people but never quite knew exactly how and in what capacity. I considered multiple health care careers and stumbled upon therapeutic recreation as I entered my first year of undergraduate school at East Carolina University. I remember hearing about therapeutic recreation and thinking, "Wow—this profession is made for me!" I quickly knew that therapeutic recreation was what I had been seeking, and I have never really looked back.

I started my professional career working with the geriatric population in a skilled nursing facility, where I worked as the activity director for just a few years, until I discovered my love for behavioral health. I accepted a position as therapeutic recreation specialist at a state psychiatric hospital, where I worked for five years on the adult acute admissions unit. I strongly feel that this position taught me invaluable clinical skills, because the acuity of the patient population was significant and led to the need to sharpen my therapeutic intervention skills and ability to assess, evaluate, and treat a variety of challenging mental health disorders. In this position, I learned much in the way of program development, group facilitation technique, and clinical documentation, as well as the benefit of adherence to a standard of practice for the therapeutic recreation profession. I was also able to work my way up to a supervisor position in which I gained skills in program and employee management. I also worked closely in mentorship and supervision of practicum students as well as interns, which was highly rewarding and something I feel is critical to the ongoing growth of the profession.

The next step in my career came in response to my relocation back to the Midwest, where I continued in the behavioral health field as the recreation therapist on a psychiatric unit in a medical hospital, until I found my current position as the therapeutic recreation coordinator at Rosecrance Health Network in Rockford, Illinois, where I have worked for 10 years. I was lucky enough to have the opportunity to build an experiential therapies program for an adult residential substance abuse program from the ground up, and today I oversee a department of experiential specialists across various levels of care, including both mental health and substance abuse programs for adults and adolescents. The services I am blessed to lead include fitness and wellness programming, mindfulness and meditation, therapeutic drumming, use of a labyrinth, team building, therapeutic horticulture and nature-based programming, leisure education, and art therapy. In this position, I have worked closely with the clinical leadership team and have served as cochair of the company's client care continuum committee, which oversees our clinical operations, including program development, evidence-based practices, outcome measures, and performance improvement.

My Advice To You

I feel that one of the best lessons I have learned in my 18 years in the therapeutic recreation field is that often our biggest "hat" we often wear is that of advocate. I have found the most rewarding parts of my career have been in advocating for my clients, for our field, and for the staff whom I have supervised. I have found the most success in the growth of my programs when I went the extra mile, over and over again, to prove our role on the treatment team and when I found ways to illustrate solid, specific outcomes from our services. I have always been recognized for my passion for the work we do, and I wholeheartedly believe those who choose the therapeutic recreation field lead with their hearts. Seek ways to shout it from the rooftops and put a spotlight on the work we do. Present meaningful trainings on our services within and outside of your agency, present at conferences, and just be heard!

Living Our Legacy: Some of Our Pictures in Time

During 2019, at least three related modern-era national professional organizations celebrated significant anniversaries: 34 years for the Alberta Therapeutic Recreation Association and the American Therapeutic Recreation Association (ATRA), both founded in 1985, and 38 years for the National Council on Therapeutic Recreation Certification (NCTRC), founded in 1981.

The year 2019 marked the 48th anniversary of the Midwest Symposium on Therapeutic Recreation and the 43rd anniversary of the Mideastern Symposium on Therapeutic Recreation. Although these regional symposiums are not organizations, they are two of the best-attended conferences on therapeutic recreation in the world, and the individuals participating in them have made significant contributions to our profession for many years.

As of 2019, four states (New Hampshire, North Carolina, Oklahoma, and Utah) and the District of Columbia (Washington, DC) require a professional license to practice therapeutic recreation. In fact, 2019 marks the 43rd consecutive year that the state of Utah has maintained its therapeutic recreation licensure law. Utah was the first state to pass such a law (S. Post, personal communication, October 14, 2006). The law provided governmental permission for those properly prepared and duly qualified in our profession to practice within the state. Also, 2018 was the 12th year that a licensure law has been in place for those working in New Hampshire and the 13th year for a licensure law in North Carolina. The states of California and Texas also have their own state certification credentials and processes in place. Unique to these two states is that, based on a reciprocity agreement between them, anyone currently certified in either state is also considered concurrently certified in the other state.

Final examples of our profession's relatively short but effective and diverse professional contribution to modern society are in the area of state and community-based programs and services. The year of 2019 marks the 24th year of the Therapeutic Recreation Summit. The Therapeutic Recreation Summit is held annually in conjunction with the Texas Recreation and Park Society (TRAPS) and is a conference combining lectures and hands-on training in the field of recreation and leisure. Also, 2019 is the 42nd year of community-based therapeutic recreation services for the city of Eugene, Oregon, and the 43rd year for therapeutic recreation services provision in Roanoke, Virginia. In 2019, the Recreation Therapy section of the California Park and Recreation Society will be celebrating its 50th anniversary, and the Florida Disabled Outdoors Association (founded in 1990), a model community-based program focused on an individual's interests, ability, and active participation, will be celebrating its 29th year. And right now, you are taking a class (or reading this book) to help prepare yourself to be a therapeutic recreation specialist! Where do you see yourself in 5 years? How about 10 years? Where will you be working and with whom? Will any of the above-mentioned historical examples be able to help you with your future? Will you create something new and different? What about in other countries? Your history is important, just as the profession's history is, but what about the future?

Using Change

All these organizations, symposia, conferences, and municipalities have experienced changes during their existence—changes in leadership, focus, services, policies, membership, and effectiveness. Change should be expected and planned for. Change, however, is often viewed as a surprise and a threat. Sometimes, those who are trying to maintain or manage organizations, households, or personal situations view change as negative. Others view change as positive, as growth or movement to remain current. The struggle is to achieve balance between the two perspectives: consistency (absence of change), which helps build or establish identity (thus, recognition, brand identity, specialization, standardization, and strength), and change, which helps build relevance (meeting new, expanding, or changing markets and needs).

So as you consider your future and the future of this profession, you should think about your comfort level with these concepts (consistency vs. change), both personally and professionally (or academically). Do you have a growth mindset, or do you want to develop one? No matter how you answered these questions, you need to think about the short term (the situation right now, your first internship and/or your first job) and then, about the long term (your goals for 2 years from now, your 5- or 10-year goals, and maybe even your 50-year goals or expectations). You will have many choices as you move through your life, and the decision to make your career within this profession is just the beginning.

Let us look at a couple of scenarios of how change has occurred in the practice of other professions and how those changes have been considered both good and bad. They are familiar change agents to many of you. The younger you are, the less you may know about their history.

Take a minute and think about computers and how big (or small) they are and how you use them. Now, take a moment and think about phones and how big (or small) they are and how you use them. Believe it or not, these two things were at one time completely separate entities and provided completely separate experiences and opportunities for both the professionals involved in their development and use and their consumers and users. Originally, they were not directly related to each other, but they did share some common knowledge and technology. Now, they are so intertwined that it would be difficult for most of you to think of them as separate or unconnected to each other.

The common knowledge base (electronics) combined with a common purpose (communication verbally, numerically, or graphically) and an open and willing consumer base (real or perceived demand) created the right atmosphere for cultural change agents (belief systems, use patterns, expectations, etc.) to develop in both industries and allow them to grow. These changes were experienced individually at first and then together in ways beyond many providers' imaginations. In both cases, however, these changes were viewed skeptically by some and with fear by others, and some people experienced job losses in the old industries while others found jobs in the new industries.

If you are confused, let's slow down and approach this from a different perspective. To begin with, you need to think historically about each of these areas of technology (computers and telephones) and note that all of these changes have happened within the past 40 to 100 years, depending on where you live.

First, examine the items in table 13.1. Then, think about the development and changes in personal communication hardware options from the current technology back to past practices or services. Note that these two technologies are essentially now integrated into one so that now, everyone thinks of them as the same thing and expects things to get more, not less, integrated. Think about what your parents or grandparents would have thought if you had told them as teenagers about this synergy.

Depending on when you first encountered either of these technologies and how and why you used them, you may view them as either helping people become more connected to each other or separating people as we struggle to keep up with change. For example, some senior citizens love email because it allows them to do things such as communicate

Table 13.1 Evolution of Technology in Popular Culture

Time period	The telephone	The computer
Good ol' days	Smoke signals Pony Express Telegraph Party lines	Cave drawings (records) Abacus (calculations) Dictionary (information) Encyclopedia (information)
1960s	Rotary phones	Room-sized computers
1970s	Push-button phones	Desktops
1980s	Bag phones	Internet
1990s	Pocket cell phones	Laptops
2000s	Cell phones, watches, glasses	Cell phones, watches, glasses
21st Century	Multiple integrated technology devices, such as TVs, smart cars, homes, appliances, bio-memory, prosthetics (stored and accessed via the cloud or other specific wireless systems)	

with distant family and friends or shop online when "getting out" might be difficult. But others are intimidated by the prospect of learning how to use computers or fear that online shopping is dangerous because of the risk of identity theft. The latter group would much rather use a telephone or have an "in-person" experience, and when societal demands discourage this, they feel disconnected. Thus, differing levels of technological knowledge and use can both separate and connect us with family, friends, and society in general.

Ultimately, changes in familiar technologies such as these can be viewed as factors affecting cultures worldwide. How these changes affect us, whether they harm or hurt us and how society should react, is a debatable point that should be considered. The final thing to notice about the example provided here is that these (at one-time) seemingly completely different professions did end up working together. This **interprofessional** (or multidisciplinary) approach helped with solving problems and made both technologies more efficient, effective, user friendly, and desirable. In fact, this interprofessional approach has become an expectation for most people worldwide and even considered an essential part of one's standard of living. *Who'da thunk it?*

The Emergence of a Global Society

Significant changes in culture and interdependent belief systems are happening all around us. These cultural changes are occurring worldwide, not just in the United States or North America. Furthermore, change is occurring faster than it did in the past largely because of technology. We are becoming a more global; mobile; and in some ways, dissatisfied and segregated society—economically, socially, educationally, politically, ethnically, and in terms of health status, human rights, and quality of life (Putnam, 2000; Veblen, 1899). The eventuality of a one-world economy has been discussed and debated for years. The European Union, the World Bank, the United Nations, the World Health Organization, the expansion of **capitalism**, the growth of multinational organizations, the increase in **outsourcing**, the growth of collaborative relief and aid work, and the application of democracy and free enterprise to other countries are all evidence of efforts to create or control economic and political systems worldwide. Embedded within these change agents are fundamental issues that also need to be addressed—race, religion, age, gender, language, terminology, cross-cultural concerns, immigration versus refugee status, and best or better practices in serving those affected by these changes.

So where and how do these situations, groups, organizations, efforts, or changes affect our profession and those whom we serve now and will serve in the future? Are we connected to any one of these potential influencers? If not, could or should we be connected? If so, how and why should we be connected? Are we influencers? If we are, at what level and how widespread is our influence? Are we players or influencers in our own country or state, within our community, or within our place of employment? Are you currently working with other types of professionals (i.e., interprofessionally/multidisciplinarily)? Remember the previous "who'da thunk it" example with telephones and computers? Now think about what you have read in previous chapters and consider the other disciplines we currently work with, the settings and populations that we serve and then ask yourself, who else can or should we work with? Who else can we help? Who can help us improve our practice, our profession and thus the quality of life for those we serve? Are there other disciplines, technologies, or techniques that others are using that we should be using? Are there other disciplines using or possibly sharing clinical pathways using a framework such as the *International Classification of Functioning, Disability and Health*, or *ICF* model? You and your instructor should recognize these questions as being rhetorical. Each question also contains a **problatunity**—a problem and an opportunity.

Acknowledging that our world is ever changing and will evolve with or without our involvement is critical. The challenge before you as both an individual and a member of a group of potential professionals is to start thinking globally and then, plan to act locally. It has been said that if you control the questions, then you also control the answers. So what should be on the scoreboard (criteria) to determine how much, or even if, we contribute to the global society? What must we do to influence policy, legislation, regulations, the practice of the profession, and day-to-day services so that ultimately we can meet the needs of our society?

For an example, consider that the United Nations Development Program's **human development index** (2018) identified Norway as the best place in the world to live, followed by Switzerland; Australia; Ireland; Germany; Iceland; Hong Kong, China (SAR); Sweden; Singapore; and then the Netherlands as the top 10. The next five included Denmark, followed by Canada, the United States, the United Kingdom, and Finland. According to the article, 2018 was the eighteenth consecutive year for Norway to be ranked first by the United Nations. Some of the indicators (criteria) used in support of this top ranking were that Norwegians earn 40 times more than those who live in the lowest-ranked countries (the lowest-scoring countries were Niger and the Central African Republic, South Sudan, Chad, Burundi, and Sierra Leone) and Norwegians live almost twice as long and have a literacy rate that is nearly five times higher than those who live in the lower-scoring countries. Norway is also an oil-rich country. The report was not able to rank 17 countries, including Iraq, Afghanistan, and Somalia, because of insufficient or missing data. How many of these indicators are also tied to quality of life? How many of those living in these countries consider leisure or recreation an important or essential part of life? Which countries have viable therapeutic recreation specialists practicing or providing services in them now?

Which countries would be open to our services and why? Which countries could benefit the most from our profession and why?

We have considered enough broad questions for now. Next, we need to consider the future of our profession and help you decide on the direction and methodologies that you can use to get you where you want to be.

The Future of Therapeutic Recreation as a Profession

According to Carter, Robb, and Van Andel (2019), therapeutic recreation is considered to be one the emergent health care professions in the field of human services in the United States. A reason for this is the ever-growing population. The U.S. Census Bureau (2018) predicted that between the years 2010 and 2050, the number of seniors who are 65 years and older would expand from 40.2 million to 88.5 million. In 2016, the American Association of Retired Persons (AARP) did a study on older Americans and pointed out that those who were 65 and older made up 13 percent of the U.S. population; therefore, AARP expected this population to grow to 19.3 percent by the year 2030 (AARP International, 2018). Furthermore, people in general are living longer largely because they are more knowledgeable about health issues; they seek early help, live healthier lifestyles, and have access to improved health services and innovations in medical technology for treatments; and heart disease and stroke have declined (Carter, Van Andel, & Robb, 2019). Vincent and Velkoff (2010) further indicated that the explosion of the population in the United States would have a dramatic effect on health care professionals. The over-65-population explosion will affect therapeutic recreation specialists because they provide services that are aimed to "treat, change, or ameliorate effects of illness and disability" (Park, 1981, p. 3). According to the Bureau of Labor Statistics (BLS; 2017), the number of therapeutic recreation specialists will grow an average of 7 percent from 2016 to 2026 as compared to other health service practitioners because the number of seniors in senior homes or independent living facilities is expected to increase. The BLS stated, "As the large baby-boom generation ages, they will need therapeutic recreation specialists to help treat age-related injuries and illnesses, such as strokes, Alzheimer's disease, and mobility-related injuries that require recreational therapy" (BLS, 2017, Job Outlook section, para. 2).

The BLS also reported,

In addition, the number of people with chronic conditions, such as diabetes and obesity, is growing. Recreational therapists will be needed to help patients maintain their mobility, to teach patients about managing their conditions, and to help patients adjust recreational activities to accommodate any physical limitations. Therapists will be needed also to plan and lead programs designed to maintain overall wellness through participation in activities such as camps, day trips, and sports.

Recreational therapists will increasingly be utilized in helping veterans manage service-related conditions such as post-traumatic stress disorder (PTSD) or injuries such as the loss of a limb. Recreational therapists can lead activities that help veterans to reintegrate into their communities and help them to adjust to any physical, social, or cognitive limitations (BLS, 2017). Wages have remained relatively stable and areas of consistent employment are identified in the report. For example, the states with the highest number of recreation therapists include: 1) New York, 2) California, 3) Pennsylvania, 4) Illinois, and Texas. The state with the highest average wage is California at $68, 510 (BLS, 2017). https://www.bls.gov/oes/current/oes291125.htm%20-%202017

Professional development is essential to all therapeutic recreation professionals. It not only ensures that they maintain their level of competency but also exposes them to the current trends, knowledge, skills, and practices in the field. It should be viewed as an ongoing process throughout their careers as therapeutic recreation services providers. The ultimate goal of continuing professional development is to maintain the safety of those receiving therapeutic recreation services.

The move to use a model based on the *ICF* (see chapter 5 for more information) and integrated with an evidence-based practice approach is clearly becoming the norm. Above all, the statistics indicate a growing need for what our profession offers. Although some specific current trends were discussed above, at this point, rather than attempting to predict exactly what the future practice of this profession will be, this chapter presents two primary tools for you to use in both navigating change and creating the future of our profession. First, a model of **professional development** is presented. You can immediately start applying this model to your

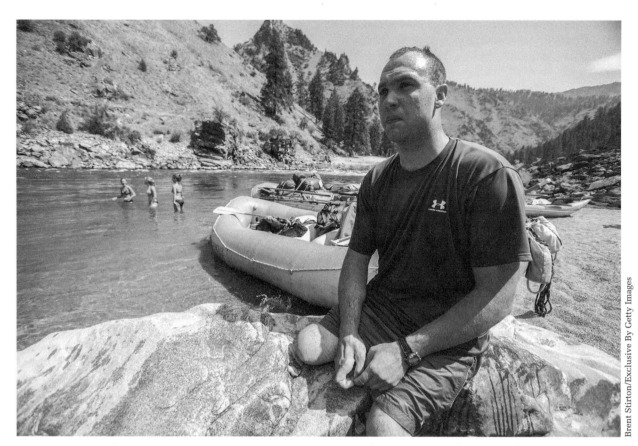

Veterans who have experienced physical and emotional trauma can benefit from therapeutic recreation services focused on recovery and return to civilian life.

professional development as a student, and later on, you can use it as a professional, which will ultimately further develop the profession. Second, six worldviews, or **paradigms**, for understanding the future of therapeutic recreation are presented. You should consider each paradigm individually and then, all of them collectively; discuss the implications of these paradigms with each other and with your instructor; and brainstorm ways to apply them within your own practice (life, current situation, occupation, and future career). You can then use them to have a positive influence on the future of our profession through your professional decision making, life choices, and personal and professional affiliations and commitments (organizational alliances; memberships; donations of time, money, or intellectual thought; and various networks).

Developing a Collective Wisdom

The collective knowledge base of a profession and its applicability to practice will influence future directions of the profession. If the knowledge base and applicability of a profession do not grow or change to meet new expectations or are not shared and used both internally and externally (settings, populations, situations, purposes, and professions), then opportunities for positive influence and the potential of our profession are limited. For that reason, besides considering the six organizational paradigms presented in this chapter, you should already be considering your personal and professional development. For instance, therapeutic recreation specialists who work in health care settings are required to practice in an environment that uses advanced skills. Aside from a wide range of general skills, there is a need to develop and acquire specific knowledge and skills in specialized areas of the population. NCTRC offers specialty certification in the areas of physical medicine/rehabilitation, geriatrics, developmental disabilities, behavioral health, and community inclusion services (NCTRC, 2015). These specialty certifications are being recognized as having a distinct level of expertise in their respective areas. Certified therapeutic recreation specialists (CTRSs) who wish to pursue one or more of these certificates must demonstrate their proficiency by completing graduate-level courses or taking continuing education hours within the designated specialty areas along with current work experience that reflects their expertise. In addition, they must submit references from a peer professional and a recent employment supervisor. Pursuing additional recognition through certification would provide a higher level of assurance in the quality of therapeutic recreation services by the means of professional development. Certification in these areas is not easily obtained because of the stringent requirements. However, those who are able to obtain these certifications are being recognized as people who possess the advanced knowledge and skills in their daily treatment. Going forward, the specialty certifications, state licensure, or other advanced credentials may potentially be required as part of the professional development to work in these specialized areas of the population. Applying the following model to your personal and professional development will ultimately enhance the collective wisdom of therapeutic recreation. Finally, you should consider interdisciplinary work via an *ICF* approach to your evidence-based practice.

A Model of Personal and Professional Development

The model of personal and professional development presented in figure 13.1 was created in the early 1990s. It was used in consulting practices with organizations and individuals and presented at the Midwest Symposium on Therapeutic Recreation (Robertson, 1993) in a session titled "The Wheel of Fortune or the Wheel of Torture? A Conceptual Model for Professional and Personal Development."

The model uses the wheel of a bike as a metaphor. We begin by imagining our professional and personal body of knowledge (what we know about our profession and its applicability to helping others and managing ourselves and our practice) as the hub of a wheel on a multigeared bicycle. The spokes are the delivery mechanisms to put our body of knowledge to work. They are the links between theory (the hub), practice or application (the tire rim), and the consumer group (the tire itself). The spokes are also a mechanism to help build or increase our individual or corporate body of knowledge. The tire rim can also represent the organization or management structure, and the tire tread can represent face-to-face, day-to-day services delivery. The size of the tire may represent your sphere of influence, community size, or the size of your role in a given job. The four spokes (reading, writing, speaking, and doing) are the minimum requirements for professionals who are trying to keep up with best practices and ahead of changes.

At first, your body of knowledge may be small, but over time and given the many opportunities that you will find in this profession, the size and shape of your spokes may change. Long and thin spokes could represent specialization; thick and short spokes may represent lots of experience but in one role, capacity, or comfort. As you seek to develop each spoke, you are adding to your knowledge base and possibly the knowledge base of the profession. If you focus on the development of a single spoke, the other spokes will be shorter or smaller, so you will need more effort to move your wheel or bike ahead (a lack of development). Of course, the four spokes are just the beginning of our analogy. You could add any number of spokes to strengthen yourself and our profession and to improve intervention efficacy. Here are a few spokes that you might add: alternative credentials, work experience in new settings or with people with other types of disabilities, involvement with other aspects of your organization or agency, new knowledge or technology, experimentation, research or evaluation of services, quality assurance, and active involvement with a related or unrelated professional organization. Of course, if you add gears, such as more education, more specialized knowledge or skills, more or higher levels of responsibility, or more time, you might move along quicker or more effectively.

Growing Pains

The model was initially called the wheel of fortune or the wheel of torture because it implies that you, and only you, are responsible for development. It also implies that if you are not active, you can become stuck in a rut; spend your time spinning your wheels; or lose a spoke and become wobbly, broken, and useless (or need a repair). You also run the risk of overdoing things and burning yourself out. On the other hand, the model could be the mechanism that leads you to growth and a satisfying, rewarding career (you determine what you find important and satisfying for yourself) and

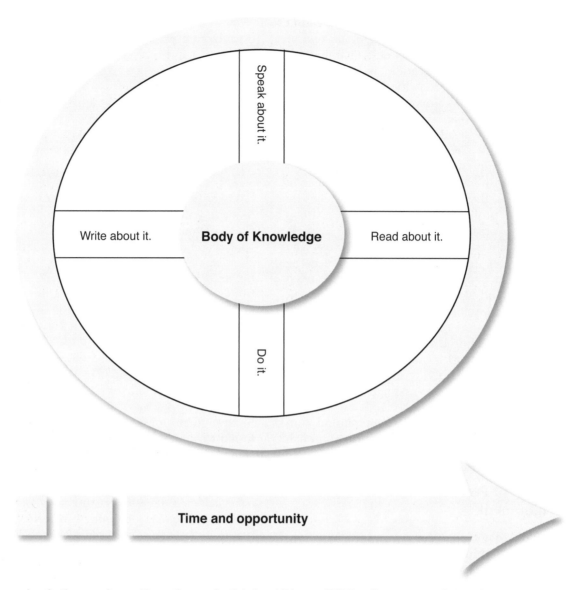

Speak about it.

Write about it.　**Body of Knowledge**　**Read about it.**

Do it.

Time and opportunity

Example of other spokes—Alternative credentials in addition to CTRS or licensure, work experience in new settings or working with folks with other types of disabilities, involvement with other aspects of your organization or agency, new knowledge or new technology, experimentation, research or evaluation of services, quality assurance, active involvement with a related or unrelated professional organization, and so on.

Example of other gears—More education, more or higher levels of responsibility, time in a given position or role, trying other disciplines or new body of knowledge to your practice, and so on.

Figure 13.1　A conceptual model of personal and professional development, previously presented as "The Wheel of Fortune or the Wheel of Torture?"

thus, your fortune. Note here that personal growth and professional development are processes, not events. They require work, focus, practice, time, and some level of competition and stress. Keep in mind the benefits and obligations of purposefully pursuing your personal and professional development. Using the model can help ensure that you experience such benefits and live up to your obligations.

Reaching Out

We, as a profession, need to be preparing potential professionals like you to meet many roles. The first step is to provide direct care services and then

A PORTRAIT OF A FUTURE EXEMPLARY PROFESSIONAL

Throughout this book, we have featured "Exemplary Professionals" as a way to help you understand what your future might entail as a therapeutic recreation specialist. For this chapter, we ask you to consider what it will take for this portrait to someday be about you. Reflect back on chapter 1, where it was suggested that this profession or any particular job opportunity it brings may not be right for everyone. In part, this is a personal choice; either you do or do not have a desire for this profession. But also, it is a matter of competence, or being adequately trained and prepared to do the job. Don't let this latter part derail your career. You can be the outstanding professional of the future if you commit yourself to working hard and seeking answers. Some suggestions follow that can help ensure your professional competence and future success. You are encouraged to create a professional development plan that addresses each of these items.

- Don't be afraid to ask questions and seek answers from the following people as often as possible.
  - Current and former students at your school and other schools
  - Professors from your school and other schools
  - Professionals from a variety of settings
  - Leaders of therapeutic recreation professional organizations
  - NCTRC or state licensure staff and representatives
- Investigate beyond what you learn in class.
  - Read books, journals, and newsletters related to therapeutic recreation.
  - Join a LISTSERV, chat room, or blog related to therapeutic recreation.
  - Regularly visit the websites of the American Therapeutic Recreation Association (ATRA), and the National Center for Therapeutic Recreation Certification (NCTRC) and other professional websites.
  - Join professional organizations—get and stay involved, and become a leader.
  - Attend professional trainings and conferences.
  - Visit therapeutic recreation programs and organizations.

- Complete as many hours of volunteer, service learning, or other hands-on experiences as you can.
  - Choose your internship(s) wisely—again, visit many sites before choosing.
- Consider how additional schooling and training might enhance your abilities.
  - Master's or doctoral degree
  - Child Life Certification (http://www.childlife .org/Certification/)
  - Training and certifications in areas such as therapeutic riding, challenge course facilitation, wilderness first responder, and aquatics
- Be prepared to meet or exceed all credentialing requirements for the state or setting that you hope to work in. These requirements could include national certification, state licensure, state registration, or any combination of the three.
- Work hard—your success is ultimately dependent on your willingness and dedication to learn and your ability to apply what you learn.
- Try and remember the **ABC's**. In this case, the **ABC's** are a long acronym: A= attitude, it all starts here as your **A**ttitude affects your **B**ehavior, which in turn affects both your **C**ommunication and **C**ommitment and, thus, the **C**onsequences of your choice in attitude and performance (behavior). The possible outcomes include one of three **S's**, **S**uccess, **S**tagnation, or **S**tinks. It is somewhat of a self-fulfilling prophesy. To help change or modify your **ABC's** consider getting D.I.R.T.Y.! D.I.R.T.Y.: **D**evelop an **I**nterest in **R**isk **T**aking (in one or all of the five domains of living and learning: social, emotional, physical, intellectual, and spiritual) and the **Y** is for you. The ABC's and the getting DIRTY acronyms are linked to a growth mindset in that willingness to grow and develop are directly related to your Attitude, your Behavior, your Communication, your Commitment, and the Consequences that follow, as well as how you or others may think about the Consequences of your performance (e.g., the S's - success, stagnation, or stinks/sucks). The ABC's and getting DIRTY (trying new things, not being afraid to fail, learn from

(continued)

your mistakes and move on) are reminders to check yourself in each area and to have the right mindset. Finally, be sure to enjoy your profession and those you work with and actually try to become a role model for those you work for, and/or for those you work with by enjoying the opportunities you are given and taking time for your own leisure and recreation.

Through this process, you will begin to develop a vision for your future, a professional philosophy, and a bond with the values of our profession. Take a second to try to imagine what your vision might look like. Where will you be and what will you have accomplished 30 years from now? Then, spend a few minutes writing an "Outstanding Professional" description of yourself in 30 years. Share what you write with others as a way to reinforce this vision for your future.

to manage or direct others to provide services. The next step is to prepare you to research and track local, state, national, and international trends and best practices and, finally, to be culturally competent. Likewise, we need to seek access to and become a positive influence on groups or organizations that are non–therapeutic recreation focused (e.g., the World Health Organization; the United Nations; state legislatures; specific advocacy groups, such as Easterseals, the Association for Adults with Developmental Disabilities (AADD), American Association on Intellectual and Developmental Disabilities (AAIDD), and the Autism Society; centers for independent living; private for-profit and nonprofit organizations; foundations; faith-based organizations; and charities). Individually, you need to feel comfortable with and be willing to take our knowledge base and apply it in many different settings and service arenas. As a profession, we need to find more ways to collaborate with like-minded organizations and professions so we can influence both policy and practice. Think back to the earlier discussion of our global community and the telecommunication and computer example. Finally, also think about a growth mindset, and as you read the following section, consider how this highly interconnected world might provide challenges and opportunities for you and our profession both inside and outside our traditional roles and realms. Again, consider both interdisciplinary and *ICF* models.

Worldviews: Finding the Optimal Perspective

Here is where your new work begins. Introduced here are six potential **worldviews** (paradigms, perspectives, or conceptual models) that our profession might consider as we work to determine how to operate in the future. These models or ideas are not new; some are over 100 years old. They do,

however, represent differing perspectives of how one might view the world (positively, negatively, or with uncertainty), how we live and interact within it, and how we make decisions. Ultimately, these viewpoints have the potential to affect the profession and how we practice therapeutic recreation now and in the future. In the latest *Megatrends* book, Aburdene (2005) suggested that future generations should seek to work at places that are congruent with their own personal paradigms.

Social and Civic Engagement Paradigm

The social and civic engagement perspective asserts that everything is framed and dealt with through the art and science of citizenship, politics, and democracy to identify and deal with issues such as social capital, social equity, and social justice. Access equals influence, so the development and use of social and professional networks, connectivity, and collaborative approaches to planning and problem solving is important. Service learning, community service, and other community-focused agendas are also used. This paradigm could also simply be considered a grassroots or political approach (Bennett, 1999; Dustin, 1993; Putnam, 2000; Putnam & Feldstein, 2003; Veblen,1899).

Consumer, or Economic, Paradigm

An alternative approach is to view the dynamics of our world within the context of economic models (i.e., supply and demand, cost–benefit modeling, profit generation, market-share value, and cost recovery), which typically assert that decisions are money driven and made from either a micro- or macroeconomic perspective. This perspective may entail simple supply versus demand approaches, market-share value versus market-share total approaches, or value-added approaches. Potential issues from this perspective might include the effect of minimum wage on

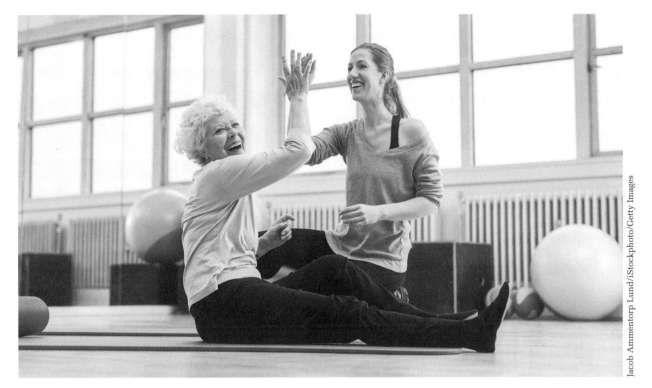

You must learn to analyze your world through many different viewpoints so that when you are helping clients, you can more easily see into theirs.

industry, education, and employment rates. This perspective might also look at the effects of collective bargaining (unions) on profit margins, general productivity, salary or position compression, merit pay versus raises based on cost of living, investment strategies, and wealth management and protection. In this "you get what you pay for" approach, margins and volumes are critical. This approach can be referred to as a marketing, or Wal-Mart versus Versace, approach (Bennett, 1999; Kelly & Warnick, 1999; Putnam, 2000; Putnam & Feldstein, 2003; Veblen, 1899).

Quality Management, or Mission and Vision, Paradigm

This perspective is based on the use of core values to shape the decision-making process. Under this philosophy, those involved in achieving the mission must believe in the values of the group that they are working with and use those shared values as a beacon to guide their work. Values are often prioritized, and strategic planning is used to achieve missions or visions. Leaders who implement such a philosophy often work hard to model agency or organizational values and the associated desired behavior. Also critical is recognizing and rewarding value-congruent behavior

demonstrated by team members. This approach could be viewed as either a ritualistic or a humanistic approach (Covey, 2005; Holtz, 1998; Loher & Schwartz, 2003; O'Neill & Conzemius, 2006).

Behavioral, or Outcomes, Paradigm

Focusing on the end product, this approach is often data driven. It could involve a combination of organizational management and marketing strategies as well as the use of the scientific method as a forecasting tool. Examples within our profession might include issues of time on task, scope and sequence, billable time versus downtime, standard operating procedures, **diagnostic related groups (DRGs)**, **risk pool insurance** systems, optimization of resources, and market share or niche approaches. The outcome is sometimes more important than the means of getting there. This approach could also simply be viewed as the segmentation–sterilization, or specialization, approach (Hubbard, 1993; Leavitt, 2006; O'Neill & Conzemius, 2006).

Change Theory Paradigm

Change theory can involve a mathematical or theoretical examination for patterns, interventions, issues, perspectives, and outliers. It can also focus on abstract or obtuse issues and the expected versus the unexpected. This approach could simply be viewed as the mathematical, experimental, or systematic pattern and outlier approach. Change theory projects futures based on trends of the past (Blanchard, Lacinak, Tompkins, & Ballard, 2002; Buckingham & Clifton 2001; Covey, 2005; Hutchens, 2000; Johnson, 1998; Senge et al., 1999).

Spirituality or Religious Systems Paradigm

This paradigm acknowledges the influence of religious systems on the world in which we live. Belief can be in a higher power (Buddhism, Christian, Judaism, or Muslim), within oneself (self-reverent thought, self-determination, or self-control), or in many things (Christian Science, holistic health, or new age beliefs). Belief may not exist or may be of an undetermined nature (agnostic, atheist, not exposed to belief systems, or have not thought about it). Faith or hope issues as well as rituals or beliefs about birth, illness, disability, gender, purpose in life, roles, families, relationships, lifestyle issues, and death all influence our world, how it works, and how we work within it (Aburdene, 2005; Buckingham & Clifton, 2001; Holtz, 1998; Lipson, Dibble, & Minarik, 1996; Zander & Zander, 2000).

Summary

National Geographic photographer Dewitt Jones has spent years finding beauty in places where most of us would never think to look. His name may not be familiar, but you probably know him through his work. I mention Dewitt here because he has realized that his ability to find what is right with the world can serve as a template for many of life's challenges. He now spends much of his time sharing this message with people and talking about how perspective is important to finding our way in life. Moving a short distance or waiting a few seconds can make a world of difference in both photography and how we see problems, opportunities, one another, and the world in general. The six paradigms serve as examples of how different perspectives suggest different pathways to the future. Each of these paradigms can be used to solve a single problem but in very different ways and often with far different results. Within the world of therapeutic recreation, we must learn to examine, critique, and apply these and other viewpoints available to us when venturing into our professional futures, individually and collectively.

DISCUSSION QUESTIONS

1. How does knowing and understanding the past help improve the future? How does it prevent or hinder improvement or change?

2. Identify the primary elements of the professional development model, and discuss which element (spoke, hub, or tire) will be the most challenging for you and why.

3. Create a plan to help you work on this element both before and after you graduate. Share this plan with at least one other person.

4. Identify at least three trends (e.g., social, economic, or cultural) that could affect the future of this profession and your potential for becoming a practicing professional.

5. Identify one new trend (e.g., technology, economic, or social) that is changing the way that you or those around you complete (or not) a routine task. Describe the trend to someone else, and then, identify how this trend could be used (positively or negatively) within this profession as you know it.

6. Identify by name or description the six paradigms presented, and then, identify how and why each paradigm could be used to assure or eliminate services to those you work with.

Glossary

accreditation—Credentialing of an academic institution and specific curriculum that meets or exceeds prescribed criteria of educational quality with regard to professional preparation curricula.

active treatment—Services designed to promote the achievement of specific therapeutic outcomes directly related to illness or disability.

activity—WHO indicator of being able to execute and complete tasks (e.g., reading, thinking, walking, dressing, voiding, solving problems, having basic interpersonal interactions, making decisions).

activity analysis—The process of breaking down an activity into the various skills and requirements (equipment and setting) necessary for successfully doing the activity.

activity goal—The objective or targeted outcome related to a game, a task, or an activity.

activity limitation—WHO indicator of difficulties experienced when attempting to perform tasks.

activity theory—Theory of aging that asserts successful aging is dependent upon the maintenance of life activities associated with such roles.

adult day facilities—Facilities in which care is provided during day hours to older adults, often with physical or intellectual impairment.

Alliance for Therapeutic Recreation—Board members of both ATRA and NTRS who meet to communicate and work in partnership on certain issues.

allied health profession—A profession made up of formally trained and credentialed health care providers who assist physicians and other members of the treatment team in providing services relevant to their expertise.

ambulation—Walking.

Americans with Disabilities Act (ADA)—Federal legislation passed in 1990 and effective in 1992 that made it illegal to discriminate against a person based on the existence of a disability.

American Therapeutic Recreation Association (ATRA)—Created in 1984. A therapeutic recreation professional organization that separated from NTRS and NRPA, which emphasizes that therapeutic recreation is treatment for therapeutic change. Further, ATRA separates its therapeutic recreation historical roots and alignment to parks and recreation and its distinct association with leisure.

aneurism—Dilation, or ballooning, of a blood vessel by more than 50 percent of its normal diameter, sometimes resulting in bursting and internal bleeding.

anomie—A dysfunctional state of alienation and isolation from economic, cultural, political, and primary socialization group systems.

aphasia—Impairment or inability to speak, comprehend, read, or write, resulting from damage to the brain.

art therapists—Master's-level psychotherapists who are trained in both psychology and art.

assessment—An information gathering process intended to identify client needs, desires, interest, resources, and overall level of functioning.

assessment report—A document summarizing results and recommendations from a completed assessment.

assisted living facilities—Nonmedical living facilities for people who are unable to live on their own but do not need continuous nursing care.

atlantoaxial instability—Laxity between the ligaments and muscles surrounding the joint between vertebrae C1 and C2, which may slip out of alignment and result in spinal cord injury.

at risk—Refers to a set of presumed cause–effect dynamics that place a child or adolescent in danger of future negative outcomes.

autism—A neurological disorder that affects a person's ability to communicate, understand language, play, and relate to others. A diagnosis of autism is given when a person exhibits 6 of more of 12 symptoms listed across three major areas: social interaction, communication, and behavior.

autonomic dysreflexia (AD)—An excessive rise in blood pressure that could be life threatening.

Baby Boomers—The generation born between 1946 and 1964.

behavior modification—The use of positive and negative reinforcers to reduce negative and increase positive behaviors.

bibliotherapy—Uses reading materials, such as novels, plays, short stories, booklets, and pamphlets, to help clients become aware that other people have similar problems, become aware of new insights, and structure their lives.

biofeedback—Involves measuring body functions such as heart rate or temperature and then using this information to master conscious control of the associated function.

biopsychosocial model—A broad model that attributes level of health to an interaction of biological factors, psychological factors, and social factors.

blood pressure—A measure of the pressure of the blood on the arterial walls that consists of two values: systolic blood pressure, as the heart contracts or pumps the blood to the circulatory system (90 to 140 mmHg), and diastolic blood pressure, as the heart fills up with blood following a contraction (60 to 90 mmHg).

briefing—The process of providing information related to goals, expectations, and events of an upcoming therapeutic recreation session.

Canadian federalism—Refers to Canadian political ideology that emphasizes expression of both diversity and unity.

capacity qualifier—WHO indicator of a person's highest probable level of functioning can be indicated and differentiated depending on whether activity and participation are occurring with or without assistance.

capitalism—Economic system characterized by a free market and private and corporate business ownership.

cardiovascular—Refers to the circulatory system: heart, arteries, and veins.

career resilience—Taking control of one's own future by taking responsibility to seek out appropriate training, at one's own expense if necessary, to position oneself for a desired career track; to promote oneself.

causal attributions—Beliefs held about the causes of the events that occur in life.

cerebral palsy (CP)—A group of disorders characterized by an inability to control muscular and postural movements resulting from damage to the brain before age 12.

cerebrovascular accident (CVA)—An acute neurological injury resulting from disruption of blood flow to the brain because of blockage or bleeding of blood vessels.

certification—A form of voluntary credentialing that ensures that a person has met specific standards or criteria with regard to education, experience, and continuing professional development through an application process and required exam.

chaining—Teaching small parts or simplified versions of a behavior by having each lesson build on the previously taught information.

change theory—The examination of data (behavioral, numeric, thematic, logical, or philosophical) for patterns, changes in patterns, normalcy and abnormality, and causes of patterns, followed by the real, perceived, or theoretical understanding of the cause of the pattern and, finally, the knowledge of how to change said pattern.

chronic—A persistent or lasting medical condition or disease.

clinical pathways—A standardized process used to direct patient care within the health care system, specifying the role of various professionals at various levels and stages of care.

closed neural tube defect—A form of spina bifida in which the spinal cord is marked by a malformation of fat, bone or membranes, with disability ranging from no symptoms to partial paralysis and bowel and bladder difficulties.

code of ethics—The official moral ideology of a professional group; within helping professions, a code of ethics is a basic requirement for recognition as a professional body.

cognitive plasticity—The ability to acquire or improve cognitive skills.

compulsions—Repetitive behaviors or mental acts performed to prevent or reduce anxiety or distress.

congenital—A condition present at birth.

construct—A nonobservable trait that cannot be directly measured, such as happiness or satisfaction.

constructivism—Learning theory that focuses on the importance of learning through experience rather than lecture and memorization.

continuity theory—Theory of aging that states that successful aging is based on one's ability to maintain the same activities, behaviors, relationships as they did in their earlier years of life.

contracture—Permanent shortening of muscle groups and connective tissues surrounding the joint.

contraindication—A condition or indication against a particular line of treatment or activity.

convoy model of social relationships—Contemporary framework for aging that focuses on the importance of social networks as people age.

countertransference—Situation in which a therapist begins to associate his or her own feelings, sometimes repressed, toward a client.

crisis care—Level of psychiatric care in which a client receives supervision 24 hours a day for a short time, typically 30 days or less.

critical force—A factor that can influence the entire experience.

cumulative inequality theory—Systematic explanation of how inequalities develop and influence the quality of life.

day treatment—Level of care in which a client resides at home but attends treatment-related activities at a treatment facility throughout the day.

debriefing—Skillful questioning of a client or group of clients to enhance understanding, learning, or insight.

decubitus ulcers—Damage to the skin and possibly underlying tissues resulting from prolonged pressure on bony weight-bearing areas of the body or excessive sweating or pressure on an area of the body during a fall.

defense mechanisms—Unconscious behaviors aimed at reducing anxiety.

degenerative—Refers to a condition in which tissues or organs progressively deteriorate over time.

delusions—False beliefs related to one's perceptions or experiences.

dementia—Progressive decline in cognitive function characterized by disturbances in memory, attention, language, and problem solving.

Dementia care facility—Provides residential care and support for individuals who are experiencing the challenges that come with memory loss and disorientation.

demyelinating disease—Disease that affects the myelin sheath of nerves, which insulates them and allows them to conduct impulses or signals to and from the brain.

developmental delay—Markedly late achievement of a typical developmental milestone.

developmental disability—Severe, chronic disability originating before age 22 and resulting in substantial functional mental or physical impairments in two or more of the following areas of major life activity: self-care, receptive and expressive language, learning, mobility, self-direction, capacity for independent living, and economic self-sufficiency.

diagnostic related groups (DRGs)—A hospital classification system developed by the Centers for Medicare & Medicaid Services that categorizes patient cases based on expected resource use.

dietitian—A professional who promotes health through sound eating habits by assessing the nutritional needs of clients and planning and managing dietary intake.

disengagement theory—Theory of aging that states that withdrawal from activities and society is normal and acceptable with age.

diversional therapy—A client centered practice, typically practiced in Australia, that recognizes that leisure and recreational experiences are the right of all individuals.

Down syndrome—A chromosomal developmental disability and a form of intellectual impairment resulting from the production of an extra chromosome during cell development.

Duchenne muscular dystrophy—A genetic disorder characterized by progressive muscle degeneration and weakness.

dysarthria—Neurologically based disruption of tongue, throat, lip, or lung function that affects speech.

ecological approach—A theoretical approach that considers the interaction between an individual and the surrounding environment.

ecological model of disability—A view of disability as being reciprocal in nature; a change that occurs within the community will change not only that system but also the individuals, directly or indirectly.

ecological system—The interaction between people (including personal characteristics, behaviors, and physiological factors) and their environments. The environment encompasses immediate settings or people (home, classroom, neighborhood, family, teacher, counselor, and peer groups) as well as larger contexts in which these settings or people are embedded (cultural, political, educational, and community institutions).

elder orphans—Elderly individuals who have no adult children, spouse or companion to depend on for support.

ethics—Deals with the duties and obligations of professionals to their consumers (service recipients), the profession, and the wider public.

etiological—Refers to the cause or the source of a disease or disability.

evaluation—The process of determining the effectiveness of therapeutic recreation programs in addressing client goals.

excess disability—When a person with a disability loses additional abilities as a result of factors other than the disability itself.

expressive arts—The employment of visual arts, music, dance, or drama techniques with the intent to produce and achieve a final product.

facilitation skills—Related to the interpersonal interactions that the therapist has with clients; sometimes referred to as soft skills.

fasciculations—Brief, spontaneous contractions affecting a small number of muscle fibers, which can cause a flicker of movement under the skin.

flaccidity—A complete loss of muscle tone.

Florence Nightingale—Cited as an early medical expert (nurse) who highlighted the therapeutic effects of recreation while working in British hospitals during the Crimean War (1854-1856).

forensic—Indicates that a treatment program is somehow related to the legal system typically because of the influence of a mental condition on a person's criminal behavior or ability to stand trial.

functional intervention (FI)—Component that focuses on correcting functional deficits in the physical, mental, emotional, and social domains.

galactosemia—A genetic condition that results in a deficiency in an enzyme responsible for processing galactose, a sugar found in many common foods.

Glasgow Coma Scale—A scale used to determine the conscious state of a person.

goals—General outcomes expected to result from participation in a therapeutic recreation program.

Halliwick method—A 10-step process for teaching swimming to people with significant physical disabilities with the primary goal of achieving total client independence in the water.

hallucinations—Perceived sensory experiences that do not really exist.

health—A state of complete physical, mental, and social well-being and not merely the absence of disease or infirmity.

health condition—The current health status of a person, regardless of whether a disease, disorder, or trauma exists.

health protection/health promotion model—A practice model meant to be used to guide therapeutic recreation clients toward achieving health and self-actualization; contains three components: prescriptive activities, recreation, and leisure.

hemiplegia—Paralysis of one vertical half of the body.

hippotherapy—A form of animal-assisted therapy in which the movement created by the gait of a horse is used as a therapeutic tool for a variety of orthopedic conditions; requires extensive training and is typically conducted by a physical therapist.

holistic—Considering all aspects or properties of a given phenomenon, system, situation, or problem.

hospital recreation—Antecedent term to therapeutic recreation. The Red Cross hired recreation workers in hospital settings during both world wars. Further, hospital recreation had a specific section in the American Recreation Society (1938-1965).

Hull-House—A settlement house in a poor district of Chicago, which was established by Jane Addams, Ellen Gates Starr, and Mary Keyser in September 1889. Hull-House established agencies in the worst slums of Chicago (13th Ward), where Hull-House residents provided human services and engaged in social action on behalf of people with special needs (e.g., art, education, citizenship classes, community development, immigration protection, recreation programming).

human development index—A comparative measure of life expectancy, literacy, education, and standards of living for countries worldwide.

humanitarian treatment movement—A social movement that swept through Europe in the late 1700s and early 1800s regarding the treatment of people with special needs (e.g., people with mental illness, people with disabilities). Paramount aspects to this movement were removing patients from dungeons and allowing them to move freely on hospital grounds outside mainstream communities.

hydrocephalus—A condition resulting in an enlarged head that is caused by an abnormal accumulation of cerebrospinal fluid.

hypertension—High blood pressure.

hypertonia—Increased amount of tone in a muscle group.

hyporeflexia—Below normal or absent reflexes

hypotonia—Decreased amount of tone in a muscle group.

impairment—A significant deviation, loss, or problem in a body function or structure.

implementation—The process of administering planned therapeutic recreation programs.

inclusive recreation—Recreation opportunities designed so that people with disabilities can experience leisure in mainstream society. Three venues of inclusive recreation are community reintegration programs, community integration programs, and community development programs.

individualized education program (IEP)—A legal document created for a child with a disability that outlines the educational and related service goals, including evaluation of those services. It is reviewed and updated once a year.

individualized program plan (IPP)—A plan of action regarding the provision of services to a particular therapeutic recreation client; also known as a treatment plan or a care plan.

Individuals with Disabilities Education Act (IDEA)—Federal law passed in 1974 that requires free and appropriate education of all children, regardless of disability, and provides about 10 percent of the annual cost of educating a child with a disability.

Inkerman Cafe—Created by Florence Nightingale in September 1855 as a small wooden hut that was located at the center of the hospital complex. The structure had a recreation room and a coffeehouse. The cafe provided a safe place where soldiers could escape their problems and find friendship.

intellectual disability—An impairment of intellectual functioning that onsets before the age of 18 and impacts adaptive functioning in a significant way.

intellectual impairment—Significant impairment of intellectual skills such as reasoning, problem-solving, planning, abstract thinking, judgment, academic learning and learning from experience.

interdependence—Participation that involves reciprocal interaction between people.

interorganizational networking—An aspect of organizational networking that refers to the networking between organizations with similar characteristics.

interprofessional—Professional practice or initiatives involving professionals from multiple disciplines.

intraorganizational networking—An aspect of organizational networking that focuses on the networks that operate, individually and collectively, within an organization for a shared goal and ultimately the betterment of the organization.

job—A regular remunerative position.

Labor Museum—A community leisure education program developed at Hull-House that provided a developmental process in which groups of people increased their understanding of leisure and the relationship among leisure, lifestyle, culture, and society. The Labor Museum developed from Jane Addams' concern for (1) the disdainful attitudes that immigrant children had toward their parents' old-world traditions and culture and (2) the contemptuous attitudes that Americans had toward poverty-stricken immigrants living in Chicago.

learning disability—A general classification given for significant problems with language or mathematical calculations not related to intellectual impairment or emotional or psychological problems in children.

least restrictive environment—A setting that allows maximum integration with the larger community. In the case of children with developmental disabilities, this includes educating and providing services in the same setting with children without disabilities.

leisure ability model—A practice model that describes the ultimate goal of therapeutic recreation services to be an enhanced leisure lifestyle and includes three components: functional intervention, leisure education, and recreation participation.

leisure education—A developmental process through which a person or group of people increase their understanding of leisure and the relationship among leisure, lifestyle, and society.

leisure orientation to therapeutic recreation—Belief that the distinctness of therapeutic recreation is its clear association with programming recreation and leisure services. As such, leisure is an end unto itself, which creates freedom and choice among people with special needs.

licensure—A form of professional credentialing required by state law. Anyone wishing to practice the profession within the given state must be licensed.

life-span development—The study of growth over the entire life of a person.

manic (mania)—Elevated level of mood involving symptoms such as distractibility, indiscretion, grandiosity, flight of ideas, increased activity, sleep deficit, and talkativeness.

maximum heart rate—Defined as a person's age subtracted from 220. For example, a 40-year-old person would have a maximum heart rate of 180 (220 − 40 = 180).

Medicaid—Insurance program sponsored by the federal government for people with disabilities. Each state sets its own guidelines for, administers, and partly funds Medicaid.

medical model of disability—A perspective that views disabilities as being physiological, cognitive, social, or psychological and in need of remediation.

meditation—The practice of focusing the mind.

moral character—What sort of person one ought to be.

moral community—How society should be constructed to enable ethical people to act ethically.

moral conduct—How one should act.

multi-infarct dementia—Refers to a group of syndromes caused by different mechanisms, all resulting in vascular lesions in the brain.

muscular dystrophy (MD)—Refers to a group of genetically linked diseases that cause progressive muscle weakness and loss of muscle mass.

myelomeningocele—A form of spina bifida in which a defect in the spinal column causes the spinal cord and vertebral sac to protrude through the vertebra, resulting in partial or full paralysis below the spinal opening.

National Association of Recreation Therapists (NART)—Created in 1953 (1) so that the therapy orientation to therapeutic recreation would have even greater distance from the recreation and physical education curriculum of AAHPER and (2) to bring greater importance to clinical outcomes and the role of recreation in bringing functional improvements in clients. NART eventually merged with three other professional organizations to develop the National Therapeutic Recreation Society, a branch of the National Recreation and Park Association, in 1966.

National Council for Therapeutic Recreation Certification (NCTRC)—An independent credentialing agency created in 1981 that oversees the national certification program in therapeutic recreation in the United States.

National Recreation and Park Association (NRPA)—Made up of five recreation and leisure professional organizations that merged in 1966. Today, NRPA is a parks and recreation professional organization with a mission to advance parks, recreation, leisure, and environmental conservation.

National Therapeutic Recreation Society (NTRS)—A branch of the NRPA created in 1966 to enhance the competencies of therapeutic recreation specialists. Four therapeutic recreation professional organizations merged to form NTRS (Hospital Recreation

Section of the American Recreation Society; Recreation Therapist Section of the American Association of Health, Physical Education, Recreation, and Dance; National Association of Recreation Therapists; and Recreation Services for the Handicapped Section of the National Recreation Association).

networking—The ability to create and maintain an effective and diverse system of resources, made possible by using relevant information, having good working relations, and maintaining and communicating a good track record.

normalization principle—A theoretical framework developed by the Scandinavian academic Bengt Nirje to help people with disabilities become included in mainstream society. Makes available to persons with disabilities patterns of life and conditions of everyday living that are as close as possible or indeed the same as the regular circumstances and ways of life of their communities.

nurse—A licensed medical professional who assists individuals, families, and communities to attain, re-attain, and maintain optimal health and functioning by observing patients, assessing symptoms, and documenting progress.

nursing home facilities—Residential facilities for people who require constant nursing care.

objectives—Specific indicators of goal achievement, characterized by identification of an expected behavior, a condition under which the behavior will occur, and a criteria for determining whether the behavior has occurred.

obsessions—Persistent thoughts, ideas, impulses, or images that are experienced as intrusive and inappropriate and that cause marked anxiety or distress.

orthopedic impairment—Condition caused by disruption of the musculoskeletal system.

orthostatic hypotension—A decrease, or drop, in blood pressure because of the pooling of blood in the lower extremities and abdominal area.

osteoarthritis (OA)—Arthritis that results from wear and tear on joints over a person's life span.

outcome—Observed change in client's status as a result of intervention or interaction.

outpatient care—Level of care in which clients reside at home but attend regular therapy sessions at the care facility.

outsourcing—Delegating non-core business operations to outside agencies, sometimes across national boundaries (offshore outsourcing).

paradigm—A thought pattern, set of practices, or conceptual model used for explanation.

paraplegia—Complete or partial impairment of movement or sensation affecting the involvement of both legs.

Parkinson's disease (PD)—A central nervous system disorder that affects muscle control.

participation—WHO indicator of involvement in meaningful life situations (e.g., going shopping, spending time on a hobby, dating, completing work tasks, volunteering, attending sporting events).

pathological reflex—Reflex responses that persist beyond the normal developmental time period.

performance qualifier—WHO indicator of what a person does in his or her current environment.

pericarditis—Inflammation of the lining of the heart.

person-centered care—Care that actively engages the patient or client in their treatment, acknowledging their presence in and ownership of the care process.

person-first terminology—Language that refers to all people as individuals first and as personal characteristics second.

pervasive developmental disorder (PDD)—A neurological disorder that affects a person's ability to communicate, understand language, play, and relate to others. The diagnosis of PDD-NOS (not otherwise specified) is given when a child displays behaviors similar to autism but to a lesser extent.

phenylketonuria (PKU)—An inherited condition caused by a defect in the gene that helps create an enzyme needed to break down phenylalanine, which untreated can result in intellectual disability and other impairments.

physical activity—All forms of bodily movement produced by the contractions of skeletal muscles that substantially increase energy expenditure.

planning—The process of developing and organizing therapeutic recreation services for a client based on assessment results.

positive psychology—The branch of psychology that uses scientific understanding and effective intervention to aid in the achievement of a satisfactory life, rather than treating mental illness.

positive youth development—A service approach focusing on children's unique talents, strengths, interests, and potential.

precaution—Measure taken to avoid injury or a potential problem.

presenting problem—A client's primary reason for receiving treatment.

primary prevention—The reduction of the number of new cases of identified problems or conditions occurring within a population; targets the promotion of health and development.

problatunity—Refers to a perspective that a problem and an opportunity can reside in the same time and space, essentially being one and the same.

profession—Efforts of the person are directed toward service rather than simply financial remuneration.

professional authority—The ability of a profession to hold its members accountable.

professional credentialing—Evidence that a professional has acquired a body of knowledge that includes theory, philosophy, and practice within a given field.

professional culture—Made up of the customary beliefs, norms, or traits of the profession; often defined by professional associations.

professional development—The exchange and transmission of professional knowledge through professional associations' conferences, workshops, and publications.

professionalism—The conduct, aims, or qualities that characterize a profession or professional person and includes both professional and personal advocacy.

professional standards of practice—A set of guidelines for providing quality and effective services that are continually updated and refined by experienced professionals.

progressive relaxation—Stress management technique involving progressive tensing and relaxing of muscles throughout the body.

progress notes—Formal documentation procedure for recording the progression or regression of clients over time.

prosthetic device—Artificial limb designed for an amputated extremity.

psychiatrist—Medical doctor who prescribes medications to treat various forms of mental illness and is extensively trained in diagnosis and treatment modalities for mental illness.

psychologist—A social scientist who studies psychology, which is the study of the human mind and human behavior.

pulmonary—Refers to the lungs.

registration—A form of professional credentialing that is voluntary and generally provides a list of people who have met a minimum standard with regard to education and experience within a specific field.

rehabilitation hospital—Health care facility that specializes in longer-term treatment of medical conditions, often after clients have already received treatment from acute care facilities.

residential care—Level of care in which clients reside at the treatment facility.

rest cures—The use of rest and recreation to help restore mental health. Used as a medical strategy during the medicalization of spas and thermal baths (1800 to mid-1900s).

rheumatism—An older term used for arthritis.

rheumatoid arthritis (RA)—Involves inflammation of the lining of joints and is believed to be related to an attack on the body by the immune system.

risk pool insurance—Partnerships, or pools, formed by insurance companies to reduce potential risk of catastrophic events.

secondary condition—Medical, social, emotional, family, or community problem that a person with a primary disabling condition likely experiences.

secondary prevention—Reducing the number of existing problem cases and lowering the prevalence of the manifested problems or conditions in the population.

seizure—An abnormality in the electric activity in the brain.

selective optimization with compensation (SOC) theory—Suggests that seniors select and optimize their best abilities and most intact functions while compensating for declines and losses.

self-advocacy—The ability of people with disabilities to promote for their own rights.

self-determination theory—A theory of motivation that focuses on the degree to which an individual's behavior is self-motivated and self-determined.

self-efficacy—The belief that one has about his or her capabilities to perform a particular task or manage a situation successfully.

separatist mentality (in therapeutic recreation)—Mindset adopted by members of the NTRS in the early 1980s who separated themselves from NTRS and NRPA so that they could follow a therapy orientation to therapeutic recreation. This group eventually created the American Therapeutic Recreation Association.

sequencing—Arranging the elements of a therapeutic recreation session or series of therapeutic recreation sessions in an order that facilitates successful performance.

settlement house—Established human services agency developed purposely in city slums where human services workers provided human services (e.g., education, citizenship classes, community development, immigration protection, recreation) and engaged in social action on behalf of the poor living in the area.

severe combined immune deficiency (SCID)—A primary immune deficiency that usually results in a severe defect in both the T- & B-lymphocyte systems, and the onset of serious infections within the first few months of life.

shaping—Teaching small parts or simplified versions of a behavior with each lesson slightly modifying the previously taught information.

social capital—The collective value of all social networks and the tendencies that arise from these networks to do things for each other. Networks that build social capital are characterized by reciprocity and trust.

social inclusion—Valuing the participation of all people in social aspects of community activities.

social model of disability—A perspective of disability that focuses on barriers being attributed to physical, cognitive, social, or emotional aspects of a society.

social worker—A professional who helps people function in the healthiest way possible in the environment, manage their relationships, and solve personal and family problems.

socioemotional selectivity (SES) theory—A theory of aging that asserts that, as an individual ages, she becomes more selective about how to spend resources such as time and money, focusing in on activities that provide emotional support.

spasticity—Involuntary increase in muscle tone.

specifier—A descriptor used to specify characteristics, course of prognosis, and severity of a *DSM-5* diagnosis.

speech-language pathologist—Professional trained in disorders related to speech, language, cognitive communication, and swallowing skills.

spina bifida—A condition in which the spinal column does not close during gestation.

spina bifida occulta—A mild form of spina bifida that typically is asymptomatic.

spiral goals—Goals that are expressed outside the group, in the real world.

stages of playful behavior—Suggested by Piaget; include sensorimotor play, symbolic play, and cooperative play.

strengths—Capabilities and resources possessed by a client or available through the surrounding environment.

strengths-based approach—Approach that focuses first on capabilities when working with a client.

strength training—Exercise or activity that maintains or improves skeletal muscle strength and endurance.

stroke—See *cerebrovascular accident*.

subtype—A specific subgroup within a *DSM-5* diagnosis.

syndrome—A group of symptoms or abnormalities that indicate a particular trait or disease.

systematic desensitization—A therapy technique in which the client maintains a relaxed state while being subjected to a hierarchy of fear- or anxiety-producing stimuli.

task analysis—The breaking down of a specific skill into its component parts.

technical skills—Tasks of a noninterpersonal nature associated with job responsibilities, such as completing documentation or preparing equipment; sometimes referred to as hard skills.

terminal—A progressive disease expected to cause death.

terminal values—A perspective used to generalize a feeling and affiliate people for group action.

tertiary prevention—The reduction of harmful effects and complications that occur within an existing disorder and identified condition; may also be referred to as treatment or rehabilitation.

tetraplegia (also, quadriplegia)—Complete or partial impairment of movement or sensation affecting the involvement of all four limbs.

therapeutic recreation—The purposeful use and enhancement of leisure as a means of maximizing a person's overall health, well-being, and quality of life.

therapeutic recreation process—The overall process of assessing, planning, implementing, and evaluating therapeutic recreation programs.

therapeutic riding—Use of horseback riding as an alternative therapy for a variety of psychological, social, or physical conditions.

therapy orientation of therapeutic recreation—Belief that the essence of therapeutic recreation is to use or prescribe recreation and leisure for medical purposes. As such, recreation and leisure are a means to an end (treatment).

thermal injuries—Injuries resulting from exposure to temperature extremes.

thermoregulation—Regulation of body temperature.

transference—Unconscious redirection of feelings from one person to another, often occurring in therapy when the client redirects feelings toward the therapist.

transient ischemic attack (TIA)—Temporary disturbance of blood flow to the brain, resulting in short-term neurological dysfunction; also known as ministrokes.

treatment modality—Activities used to help clients meet therapeutic goals.

treatment protocols—A standardized process for providing consistent treatment for a particular client group or within a particular form of treatment.

unconditional positive regard (UPR)—Accepting a client as worthy and capable, although the client may not act or feel that way. UPR is one of the three necessary conditions for positive change in therapy along with genuineness and empathy.

utopian years of therapeutic recreation—A social movement that began in the early 1960s to unite all leisure-oriented professionals and therapeutic recreation organizations together into one loosely structured organization.

values clarification—Technique that can help clients examine their personal behavior, identify the values that are driving this behavior, determine whether these values are in line with their core personal values, and shift behavior to be congruent with personal core values.

V code—An *ICD-9* clinical notation used to indicate the presence of specific social and environmental factors that affect a client's treatment.

well-being—A state of successful, satisfying and productive engagement with one's life and the realization of one's full physical, cognitive, and social-emotional potential.

worldview—The lens, or perspective, through which one sees the world and interacts with it.

Z code—An *ICD-10* clinical notation used to indicate the presence of specific social and environmental factors that affect a client's treatment.

References

AARP International (2018). The Aging Readiness and Competitiveness Report. Retrieved from http://arc.aarpinternational.org/countries/united-states

Abramson, L.Y., Seligman, M.E., & Teasdale, J.D. (1978). Learned helplessness in humans: Critique and reformulation. *Journal of Abnormal Psychology, 87,* 49-74.

Aburdene, P. (2005). *Megatrends 2010: The rise of conscious capitalism.* Charlottesville, VA: Hampton Roads Publishing.

Addams, J. (1895/1990). Art work. In M.L. McCree Bryan & A.F. Davis (Eds.), *100 years at Hull-House* (pp. 39-41). Bloomington, IN: Indiana University Press. (Reprinted from *Forum*, July 1895, pp. 614-617).

Addams, J. (1905/1990). Hull-House woman's club anthem. In M.L. McCree Bryan & A.F. Davis (Eds.), *100 years at Hull-House* (p. 108). Bloomington, IN: Indiana University Press. (Reprinted from *The Commons*, April 1905, p. 225).

Addams, J. (1909/1972). *The spirit of youth and the city streets.* Urbana, IL: University of Illinois Press.

Addams, J. (1910/1981). *Twenty years at Hull-House.* New York, NY: Signet.

Administration on Aging (AoA). (2016). A profile of older Americans. Retrieved from www.acl.gov/aging-and-disability-in-america/data-and-research/profile-older-americans

Administration on Developmental Disabilities. (2018). ADD fact sheet. Retrieved from https://web.archive.org/web/20080103041344/http:/www.acf.hhs.gov:80/programs/add/Factsheet.html

Akiyama, H. (2000). How persons with mental illness lived in the 20th century. *Normalization: Welfare for Persons with Disabilities, 20*(7), 9-14.

Alberta Therapeutic Recreation Association. (2010). *Membership directory.* Calgary, AB: ATRA.

Algase, D.L., Beck, C., Kolanowski, A., Whall, A., Berent, S., Richards, K., & Beattie, E. (1996). Need-driven dementia-compromised behavior: An alternative view of disruptive behavior. *American Journal of Alzheimer's Disease, 11*(6), 10-19.

Allen, B., & Allen, S. (1995). The process of a social construction of mental retardation: Toward value-based interaction. *The Journal of the Association for Persons With Severe Handicaps, 20,* 158-160.

Allen, L.R., Paisley, K., Stevens, B., & Harwell, R. (1998). The top 10 ways to impact at-risk youth in recreation programming. *Parks and Recreation, 33*(3), 80-85.

Alzheimer's Association. (2017). Memories in the making. Retrieved from www.alz.org/sewi/in_my_community_20372.asp

American College of Sports Medicine and the American Heart Association. *Circulation, 116*(9), 1081-1093.

American Hospital Association. (2017). Fast facts on U.S. hospitals. Retrieved from www.aha.org/research/rc/stat-studeies/fast-facts.shtml

American Psychiatric Association. (2013). *Diagnostic and statistical manual of mental disorders* (5th ed.). Arlington, VA: Author.

Americans with Disabilities Act of 1990, Pub. L. No. 101-336, § 2, 104 Stat. 328 (1991).

Anderson, L.S., & Heyne, L.A. (2012a). Flourishing through leisure: An ecological extension of leisure and well-being model in therapeutic recreation strengths-based practice. *Therapeutic Recreation Journal, 46*(2), 129-152.

Anderson, L.S., & Heyne, L.A. (2012b). *Therapeutic recreation practice: A strengths approach.* State College, PA: Venture.

Anderson, L.S., & Heyne, L.A. (2016). Flourishing Through Leisure and the Upward Spiral Theory of Lifestyle Change. *Therapeutic Recreation Journal, 50*(2), 118.

Antonucci, T., Birditt, L., & Akiyama, H. (2009). Convoys of social relations: An interdisciplinary approach. In V. Bengtson, D. Gans, N. Putney, & M. Silverstein (Eds.), *Handbook of theories of aging* (2nd ed.). New York, NY: Springer.

Arai, S.M., Berbary, L.A., & Dupuis, S.L. (2015). Dialogues for re-imagined praxis: using theory in practice to transform structural, ideological, and discursive "realities" with/in communities. *Leisure/Loisir, 39*(2), 299-321.

Archie, V.W., & Sherrill, C. (1989). Attitudes toward handicapped peers of mainstreamed and nonmainstreamed children in physical education. *Perceptual and Motor Skills, 69,* 319-322.

Association for Experiential Education. (2018). Accreditation for adventure and outdoor behavioral healthcare programs. Retrieved from www.aee.org/standards2

American Therapeutic Recreation Association (2013). *ATRA standards of practice.* Reston, VA: Author.

Austin, D.R. (1998). The health protection/health promotion model. *Therapeutic Recreation Journal, 32*(2), 109-117.

Austin, D.R. (2001). *Glossary of recreation therapy and occupational therapy.* State College, PA: Venture.

Austin, D.R. (2002). A third revolution in therapeutic recreation. In D.R. Austin, J. Dattilo, & B.P. McCormick (Eds.), *Conceptual foundations for therapeutic recreation* (pp. 273-288). State College, PA: Venture.

Austin, D.R. (2004). *Therapeutic recreation: Processes and techniques* (5th ed.). Champaign, IL: Sagamore.

Austin, D.R. (2011). Reformation of the Health Protection/Health Promotion Model. *American Journal of Recreation Therapy, 10*(3), 19-26

Austin, D.R. (2013). *Therapeutic recreation processes and techniques: Evidenced-based recreational therapy* (7th ed.). Urbana, IL: Sagamore Publishing.

Austin, D.R., & Crawford, M.E. (1996). Therapeutic recreation: An introduction. Needham Heights, MA: Allyn and Bacon.

Austin, D.R., Crawford, M.E., McCormick, B.P., & Van Puymbroeck, M. (2015). Recreational therapy: An introduction (5th ed.). Urbana, IL: Sagamore Publishing.

Australian Institute of Health and Welfare (AIHW). (2016). *Australia's health.* Canberra, Australia: AIHW.

Australian Sports Commission (ASC). (2016). *AusPlay participation data for the sports sector: Summary of key national findings October 2015 to September 2016 data.* Canberra, Australia: ASC.

Autry, C.E. (2001). Adventure therapy with girls at-risk: Responses to outdoor experiential activities. *Therapeutic Recreation Journal, 35*(4), 289-306.

Auxter, D., Pyfer, J., & Huettig, C. (2005). *Principles and methods of adapted physical education and recreation* (10th ed.). New York, NY: McGraw-Hill.

Avedon, E.M. (1974). *Therapeutic recreation services: An applied behavior science approach.* Englewood, NJ: Prentice Hall.

Ayllon, T. (1999). *How to use token economy and point systems* (2nd ed.). Austin, TX: PRO-ED.

Azrin, N.H., & Besalel, V.A. (1999). *How to use positive practice, self-correction, and overcorrection* (2nd ed.). Austin, TX: PRO-ED.

Baio, J., Wiggins, L., Christensen, D.L., Maenner, M.J., Daniels, J., Warren, Z., . . . Dowling, N.F. (2018). Prevalence of autism spectrum disorder among children aged 8 years – Autism and Developmental Disabilities Monitoring Network, 11 sites, United States, 2014. *Morbidity and Mortality Weekly Report, 67*(6), 1-23. doi:10.15585/mmwr.ss6706a1

Bandura, A. (1986). *Social foundations for thought and action: A social cognitive theory.* Englewood Cliffs, NJ: Prentice Hall.

Bartko, W.T., & Eccles, J.S. (2003). Adolescent participation in structured and unstructured activities: A person-oriented analysis. *Journal of Youth and Adolescence, 32*(4), 233-241.

Bedini, L.A. (1995). The "play ladies": The first therapeutic recreation specialists. *Journal of Physical Education, Recreation and Dance, 66*(8), 32-35.

Bedini, L.A. (2000). "Just sit down so we can talk": Perceived stigma and community recreation pursuits by people with disabilities. *Therapeutic Recreation Journal, 34,* 55-68.

Bedini, L.A., & Henderson, K.A. (1994). Women with disabilities and the challenges to leisure service providers. *Journal of Park and Recreation Administration, 12*(1), 17-34.

Belza, B., & PRC-HAN Physical Activity Conference Planning Workgroup. (2007). *Moving ahead: Strategies and tools to plan, conduct, and maintain effective community-based physical activity programs for older adults.* Atlanta, GA: Centers for Disease Control and Prevention. Retrieved from www.cdc.gov/aging/pdf/community-based_physical_activity_programs_for_older_adults.pdf

Bennett, W.J. (1999). *The index of leading cultural indicators: American society at the end of the twentieth century.* New York, NY: Random House.

Berry, L.L., & Seltman, K.D. (2008). *Management lessons from Mayo Clinic: Inside one of the worlds most admired service organizations.* New York, NY: McGraw-Hill.

Bhat, S., Varambally, S., Karmani, S., Govindaraj, R., & Gangadhar, B.N. (2016). Designing and validation of a yoga-based intervention for obsessive compulsive disorder. *International Review of Psychiatry, 28*(3), 327-333.

Bielak, A.A., Anstey, K.J., Christensen, H., & Windsor, T.D. (2012). Activity engagement is related to level, but not change in cognitive ability across adulthood. *Psychology and Aging, 27*(1), 219.

Blanchard, K., Lacinak, T., Tompkins, C., & Ballard, J. (2002). *Whale done! The power of positive relationships.* New York, NY: Simon & Schuster.

Blumenfeld, H. (2010). *The basal ganglia: Neuroanatomy through clinical cases* (2nd ed). Sunderland, MA: Sinauer Associates, Inc.

Boat, T.F., & Wu, J.T. (2015). Mental disorders and disabilities among low-income children. Retrieved from www.ncbi.nlm.nih.gov/books/NBK332877/

Boccaro, J., & Outley, C. (2005, October). *Developing effective relationships in recreation youth programs.* Paper presented at the National Recreation and Park Association Annual Congress, San Antonio, TX.

Bogdan, R., & Taylor, S.J. (1992). The social construction of humanness. In P.M. Ferguson, D.M. Ferguson, & S.J. Taylor (Eds.), *Interpreting disability* (pp. 275-296). New York, NY: Teachers College Press.

Bolandzadeh, N., Tam, R., Handy, T.C., Nagamatsu, L.S., Hsu, C.L., Davis, J.C., . . . Liu Ambrose, T. (2015). Resistance training and white matter lesion progression in older women: Exploratory analysis of a 12-month randomized controlled trial. *Journal of the American Geriatrics Society, 63*(10), 2052-2060. doi:10.1111/jgs.13644

Brody, E.M., Kleban, M.H., Lawton, M.P., & Silverman, H.A. (1971). Excess disabilities of mentally impaired aged: Impact of individualized treatment. *The gerontologist, 11*(2_Part_1), 124-133.

Broida, J.K. (2000). *Therapeutic recreation—the benefits are endless.* Ashburn, VA: National Recreation and Park Association.

Bronfenbrenner, U. (1989). Ecological systems theory. In R. Vasta (Ed.), *Annals of child development: Vol. 6. Six theories of child development: Revised formulations and current issues* (pp. 187-249). Greenwich, CT: Jai Press.

Brooks, S. (2000). *Canadian democracy: An introduction* (3rd ed.). Don Mills, ON: Oxford University Press.

Bryan, M.L.M., & Davis, A.F. (Eds.). (1990). *100 years at Hull-House.* Bloomington, IN: Indiana University Press.

Buckingham, M., & Clifton, D. (2001). *Now, discover your strengths.* New York, NY: Simon & Schuster.

Bucolo, J.A. (2003). *Re-inventing yourself: The key to today's career success.* Paper presented at the Life Services Network 2003 Annual Convention and Expo. Chicago, IL.

Buettner, L., & Fitzsimmons, S. (2003). *Dementia practice guidelines for recreational therapy: Treatment of disturbing behaviors.* Alexandria, VA: American Therapeutic Recreation Association.

Bullock, C.C., & Mahon, M.J. (2000). *Introduction to recreation services for people with disabilities: A person-centered approach* (2nd ed.). Champaign, IL: Sagamore.

Bureau of Labor Statistics (BLS), U.S. Department of Labor. (2017). *Occupational outlook handbook: Recreational therapists* (2014-2015 ed.). Retrieved July 3, 2017, from www.bls.gov/ooh/healthcare/recreational-therapists.htm

Burgstahler, S., & Doe, T. (2006). Improving postsecondary outcomes for students with disabilities: Designing professional development for faculty. *Journal of Postsecondary Education and Disability, 18*(2), 135-145.

Burlingame, J., & Blaschko, T.M. (2010). *Assessment tools for recreational therapy and related fields* (4th ed.). Ravendsdale, WA: Idyll Arbor.

Cachioni, M., Nascimento Ordonez, T., da Silva, T.B.L., Tavares Batistoni, S.S., Sanches Yassuda, M., Caldeira Melo, R., ... & Lopes, A. (2014). Motivational factors and predictors for attending a continuing education program for older adults. *Educational Gerontology, 40*(8), 584-596.

Cameron, D., & Valentine, F. (2001). *Disability and federalism: Comparing different approaches to full participation.* Montreal, QC, and Kingston, ON: McGill-Queen's University Press.

Campbell, W.J. (1997). *The book of great books: A guide to 100 world classics.* New York, NY: Metrobooks.

Carbonneau, H., St-Onge, M., Morier, J., Roult, R., Cantin, R., & Berthiaume, R. (2015). Quebec's recreation intervention model in health care and social services and its implications for the National Council for Therapeutic Recreation Certification's standards. *World Leisure Journal, 57*(1), 6-18.

Cardenas, D., Henderson, K.A., & Wilson, B.E. (2009). Experiences of participation in senior games among older adults. *Journal of Leisure Research, 41*(1), 41-56.

Carruthers C., & Hood C.D. (2007). Building a life of meaning through therapeutic recreation: The leisure and well-being model, part 1. *Therapeutic Recreation Journal, 41*(4), 276-297.

Carter, M., Robb, G., & Van Andel, G. (1988). *Therapeutic recreation: A practical approach.* St. Louis, MO: Times Mirror/Mosby.

Carter, M.J., & Van Andel, G.E. (2011). *Therapeutic recreation: A practical approach* (4th ed.). Long Grove, IL: Waveland Press.

Carter, M.J., Van Andel, G.E., & Robb, G.M. (2019). *Therapeutic recreation: A practical approach* (4th ed.). Long Grove, IL: Waveland Press.

Centers for Disease Control and Prevention (CDC). (1992). Recommendations for the use of folic acid to reduce the number of cases of spina bifida and other neural tube defects. *MMWR*, 41(No. RR-14), inclusive page numbers. Retrieved from https://www.cdc.gov/mmwr/preview/mmwrhtml/00019479.htm

Centers for Disease Control and Prevention (CDC). (2004). Suicide attempts and physical fighting among high school students—United States 2001. *Morbidity and Mortality Weekly Report, 52*(22), 474-476.

Centers for Disease Control and Prevention (CDC). (2005). Social support and health-related quality of life among older adults—Missouri, 2000. *Morbidity and Mortality Weekly Report, 54*(17), 433-437.

Centers for Disease Control and Prevention (CDC). (2013). The state of aging and health in America 2013. Retrieved from www.cdc.gov/aging/pdf/State-Aging-Health-in-America-2013.pdf

Centers for Medicare & Medicaid Services (CMS). (2016). Memorandum: State operations manual (SOM) surveyor guidance revisions related to psychosocial harm in nursing homes. Retrieved from www.cms.gov/Medicare/Provider-Enrollment-and-Certification/SurveyCertificationGenInfo/Downloads/Survey-and-Cert-Letter-16-15.pdf

Center for Medicare & Medicaid Services (CMS). (2018). Pace fact sheet. Retrieved from https://www.cms.gov/Medicare/Health-Plans/pace/downloads/PACE-FactSheet.pdf

Chamberlin, R.W. (1994). Primary prevention: The missing piece in child development legislation. In R.J. Simeonsson (Ed.), *Risk, resilience and prevention: Promoting the well-being of all children* (pp. 33-52). Baltimore, MD: Brooks.

Chang, Y.S., Owens, J.P., Desai, S.S., Hill, S.S., Arnet, A.B., Harris, J., & Mukherjee, P. (2014). Autism and sensory processing disorders: Shared white matter disruption in sensory pathways but divergent connectivity in social-emotional pathways. *PloS One, 9*(7).

Cherniack, E.P., & Cherniack, A.R. (2014). The benefit of pets and animal-assisted therapy to the health of older individuals. *Current Gerontology and Geriatrics Research.* http://dx.doi.org/10.1155/2014/623203

Chodzko-Zajko, W., Proctor, D., Fiatarone Singh M., Minson, C., Nigg, C., Salem, G., & Skinner, J. (2009). American College of Sports Medicine position stand: Exercise and physical activity for older adults. *Medicine & Science in Sports & Exercise, 41*(7), 1510-1530. doi:10.1249/MSS.0b013e3181a0c95c

Choi, N.G., Ransom, S., & Wyllie, R.J. (2008). Depression in older nursing home residents: The influence of nursing home environmental stressors, coping, and acceptance of group and individual therapy. *Aging and Mental health, 12*(5), 536-547.

Clapesattle, H. (1969). *The doctors Mayo* (5th ed.). Rochester, MN: Mayo Foundation for Medical Education and Research.

Combs, S.A., Diehl, M.D., Staples, W.H., Conn, L., Davis, K., Lewis, N., & Schaneman, K. (2011). Boxing training for patients with Parkinson disease: a case series. *Physical therapy, 91*(1), 132-142.

Compton, D.M. (1997). Where in the world are we going? Armageddon and utopia revisited. In D.M. Compton (Ed.), *Issues in therapeutic recreation: Toward the new millennium* (pp. 39-50). Champaign, IL: Sagamore.

Conzemius, A., & O'Neill, J. (2002). *The handbook for SMART school teams.* Bloomington, IN: National Education Services.

Corey, G. (2004). *Theory and practice of counseling and psychotherapy* (7th ed.). Pacific Grove, CA: Wadsworth.

Council for Higher Education Accreditation. (CHEA). (2012). *Fact sheet #1 profile of accreditation.* Washington, DC: Author.

Council on Accreditation Park Recreation and Tourism and Related Professions (COAPRT). (2012). *Guidelines for learning outcomes for therapeutic recreation education.* Washington, DC: Author.

Covey, S.R. (2005). *The 8th habit: From effectiveness to greatness* [book and corresponding DVD]. New York, NY: Simon & Schuster.

Coyle, C., Kinney, W., Riley, B., & Shank, J. (Eds.). (1991). *Benefits of therapeutic recreation: A consensus view.* Ravensdale, WA: Idyll Arbor.

Crawford, M.E. (2001). Issues and trends. In D.R. Austin & M.E. Crawford (Eds.), *Therapeutic recreation: An introduction.* (2nd ed.). (pp. 333-359). Boston, MA: Allyn & Bacon.

Csikszentmihalyi, M. (1993). *The evolving self.* New York, NY: HarperCollins.

Csikszentmihalyi, M. (1997). *Finding flow: The psychology of engagement with everyday life.* New York, NY: Basic Books.

Csikszentmihalyi, M., & Larson, R. (1984). *Being adolescent: Conflict and growth in the teenage years.* New York, NY: Basic Books.

Cullen, F.T., & Wright, J.P. (1997). Liberating the anomie-strain paradigm: Implications from social support theory. In N. Passas & R. Agnew (Eds.), *The future of anomie theory* (pp. 187-206). Boston, MA: Northeastern University Press.

Cumming, E., & Henry, W.E. (1961). *Growing old.* New York: Basic.

Cunningham Children's Home. (2016). About us. Retrieved from www.cunninghamhome.org/about-us

Cunningham, P. (n.d.). Java Music Club: Mutual support for cognitively impaired at risk adults. Retrieved from: http://hosting.uaa.alaska.edu/afpmc/JavaMusicClub.pdf

Czaja, S.J., Loewenstein, D., Schulz, R., Nair, S.N., & Perdomo, D. (2013). A videophone psychosocial intervention for dementia caregivers. *The American Journal of Geriatric Psychiatry, 21*(11), 1071-1081. doi:10.1016/j.jagp.2013.02.019

Damon, W. (2004). What is positive youth development? *The Annals of the American Academy of Political and Social Science, 591,* 13-24.

Dattilo, J. (2000). *Facilitation techniques in therapeutic recreation.* State College, PA: Venture.

Dattilo, J. (2015). Positive psychology and leisure education. *Therapeutic Recreation Journal, 49*(2), 148-165.

Dattilo, J., & McKenney, A. (Eds.). (2011). *Facilitation techniques in therapeutic recreation* (2nd ed.). State College, PA: Venture.

Davis-Berman, J., & Berman, D. (1999). The use of adventure-based programs with at-risk youth. In J.C. Miles & S. Priest (Eds.), *Adventure programming.* State College, PA: Venture.

DeBord, K. (1996). *Childhood years: Ages six through twelve.* Raleigh, NC: North Carolina Cooperative Extension Service.

Department of Health. (2014). National framework for recovery-oriented mental health services. Retrieved from www.health.gov.au/internet/main/publishing.nsf/Content/mental-pubs-n-recovfra

Department of Health and Ageing. (2003). *Aged care in Australia.* Canberra, Australia: Author.

De Shazer, S. (1985). *Keys to solution in brief therapy.* New York, NY: Guilford Press.

Detels, R., Visscher, B.R., Haile, R.W., Malmgren, R.M., Dudley, J.P., & Coulson, A.H. (1978). Multiple sclerosis and age at migration. *American Journal of Epidemiology, 108*(5), 386-393.

Devine, M.A. (2004). From connector to distancer: The role of inclusive leisure contexts in determining social acceptance for people with disabilities. *Journal of Leisure Research, 36*(2), 137-159.

Devine, M.A., & Dattilo, J. (2000). Expressive arts as therapeutic media. In J. Dattilo (Ed.), *Facilitation techniques in therapeutic recreation* (pp. 133-164). State College, PA: Venture.

Devine, M.A., & Lashua B. (2002). Constructing social acceptance in inclusive leisure contexts: The role of individuals with disabilities. *Therapeutic Recreation Journal, 36*, 65-83.

Devine, M.A., & McGovern, J. (2001). Inclusion of individuals with disabilities in public park and recreation programs: Are agencies ready? *Journal of Park and Recreation Administration, 19*(4), 60-82.

Devine, M.A., & Sylvester, C. (2005). Disabling defenders? The social construction of disability in therapeutic recreation. In C. Sylvester (Ed.), *Philosophy of therapeutic recreation: Ideas and issues* (vol. III; pp. 22-35). National Therapeutic Recreation Society: Ashburn, VA.

Devine, M.A., & Wilhite, B. (2000). The meaning of disability: Implications for inclusive leisure services for youth with and without disabilities. *Journal of Park and Recreation Administration, 18*(3), 35-52.

Dieser, R.B. (2002a, May). *Accreditation, certification, registration—What should we do? Outlining a Canadian vision for therapeutic recreation professionalism.* Keynote address at the Canadian Therapeutic Recreation Association Annual Conference, Calgary, AB, Canada.

Dieser, R.B. (2002b). A personal narrative of a cross-cultural experience in therapeutic recreation: Unmasking the masked. *Therapeutic Recreation Journal, 36*(1), 84-96.

Dieser, R.B. (2004a, September). *Jane Addams and Hull-House programs: Forgotten pioneers in therapeutic recreation.* Paper presented at the American Therapeutic Recreation Association Research Institute, Kansas City, Missouri.

Dieser, R.B. (2004b, Fall). Outlining a Canadian framework for therapeutic recreation professionalism: A mosaic certification framework part I. *Tribune,* 6-7. [Newsletter of the Canadian Therapeutic Recreation Association].

Dieser, R.B. (2005a). A genealogy of the United States therapeutic recreation certification framework. *Leisure Studies, 24*(1), 61-79.

Dieser, R.B. (2005b, Winter). Outlining a Canadian framework for therapeutic recreation professionalism: A mosaic certification framework part II (planting seeds). *Tribune,* 7-9. [Newsletter of the Canadian Therapeutic Recreation Association].

Dieser, R.B. (2005c). Understanding how Jane Addams and Hull-House programs bridged cross-cultural differences: Leisure programs and contact theory. *Human Service Education, 25*(1), 53-63.

Dieser, R.B. (2005/2006). Explaining the mosaic certification framework to an American audience. *Annual in Therapeutic Recreation, 14*, 42-58.

Dieser, R.B. (2012, Fall). Concerns regarding the CTRA-NCTRC partnerships: Could this be the beginning of a future divided therapeutic recreation profession in Canada? *ATRAbute,* 3-6, 14.

Dieser, R.B. (2013). *Leisure education: A person-centered, system-directed, social policy perspective.* Urbana, IL: Sagamore.

Dieser, R.B. (2014, Winter). A reply to Tanea Goncalvess response regarding the CTRA-NCTRA partnership. *ATRAbute, 1*(1), 4-7.

Dieser, R.B. Edginton, C.R., & Ziemer, R. (2017). Decreasing patient stress and physician/medical-workforce burnout through healthcare environments: Uncovering the serious leisure perspective at the Mayo Clinic Rochester campus. *Mayo Clinic Proceedings, 92*(7), 1-8.

Diversional & Recreation Therapy Australia. (DRTA). (2017). What is diversional therapy? Retrieved from http://diversionaltherapy.org.au/About-DTA/What-is-DT

Diversional Therapy Association of Australia. (DTAA). (2003). *25th annual convention workbook and DTAA history.* Sydney, Australia: Author.

Diversional Therapy Association of Australia. (DTAA). (2005). The Diversional Therapy Association of

Australia 1976-1996. Retrieved November 29, 2005, from www.diversionaltherapy.org.au/h.htm

Duckworth, K. (2015). Science meets the human experience: Integrating the medical and recovery models. Retrieved from www.nami.org/Blogs/NAMI-Blog/April-2015/Science-Meets-the-Human-Experience-Integrating-th

Duncan, M. (1991). Back to our radical roots. In T.L. Goodale & P.A. Witt (Eds.), *Recreation and leisure: Issues in an era of change* (3rd ed., pp. 331-338). State College, PA: Venture.

Durstine, J.L., Moore, G.E., Painter, P.L., & Roberts, S.O. (Eds.). (2009). *ACSM's exercise management for persons with chronic diseases and disabilities.* (3rd ed.). Champaign: Human Kinetics.

Dustin, D. (Ed.). (1993). *For the good of the order: Administering academic programs in higher education.* San Diego, CA: Institute for Leisure Behavior, San Diego State University.

Eales, L., & Goodwin, D. (2015). "We all carry each other, sometimes": care-sharing as social justice practice in integrated dance. *Leisure/Loisir, 39*(2), 277-298.

Edginton, C.R., Compton, D.M. & Hanson, C.J. (1989). *Recreation and leisure programming: A guide for the professional.* Dubuque: Wm. C. Brown.

Edginton, C.R., Hudson, S.D., & Scholl, K.G. (2005) *Leadership for recreation, parks and leisure services* (3rd ed.) Champaign, IL: Sagamore.

Edginton, C.R., Lankford, S.V., Dieser, R.B., & Kowalski, C.L. (2017). *Community parks and recreation: An introduction.* Urbana, IL: Sagamore.

Eisenman, R. (2014, July 14). Mayo Clinic earns no. 1 rank on U.S. News & World Report's honor roll. Retrieved from http://newsnetwork.mayoclinic.org/discussion/mayo-clinic-earns-no-1-rank-in-the-nation-on-u-s-news-world-reports-honor-roll/

Elshtain, J.B. (2002). *Jane Addams and the dream of American democracy.* New York, NY: Basic Books.

Engel G. (1977). The need for a new medical model: A challenge for biomedicine. *Science, 196,* 129-136.

Erdmann, A., & Schnepp, W. (2014). Conditions, components and outcomes of integrative validation therapy in a long-term care facility for people with dementia: A qualitative evaluation study. *Dementia, 15*(5). doi:10.1177/1471301214556489

Ervin, D.A., Hennen, B., Merrick J., & Morad, M. (2014). Healthcare for persons with intellectual and developmental disability in the community. *Frontiers in Public Health, 2*(83). doi:10.3389/fpubh.2014.00083

Esveldt-Dawson, K., & Kazdin, A.E. (1998). *How to maintain behavior.* Austin, TX: PRO-ED.

Eyre, H.A., Acevedo, B., Yang, H., Siddarth, P., Van Dyk, K., Ercoli, L., ... & Khalsa, D.S. (2016). Changes in neural connectivity and memory following a yoga intervention for older adults: a pilot study. *Journal of Alzheimer's Disease, 52*(2), 673-684.

Farley, B., & Koshland, G.F. (2005). Training BIG to move faster: The application of the speed-amplitude relation as a rehabilitation strategy for people with Parkinson's disease. *Experimental Brain Research, 167*(3), 462-467.

Farmer, J.E. (1997). Epilogue: An ecological systems approach to childhood traumatic brain injury. In E.D. Bigler, E. Clark, & J.E. Farmer (Eds.), *Childhood traumatic brain injury: Diagnosis, assessment, and intervention.* Austin, TX: PRO-ED.

Ferraro, K., Shippee, T.P., & Schafer, M.H. (2009). Cumulative inequality theory for research on aging and the lifecourse. In V. Bengtson, D. Gans, N. Putney, & M. Silverstein (Eds.), *Handbook of theories of aging* (2nd ed.). New York, NY: Springer.

Fine, M., & Asch, A. (1988). Disability beyond stigma: Social interaction, discrimination, and activism. *Journal of Social Issues, 44*(1), 3-21.

Fischer, M. (2004). *On Addams.* Toronto, ON: Thomson Wadsworth.

Fisher, B.E., Wu, A.D., Salem, G.J., Song, J., Lin, C.H., Yip, J., . . . Petzinger, G. (2008). The effect of exercise training in improving motor performance and corticomotor excitability in people with early Parkinson's disease. *Archives of Physical Medicine and Rehabilitation, 89*(7), 1221-1229.

Fitzsimmons, S., Sardina, A., & Buettner, L. (2008). *Dementia practice guidelines for recreational therapists: Treatment of disturbing behaviors.* Hattiesburg, MS: American Therapeutic Recreation Association.

Fonagy, P., & Target, M. (2003). *Psychoanalytic theories: Perspectives from developmental psychopathology.* London, UK: Whurr.

Fortune, D., & Yuen, F. (2015). Transitions in identity, belonging, and citizenship and the possibilities of inclusion for women leaving prison: implications for therapeutic recreation. *Leisure/Loisir, 39*(2), 253-276.

Fosnot, C.T. (1996). Constructivism: A psychological theory of learning. In C.T. Fosnot (Ed.), *Constructivism: Theory, perspectives, and practice* (pp. 8-33). New York, NY: Teachers College Press.

Foucault, M. (1965). *Madness and civilization: A history of insanity in the age of reason* (R. Howard, Trans.). London, UK: Tavistock.

Frazzitta, G., Maestri, R., Uccellini, D., Bertotti, G., & Abelli, P. (2009). Rehabilitation treatment of gait in patients with Parkinson's disease with freezing: A comparison between two physical therapy protocols using visual and auditory cues with or without treadmill training. *Movement Disorders, 24*(8), 1139-1143.

Fredrickson, B. L. (2015). Positivity resonates. Session presented at the *4th World Congress of the International Positive Psychology Association*, Orlando, FL. Retrieved from http://www.ippanetwork.org/ (IPPA membership required to access site)

Freund, A., & Baltes, P. (2002). The adaptiveness of selection, optimization, and compensation as strategies of life management: Evidence from a preference study on proverbs. *The Journals of Gerontology: Series B, Psychological Sciences and Social Sciences, 57*(5), 426-434. doi:https://doi.org/10.1093/geronb/57.5.P426

Fritsch, T., Kwak, J., Grant, S., Lang, J., Montgomery, R.R., & Basting, A.D. (2009). Impact of TimeSlips, a creative expression intervention program, on nursing home residents with dementia and their caregivers. *The Gerontologist.* doi:10.1093/geront/gnp008

Fujiwara, J., Emmert, B., & Carney, M.T. (2015). Elder orphans: hiding in plain sight: b14. *Journal of the American Geriatrics Society, 63*, S95.

Gagnon, A.G. (1995). The political uses of federalism. In F. Rocher & M. Smith (Eds.), *New trends in Canadian federalism* (pp. 23-44). Toronto, ON: Broadview Press.

Garber, C.E., Blissmer, B., Deschenes, M.R., Franklin, B.A, Lee, I-Min, Nieman, D.C., & Swain, D.P. (2011). Quantity and quality of exercise for developing and maintaining cardiorespiratory, musculoskeletal, and neuromotor fitness in apparently healthy adults: Guidance for prescribing Exercise. *Medicine & Science in Sports & Exercise, 43*(7), 1334-1359. doi:10.1249/MSS.0b013e318213fefb

Genetics Home Reference. (2018). Galactosemia. Retrieved from https://ghr.nlm.nih.gov/condition/galactosemia

Genetics Home Reference. (2018). Phenylketonuria. Retrieved from http://ghr.nlm.nih.gov/condition/phenylketonuria

Genoe, M.R., & Whyte, C. (2015). Confronting ageism through therapeutic recreation practice. *Leisure/Loisir, 39*(2), 235-252.

Germain, C.B. (1991). *Human behavior in the social environment: An ecological view.* New York, NY: Columbia University Press.

Glenwood Academy. (2016). Welcome to Glenwood Academy. Retrieved from www.glenwoodacademy.org/

Goetz, C.G., Poewe, W., Rascol, O., Sampaio, C., Stebbins, G.T., Counsell, C., . . . Seidl, L. (2004). *Movement* Disorder Society task force report on the Hoehn and Yahr Staging Scale: Status and recommendations. *Movement Disorders, 19*(9), 1020-1028.

Goodwin, D. (2003). The meaning of social experiences in recreation settings. *Impact, 16*(2), 4-5.

Gordon, E., & Yowell, C. (1994). Cultural dissonance as a risk factor in the development of students. In R. Rossi (Ed.), *Schools and students at risk* (pp. 51-69). New York, NY: Teachers College Press.

Groff, D., and Dattilo, J. (2011). Adventure therapy. In J. Datillo and A. McKenney (Eds.), *Facilitation techniques in therapeutic recreation* (2nd ed.). State College, PA: Venture Publishing.

Gunn, S.L., & Peterson, C.A. (1978). *Therapeutic recreation program design: Principles and procedures.* Englewood Cliffs, NJ: Prentice Hall.

Gustaferre, C. (1914/1990). What kind of a home I would like to have. In M.L. McCree Bryan & A.F. Davis (Eds.), *100 years at Hull-House* (pp. 132-133). Bloomington, IN: Indiana University Press. (Reprinted from *Survey*, July 1914, p. 420).

Hackett, F. (1925/1990). Hull-House: A souvenir. In M.L. McCree Bryan & A.F. Davis (Eds.), *100 years at Hull-House* (pp. 67-73). Bloomington, IN: Indiana University Press. (Reprinted from *Survey*, July 1925, pp. 275-279).

Hagan, J., & McCarthy, B. (1997). Anomie, social capital, and street criminology. In N. Passas & R. Agnew (Eds.), *The future of anomie theory* (pp. 124-141). Boston, MA: Northeastern University Press.

Hagen, C., Malkmus, D., & Durham, P. (1979). The Rancho levels of cognitive functioning. Retrieved from http://file.lacounty.gov/SDSInter/dhs/218111_RLOCFFamilyGuideEnglish.pdf

Hahn, H. (1988). The politics of physical differences: Disability and discrimination. In M. Nagler (Ed.), *Perspectives on disability* (2nd ed., pp. 37-42). Palo Alto, CA: Health Markets Research.

Hall, V.R. (1975). *Managing behavior 2: Behavior modification—basic principles.* Lawrence, KS: H & H Enterprises.

Hall, V.R., & Hall, M.L. (1998a). *How to use planned ignoring (extinction)* (2nd ed.). Austin, TX: PRO-ED.

Hall, V.R., & Hall, M.L. (1998b). *How to use time out* (2nd ed.). Austin, TX: PRO-ED.

Harris-Kojetin, L., Sengupta, M., & Park-Lee, E. (2016). Long-term care providers and services users in the United States: Data from the National Study of Long-Term Care Providers, 2013–2014. National Center for Health Statistics. *VitalHealth Stat 3*(38). Retrieved from https://www.cdc.gov/nchs/data/series/sr_03/sr03_038.pdf.

Harvard Business Review (2018). What having a growth mindset really means. Retrieved from https://hbr.org/2016/01/what-having-a-growth-mindset-actually-means

Haskell, W.L., Lee, I-Min, Pate, R.R., Powell, K.E., Blair, S.N., Franklin, B.A., . . . Bauman, A. (2007). Physical activity and public health: Updated recommendation for adults from the

Haun, P. (1965). *Recreation: A medical viewpoint.* New York, NY: Bureau of Publications.

Hauser, S.T. (1991). *Adolescents and their families: Paths of ego development.* New York: Free Press.

Hebblethwaite, S. (2015). Commentary: The professionalization of therapeutic recreation in Quebec. *World Leisure Journal, 57*(1), 19-24.

Hemingway, J.L. (2016). History of leisure. In G.J. Walker, D. Scott, & M. Stodolska (Eds.), *Leisure matters: The state and future of leisure studies* (pp. 25-32). State College, PA: Venture.

Heyne L.A., & Anderson, L.S. (2012). Theories that support strengths-based practice in therapeutic recreation. *Therapeutic Recreation Journal, 46*(2), 106-128.

Holtz, L. (1998). *Winning every day.* New York, NY: HarperCollins.

Hood, C.D., & Carruthers C. (2007). Enhancing leisure experience and developing resources: The leisure and well-being model, part II. *Therapeutic Recreation Journal, 41*(4), 298-325.

Howe-Murphy, R., & Charboneau, B.G. (1987). *Therapeutic recreation intervention: An ecological perspective.* Englewood Cliffs, NJ: Prentice Hall.

Hubbard, D.L. (Ed.). (1993). *Continuous quality improvement: Making the transition to education.* Maryville, MO: Prescott Publishing.

Hunnicutt, B.K. (1980). To cope in autonomy: Therapeutic recreation and the limits to professionalization and intervention. In G. Hitzhusen, J. Elliott, D.J. Szymanski, and M.G. Thompson (Eds.), *Expanding horizons in therapeutic recreation VII* (pp. 121-134). Columbia: University of Missouri.

Hutchens, D. (2000). *Out learning the wolves: Surviving and thriving in a learning organization* (2nd ed.). Williston, VT: Pegasus Communications.

Hutcheon, L. (1989). *The politics of postmodernism.* New York, NY: Routledge.

Hutchison, P., & McGill, J. (1998). *Leisure, integration, and community.* (2nd ed.). Toronto, ON: Leisurability Publications.

Ishikawa, S., & Harada, H. (2012). The tendency of the research about recreations that the nurses who work in psychiatry ward. *The Bulletin of Kyoritsu Women's Junior College, 7,* 55-61.

Jacob, K.S. (2015). Recovery model of mental illness: A complementary approach to psychiatric care. *Indian Journal of Psychological Medicine, 37*(2), 117-119. http://doi.org/10.4103/0253-7176.155605

Jacobson, M., & Ruddy, M. (2004). *Open to outcome: A practical guide for facilitating and teaching experiential reflection.* Oklahoma City, OK: Wood N. Barnes.

James, A. (1998). The conceptual development of recreational therapy. In F. Brasile, T.K. Skalko, & J. Burlingame (Eds.), *Perspectives in recreational therapy: Issues of a dynamic profession* (pp. 7-38). Ravensdale, WA: Idyll Arbor.

Jäncke, L. (2008). Music, memory and emotion. *Journal of Biology, 7*(21). doi:10.1186/jbiol82

Japanese Federation for Mental Health and Welfare. (n.d.). History of sports festivals for people with mental illness. Retrieved from www.f-renmei.or.jp/sports/outline/

Japan Para-Sports Association (JPSA). (2012). The history and current situation of adapted sports in Japan. Retrieved from www.jsad.or.jp/about/pdf/jsad_ss_2011_all_0111.pdf

Japan Para-Sports Association (JPSA). (2016). Training. Retrieved from www.jsad.or.jp/training/

Jewel, D.L. (1999). *Confronting child maltreatment through recreation* (2nd ed.). Springfield, IL: Charles C Thomas.

Johnson, S. (1998). *Who moved my cheese?* New York, NY: Penguin Putnam.

Kahn, F., Turner-Stokes, L., Ng, L., Kilpatrick, T., & Amatya B. (2007). Multidisciplinary rehabilitation for adults with multiple sclerosis (review). *Cochrane Database of Systematic Reviews,* 2.

Kelly, J.R., & Godbey, G. (1992). *The sociology of leisure.* State College, PA: Venture.

Kelly, J.R., & Warnick, R.B. (1999). *Recreation trends and markets.* Champaign, IL: Sagamore.

Kelly, K. (2000). *Mary Shelley's Frankenstein.* Portland, ME: Research and Education Association.

Kentucky Department of Education. (2005). *Kentucky emotional-behavioral disability: Technical assistance manual: Behavioral examples.* Retrieved July 2005, from www.state.ky.us/agencies/behave/bi/ebdex.html

Kerr, J., Rosenberg, D., & Frank, L. (2012). The role of the built environment in healthy aging community design, physical activity, and health among older adults. *Journal of Planning Literature, 27*(1), 43-60. doi:10.1177/0885412211415283

Kim, O-J. (2000). *Introduction of leisure and recreation.* Seoul, South Korea: Taekyung Books.

Kinney, J.M., & Rentz, C.A. (2005). Observed well-being among individuals with dementia: Memories in the Making, an art program, versus other structured activity. *American Journal of Alzheimer's Disease and Other Dementias, 20*(4), 220-227.

Kinney, J.S., Kinney, T., & Witman, J. (2004). Therapeutic recreation modalities and facilitation techniques: A national study. *Annual in Therapeutic Recreation, 13,* 59-79.

Kirby, D. (2001). *Emerging answers: Research findings on programs to reduce teen pregnancy.* Washington, DC: National Campaign to Prevent Teen Pregnancy.

Kiresuk, J., & Sherman, R. (1968). Goal attainment scaling: A general method for evaluating comprehensive community mental health programs. *Community Mental Health Journal, 4*(6), 443-453.

Kiresuk, J., Smith, A., & Cardillo, J. (Eds.). (1994). *Goal attainment scaling: Applications, theory, and measurement.* Hillsdale, NJ: Lawrence Earlbaum Associates.

Klippel, J.H., Stone, J.H., Crofford, L.J., & White, P.H. (Eds.). (2008). *Primer on the rheumatic diseases* (13th ed). New York, NY: Springer.

Kloseck, M., & Crilly, R.G. (1997). *Leisure competence measure: Professional manual and user's guide.* London, ON: Leisure Competence Measure Data System.

Koch, L. (2001). Disability and difference: Balancing social and physical constructions. *Journal of Medical Ethics, 27,* 370-376.

Korean Therapeutic Recreation Association. (2006). *Korean Therapeutic Recreation Association: Introduction, history, and education.* Retrieved April 2, 2006, from www.ktra.com.

Kronick, R.F. (Ed.). (1997). *At-risk youth: Theory, practice, reform.* New York, NY: Garland.

Kurtzke, J.F. (1983). Rating neurologic impairment in multiple sclerosis: An expanded disability status scale (EDSS). *Neurology, 33*(11), 1444-1452.

Kurtzke, J.F., Gundmunsson, K.R., & Bergmann, S. (1982). Multiple sclerosis in Iceland: Evidence of postwar epidemic. *Neurology, 32*(2), 143-150.

Larson, R., Csikszentmihalyi, M., & Freeman, M. (1992). Alcohol and marijuana use in adolescents' daily lives. In M.W. deVries (Ed.), *The experience of psychopathology: Investigating mental disorders in their natural settings* (pp. 180-192). New York, NY: Cambridge University Press.

Larson, R., & Richards, M.H. (1991). Boredom in the middle school year: Blaming schools versus blaming students. *American Journal of Education, 99,* 418-443.

Laselva, S.V. (1996). *The moral foundations of Canadian federalism: Paradoxes, achievements, and tragedies of nationhood.* Kingston, ON: McGill-Queen's University Press.

Lassmann, H., van Horssen, J., & Mahad, D. (2012). Progressive multiple sclerosis: Pathology and pathogenesis (review). *Nature Reviews Neurology, 8*(11), 647-656.

Leavitt, P. (2006, November 10). Norway best place to live, according to U.N. *USA Today,* p. 7A.

Lew, M.F., & Yeung, Y. (2014). *Parkinson's Disease. Reference Module in Biomedical Sciences.* Retrieved from: https://doi.org/10.1016/B978-0-12-801238-3.00146-X

Lewinsohn, P.M., Hops, H., Roberts, R., & Seeley, J.R. (1993). Adolescent psychopathology: I. Prevalence and incidence of depression and other *DSM-III-R* disorders in high school students. *Journal of Abnormal Psychology, 102,* 110-120.

Lin, Y., Chu, H., Yang, C.Y., Chen, C.H., Chen, S.G., Chang H.J., . . . Chou, K.R. (2011). Effectiveness of group music intervention against agitated behavior in elderly persons with dementia. *International Journal of Geriatric Psychiatry, 26*(7), 670-678. doi:10.1002/gps.2580

Lipson, J.G., Dibble, S.L., & Minarik, P.A. (1996). *Culture & nursing care: A pocket guide.* San Francisco, CA: University of California at San Francisco Nursing Press.

Loher, J., & Schwartz, T. (2003). *The power of full engagement: Managing energy, not time, is the key to higher performance and personal renewal.* New York, NY: Simon & Schuster.

Long, T.D. (2000). *An ethical decision making model for therapeutic recreation.* Unpublished manuscript.

Lorig, K.R., Sobel, D.S., Ritter, P.L., Laurent, D., & Hobbs, M. (2001). Effect of a self-management program on patients with chronic disease. *Effective clinical practice: ECP, 4*(6), 256-262.

Luckner, J.L., & Nadler, R.S. (1997). *Processing the experience: Strategies to enhance and generalize learning.* Dubuque, IA: Kendall/Hunt Publishing Company.

Mackaman, D.P. (1998). *Leisure settings: Bourgeois culture, medicine, and the spa in modern France.* Chicago: University of Chicago Press.

Malkin, M.J., Coyle, C.P., & Carruthers, C. (1998). Efficacy research in recreational therapy. In F. Brasile, T.K. Skalko, & J. Burlingame (Eds.), *Perspectives in recreational therapy: Issues of a dynamic profession* (pp. 141-164). Ravensdale, WA: Idyll Arbor.

March of Dimes. (2018). Cerebral palsy. Retrieved from www.marchofdimes.org/complications/cerebral-palsy.aspx

Matsuka, K., Mathiowetz, V., & Finlayson, M. (2007). Use and perceived effectiveness of energy conservation strategies for managing multiple sclerosis fatigue. *American Journal of Occupational Therapy, 61*(1), 62-69.

Mayo Clinic. (1984). *Sculptors and sculptures: Mayo building exterior* [Brochure]. Rochester, MN: Mayo Clinic. Mayo Clinic (MHU# 0675 Folder title "Artwork"). Center for the History of Medicine & Mayo Clinic Historical Suite, Rochester, MN.

Mayo Clinic. (2001). *Gonda building fact sheet* [Pamphlet]. Rochester, MN: Mayo Clinic. Mayo Clinic (MHU# 0676 Folder title "Gonda Diagnostic Bldg"). Center for the History of Medicine & Mayo Clinic Historical Suite, Rochester, MN.

Mayo Clinic. (2006). *The Rochester carillon* [Pamphlet]. Rochester, MN: Mayo Clinic.

Mayo Clinic. (2011). *Healing places* [Mayo Today]. Rochester, MN: Mayo Clinic. Mayo Clinic (MHU# 0675 Folder title "Artwork"). Center for the History of Medicine & Mayo Clinic Historical Suite, Rochester, MN.

Mayo Foundation for Medical Education and Research. (2014). *Art & healing at Mayo Clinic.* Rochester, MN: Mayo Foundation for Medical Education and Research.

McGuire, F., Boyd, R., Janke, M., & Aybar-Damali, B. (2013). *Leisure and aging: Ulyssean living in later life* (5th ed.) Urbana, IL: Sagamore Publishing.

McWhirter, J.J., McWhirter, B.T., McWhirter, E.H., & McWhirter, R.J. (2013). *At-risk youth: A comprehensive response for counselors, teachers, psychologists, and human service professionals* (5th ed.). Belmont, CA: Brooks/Cole.

MedlinePlus. (2018). Myelomeningocele. Retrieved from https://medlineplus.gov/ency/article/001558.htm

Menninger, W.C., & McColl, I. (1937). Recreational therapy as applied in a modern psychiatric hospital. *Occupational Therapy and Rehabilitation, 16,* 15-23.

Menon, D.K., Schwab, K., Wright, D.W., & Maas, A.I. (2010). Position statement: Definition of traumatic brain injury. *Archives of Physical Medicine and Rehabilitation, 91*(11), 1637-1640.

Merrell, K.W. (2002). *School Social Behavior Scales User's Guide.* Baltimore, MD: Paul H. Brookes Publishing.

Meyer, D., Marx, T., & Ball-Seiter, V. (2011). Social isolation and telecommunication in the nursing home: A pilot study. *Gerontechnology, 10*(1), 51-58.

Meyer, L.E. (1980). *Philosophical alternatives and the professionalization of therapeutic recreation.* Arlington, VA: National Recreation and Park Association.

Mitchell, G., & Agnelli, J. (2015) Person-centred care for people with dementia: Kitwood reconsidered. *Nursing Standard.* 30, 7, 46-50. Retrieved from https://www.researchgate.net/profile/Gary_Mitchell2/publication/283244999_Person-centred_care_for_people_with_dementia_Kitwood_reconsidered/links/5666aa2508ae192bbf928b58/Person-centred-care-for-people-with-dementia-Kitwood-reconsidered.pdf

Miyoshi, H., Ueno, F., & Shimoyama, N. (1999). *Asobi-litation.* Tokyo, Japan: Kirara Syobo.

Mobily, K. (1999). New horizons in models of practice in therapeutic recreation. *Therapeutic Recreation Journal, 33*(3), 174-192.

Mobily, K. (2015). Should US recreation therapy be replicated globally? An opportunity to do better. Part II. *World Leisure Journal, 57*(1), 57-68.

Mobily, K.E., & MacNeil, R.D. (2002). *Therapeutic recreation and the nature of disabilities.* State College, PA: Venture.

Mobily, K.E., & Ostiguy, L.J. (2004). *Introduction to therapeutic recreation: US and Canadian perspectives.* State College, PA: Venture.

Monroe, H. (1912/1990). The working girl's song. In M.L. McCree Bryan & A.F. Davis (Eds.), *100 years at Hull-House* (pp. 119-120). Bloomington, IN: Indiana University Press. (Reprinted from *Life and Labor,* July 1912, p. 236).

Mori, M. (2014). Support on leisure participation in post-discharge recovery phase rehabilitation: Therapeutic recreation intervention. *Health and Recreation Research, 10,* 77-80.

Moriyama, C., & Doi, A. (2009). Leisure activities in facilities for older adults in Japan: Seeking for leisure activities to improve quality of life. *The Bulletin of Shiraume Gakuen University and Junior College, 45,* 49-67.

Morris, S., Morris, M.E., & Lansek, R. (2001). Reliability of measurements obtained with the Timed "Up & Go" test in people with Parkinson disease. *Physical Therapy. 81*(2), 810-818.

Mundy, J. (1998). *Leisure education: Theory and practice* (2nd ed.). Champaign, IL: Sagamore.

Murray, H. (2011). Research in eliciting enjoyment by therapeutic recreation support model: Application of self-determination theory based on flow theory. *Proceedings of the 59th Japanese Society for the Study of Social Welfare* (pp. 201-202). Chiba, Japan.

Muscular Dystrophy Association (MDA). (2018). About neuromuscular diseases. Retrieved from www.mda.org/disease

National Alliance on Mental Illness. (2016). Mental health facts: Children & teens. Retrieved from www.nami.org/getattachment/Learn-More/Mental-Health-by-the-Numbers/childrenmhfacts.pdf

National Center for Health Statistics. (2010). National hospital discharge survey: 2010. Retrieved from www.cdc.gov/nchs/fastats/hospital.htm

National Center for PTSD. (2018). How common is PTSD? Retrieved from https://www.ptsd.va.gov/public/PTSD-overview/basics/how-common-is-ptsd.asp

National Council for Therapeutic Recreation Certification (NCTRC). (2015). 2014 CTRS Job Analysis Report: NCTRC report on the international job analysis of certified therapeutic recreation specialists. Retrieved from https://nctrc.org/wp-content/uploads/2015/07/JobAnalysisReport.pdf

National Council for Therapeutic Recreation Certification (NCTRC). (2016). CTRS: The qualified provider. Retrieved from http://nctrc.org/about-certification/ctrs-the-qualified-provider/

National Down Syndrome Society. (2018). Down syndrome facts. Retrieved from www.ndss.org/about-down-syndrome/down-syndrome-facts/

National Fragile X Foundation. (2018). Fragile X prevalence. Retrieved from https://fragilex.org/learn/prevalencegenetics-and-inheritance/

National Institute of Neurological Disorders and Stroke (NINDS). (2018). Disorders. Retrieved from www.ninds.nih.gov/Disorders

National Institutes of Health (2016). *2016 National survey on drug use and health.* Washington, DC: Author. Retrieved from https://www.nimh.nih.gov/health/statistics/major-depression.shtml#part_155029.

National Institutes of Health (2018). What are intellectual and developmental disabilities? Retrieved from https://www.nichd.nih.gov/health/topics/idds/conditioninfo/default#f4.

National Senior Games Association. (2017). History of the NSGA. Retrieved from http://nsga.com/about

Negley, S.K. (1994). Recreation therapy as an outpatient intervention. *Therapeutic Recreation Journal, 28*(1), 35-41.

Negley, S.K. (1997). *Crossing the bridge: A journey in self-esteem, relationships, and life balance.* Emsumclaw, WA: Idyll Arbor.

Nelson, C.W. (1990). *Mayo roots: Profiling the originals of the Mayo Clinic.* Rochester, MN: Mayo Foundation.

Nelson, M.E., Rejeski, W.J., Blair, S.N., Duncan, P.W., Judge, J.O., King, A.C., . . . Castaneda-Sceppa, C. (2007). Physical activity and public health in older adults: Recommendation from the American College of Sports Medicine and the American Heart Association. *Circulation, 116*(9), 1094. doi:10.1161/CIRCULATIONAHA.107.185650

Nesbitt, J.A. (1984). The new/old American TR Association Inc.: Heroic or foolish. *Journal of Iowa Parks and Recreation, 10*(4), 14-15.

Nice, C.J. (1948). Recreation is not therapy. *The Journal of Health and Physical Education, 19,* 642-643.

Nilsagard, Y., Denison, E., & Gunnarsson, L.G. (2006). Evaluation of a single session with cooling garment for persons with multiple sclerosis: A randomized trial. *Disability and Rehabilitation: Assistive Technology, 1*(4), 225-233.

Nirje, B. (1992). *The normalization principle paper.* Uppsala, Sweden: Centre for Handicapped Research.

Nishino, H.J., Chino, H., Yoshioka, N., & Gabriella, J. (2007). Therapeutic recreation in modern Japan: Era of challenge and opportunity. *Therapeutic Recreation Journal, 41*(2), 119-131.

Noh, Y., & Lee, Y. (2004). Development of professional identity in therapeutic recreation: Suggestions for Korean therapeutic recreation profession. *Korean Therapeutic Recreation Journal, 3,* 1-28.

Northern Illinois Special Recreation Association (NISRA). (2016). Programs. Retrieved June 20, 2016, from www.nisra.org/programs.html

Nudo, R.J. (2011). Neural bases of recovery after brain injury. *Journal of Communication Disorders, 44*(5), 515-520.

O'Connor, T. (2004). An overview of juvenile justice. Retrieved from http://faculty.ncwc.edu/toconnor/111/111lect14.htm

Oliver, M. (1996). *Understanding disability: From theory to practice.* London, UK: Palgrave Macmillan.

Olsen, K.D., & Dacy, M.D. (2014). Mayo Clinic: 150 years of serving humanity through hope and healing. *Mayo Clinic Proceedings Sesquicentennial Commemorative,* 11-22.

O'Neill, J., & Conzemius, A. (with Commadore, C., & Pulfus, C.). (2006). *The power of SMART goals: Using goals to improve student learning.* Bloomington, IN: The Solution Tree.

Orrù, M. (1987). *Anomie: History and meanings.* Winchester, MA: Allen & Unwin.

Ostiguy, L., & Dieser, R. (2004). Developing a framework for therapeutic recreation certification in Canada. *Expanding Horizons in Therapeutic Recreation, 21,* 21-26.

Park, D. (1981). NTRS Philosophical issues report. Washington, DC: National Recreation and Park Association.

Parker, S.E., Mai, C.T., Canfield, M.A., Rickard, R., Wang, Y., Meyer, R.E., . . . National Birth Defects Prevention Network. (2010). Updated National Birth Prevalence estimates for selected birth defects in the United States, 2004-2006. *Birth Defects Research Part A, Clinical and Molecular Teratology, 88*(12), 1008-1016.

Parliament of Australia Senate. (2006). *A national approach to mental health—from crisis to community.* Canberra, Australia: Author.

Passas, N. (1997). Anomie, reference groups, and relative deprivation. In N. Passas & R. Agnew (Eds.), *The future of anomie theory* (pp. 27-51). Boston, MA: Northeastern University Press.

Paul, J.L., & Epanchin, B.C. (1991). *Educating emotionally disturbed children and youth: Theories and practices for teachers* (2nd ed.). New York, NY: Macmillan.

Pawelko, K.A., & Magafas, A.H. (1997). Leisure well being among adolescent groups: Time, choices and self-determination. *Parks and Recreation, 32*(7), 26-39.

Pedlar, A., & Gilbert, A. (1997). Normalization and integration: The Canadian experience. In D.M. Compton (Ed.), *Issues in therapeutic recreation: Toward the new millennium* (pp. 489-506). Champaign, IL: Sagamore.

Pegg, S., & Darcy, S. (2007). Sailing on troubled waters: Diversional therapy in Australia. *Therapeutic Recreation Journal, 41*(2), 132-140.

Pegg, S., Stumbo, N., & Bennett, J. (2017). Evidence-based practices. In N. Stumbo, B. Wolfe, & S. Pegg (Eds.), *Professional issues in therapeutic recreation* (3rd ed.; pp. 333-356). Urbana, IL: Sagamore Publishing.

Perkins, D.F., & Caldwell, L.L. (2005). Resiliency, protective processes, promotion, and community youth development. In P.A. Witt & L.L. Caldwell (Eds.), *Recreation and youth development* (pp. 149-167). State College, PA: Venture Publishing.

Peterson, C. (2000). The future of optimism. *American Psychologist, 55*(1), 44-55.

Peterson, C.A. (1984). A matter of priorities and loyalties. *Therapeutic Recreation Journal, 18*(3), 11-16.

Peterson, C.A., & Gunn, S.L. (1984). *Therapeutic recreation program design: Principles and procedures.* (2nd ed.). Englewood Cliffs, NJ: Prentice Hall.

Peterson, E.T. (1934, April). Doctor Mayo tells how to live. *Better Homes & Gardens,* 16-17, 64.

Phillips, B.E. (1952a). Hospital recreation is unique. *Journal of the American Association for Health, Physical Education and Recreation, 23*(5), 29-30, 35.

Phillips, B.E. (1952b). Recreation therapy. *Journal of the American Association for Health, Physical Education and Recreation, 23*(6), 23-24.

Phillips, B.E. (1957). Uniqueness of recreation in hospital. *Journal of Health, Physical Education, and Recreation,* 28(2), 52.

Physical Activity Guidelines Advisory Committee. (2008). Physical activity guidelines advisory committee report. Washington, DC: U.S. Department of Health and Human Services. Retrieved from www.health.gov/paguidelines/report/pdf/committeereport.pdf

Piaget, J. (1970). *Genetic epistemology.* New York, NY: Columbia University Press.

Polacheck, H.S. (1989). *I came a stranger: The story of a Hull-House girl.* Urbana, IL: University of Illinois Press.

Polman, C., Reingold, S.C., Banwell, B., Clanet, M., Cohen, J.A., Filippi, M., . . . Wolinsky, J.S. (2011). Diagnostic criteria for multiple sclerosis: 2010 revisions to the McDonald criteria. *Annals of Neurology, 69*(2), 292-302.

Powell, A. (2016). The effects of computer technology use on increasing socialization and improving mental health. Retrieved from http://leadingage.org/sites/default/files/Westminster Canterbury_on_Chesapeake_Bay_Case_Study.pdf

Project Adventure. (2016). Credentialing information. Retrieved from www.project-adventure.org/introduction-credentialing/

Putnam, R.D. (2000). *Bowling alone: The collapse and revival of American community.* New York, NY: Touchstone.

Putnam, R.D., & Feldstein, L.M. (2003). *Better together: Restoring the American community.* New York, NY: Simon and Schuster.

Rappaport, J. (1987). Terms of empowerment/exemplars of prevention: Toward a theory for community psychology. *American Journal of Community Psychology, 15,* 121-147.

Robertson, T. (1993). *The wheel of fortune or the wheel of torture?: A conceptual model for professional and personal development.* Paper presented at the Midwest Symposium on Therapeutic Recreation, St. Charles, IL.

Rodriguez-Hanley, A., & Snyder, C.R. (2000). The demise of hope: On losing positive thinking. In C.R. Snyder (Ed.), *Handbook of hope: Theory, measures, and applications* (pp. 39-54). San Diego, CA: Academic Press.

Roesler, R.C. (1987, Spring). Art and the Mayo environment. *Mayo Magazine,* 10-23.

Romney, G.O. (1945). *Off the job living.* Washington, DC: McGrath and National Recreation and Park Association.

Ross, G., & Nelson, R. (2014). Using theater and drama interventions to reduce bullying in school-aged children. *Therapeutic Recreation Journal, 48*(4), 334-336.

Rovira, A., & Leon, A. (2008). MR in the diagnosis and monitoring of multiple sclerosis: An overview. *European Journal of Radiology, 67*(3), 409-414.

Russell, K. (2002). *A longitudinal assessment of treatment outcomes in outdoor behavioral healthcare.* Technical Report 28. Moscow, ID: Idaho Forest, Wildlife, and Range Experiment Station, University of Idaho—Wilderness Research Center.

Russell, M.S., Widmer, M.A., Lundberg, N., & Ward, P. (2015). Adaptation of an adolescent coping assessment for therapeutic recreation and outdoor adventure settings. *Therapeutic Recreation Journal, 49*(1), 18-34.

Ryan, R.M., & Deci, E.L. (2000). Self-determination theory and the facilitation of intrinsic motivation, social development, and well-being. *American Psychologist, 55*(1), 68-78. doi:10.1037/0003-066X.55.1.68

Sabat, S. (1994). Excess disability and malignant social psychology: A case study of Alzheimer's disease. *Journal of Community & Applied Social Psychology, 4*(3), 157-166. doi:10.1002/casp.2450040303

SAMHSA (2018). *SAMHSA's working definition of Recovery* .Rockville, MD: Author. Retrieved from https://www.samhsa.gov/recovery

Sampson, R.J. (2001). How do communities undergird or undermine human development? Relevant contexts and social mechanisms. In A. Booth & A.C. Crouter (Eds.), *Does it take a village?* (pp. 3-30). Mahwah, NJ: Lawrence Erlbaum Associates.

Schaie, K.W., & Willis, S. (2002). *Adult development and aging.* Upper Saddle River, NJ: Prentice Hall.

Schoel, J., Prouty, D., & Radcliffe, P. (1988). *Islands of healing: A guide to adventure based counseling.* Hamilton, MA: Project Adventure.

Schoen, A., Miller, L.J., Brett-Green, B.A., & Nielsen, D.M. (2009). Physiological and behavioral difference in sensory processing: A comparison of children with autism spectrum disorder and sensory modulation disorder. *Frontiers in Integrative Neuroscience, 3,* 29.

Schram, B., & Mandell, B.R. (2012). *An introduction to human services: Policy and practice* (8th ed.). Boston, MA: Allyn and Bacon.

Schray, V. (2006). Assuring quality in higher education: Recommendations for improving accreditation. Retrieved from www.ed.gov./about/bdscomm/list/hiedfuture/reports/schray2.pdf

Scott, D., Witt, P.A., & Foss, M.G. (1996). Evaluation of the impact of the Dougherty Arts Center's club on children at-risk. *Journal of Park and Recreation Administration, 14*(3), 41-59.

Search Institute. (2004). Developmental assets profile. Retrieved from www.search-institute.org/sites/default/files/a/DAP-Sample-Survey-Page.pdf

Search Institute. (2016a). Let's talk about our aspirations: 12 discussion starters for youth and adults. Retrieved from www.search-institute.org/blog/talk-about-aspirations

Search Institute. (2016b). User guide for the developmental assets profile. Retrieved from www.search-institute.org/sites/default/files/a/Fluid-DAP-User-Guide-1-2016.pdf

Search Institute. (2018a). Choosing a youth survey. Retrieved from www.search-institute.org/surveys/our-surveys

Search Institute. (2018b). The developmental assets framework. Retrieved from www.search-institute.org/our-research/development-assets/developmental-assets-framework/

Searle, M.S., Mahon, M.J., Iso-Ahola, S.E., Sdrolias, H.A., & van Dyck, J. (1995). Enhancing a sense of independence and psychological well-being among the elderly. *Journal of Leisure Research, 27*(2), 107-124.

Searle, M.S., Mahon, M.J., Iso-Ahola, S.E., Sdrolias, H.A., & van Dyck, J. (1998). Examining the long term effects of leisure education on a sense of independence and psychological well-being among the elderly. *Journal of Leisure Research, 30*(3), 331-340.

Seligman, A.B. (1997). *The problem of trust.* Princeton, NJ: Princeton University Press.

Seligman, M.E., & Csikszentmihalyi, M. (2000). Positive psychology: An introduction. *American Psychologist, 55*(1), 5-14.

Seligman, M.E. (2002). *Authentic happiness: Using the new positive psychology to realize your full potential for lasting fulfillment.* New York, NY: Free Press.

Senge, P., Kleiner, A., Roberts, C., Ross, R., Roth, G., & Smith, B. (1999). *The dance of change: Challenges to sustaining momentum in learning organizations.* New York, NY: Random House.

Shank, J., & Coyle, C. (2002). *Therapeutic recreation in health promotion and rehabilitation.* State College, PA: Venture.

Shank, J.W., Kinney, W.B., & Coyle, C.P. (1993). Efficacy studies in therapeutic recreation research: The need, the state of the art, and future implications. In M.J. Malkin & C.Z. Howe (Eds.), *Research in therapeutic recreation: Concepts and methods* (pp. 301-335). State College, PA: Venture.

Shannahoff-Khalsa, D.S., & Beckett, L.R. (1996). Clinical case report: Efficacy of yogic techniques in the treatment of obsessive compulsive disorders. *International Journal of Neuroscience, 85*(1-2), 1-17.

Shelley, M. (1818/2003). *Frankenstein.* New York, NY: Bantam.

Shelterwood Academy. (2016). Campus life. Retrieved from www.shelterwood.org/campus-life/

Sherrill, C. (2004). *Adapted physical activity, recreation, and sport: Crossdisciplinary and life span* (6th ed.). New York, NY: McGraw-Hill.

Shorter, E. (1997). *A history of psychiatry: From the era of the asylum to the age of Prozac.* New York, NY: Wiley.

Shulewitz, R., & Zuniga, S. (1999). NISRA teams with community health providers for at risk youth. *Illinois Parks and Recreation, 20*(4), 33.

Shultz, L.E., Crompton, J.L., & Witt, P.A. (1995). A national profile of the status of public recreation services for at-risk children and youth. *Journal of Park and Recreation Administration, 13*(3), 1-25.

Silver, R.A. (1989). *Developing cognitive and creative skills through art.* Mamaroneck, NY: Albin Press.

Simeonsson, R.J. (1994). *Risk, resilience, and prevention: Promoting the well-being of all children.* Baltimore, MD: Brooks.

Simon, S.B., & Olds, S.W. (1977). *Helping your children learn right from wrong: A guide to values clarification.* New York, NY: McGraw-Hill.

Skalko, T.K. (1997). Therapeutic recreation in health care reform. In D.M. Compton (Ed.), *Issues in therapeutic recreation: Toward the new millennium* (pp. 1-16). Champaign, IL: Sagamore.

Skalko, T.K. (2013). The Committee on Accreditation of Recreational Therapy Education (CARTE): The future of academic accreditation for recreational therapy/therapeutic recreation accreditation. *Therapeutic Recreation Journal, 46*(4), 244-258.

Sklar, S.L., Anderson, S.C., & Autry, C.E. (2007). Positive youth development: A wilderness intervention. *Therapeutic Recreation Journal, 41*(3), 221-243.

Sklar, S.L., & Carter, M.J. (2016). Introduction to the special issue on strengths-based practice—Part I. *Therapeutic Recreation Journal, 50*(1), 1-3.

Sklare, G. (2014). *Brief counseling that works: A solution-focused therapy approach for school counselors and other mental health professionals.* Thousand Oaks, CA: Corwin Press.

Smith, M.L., Jiang, L., & Ory, M.G. (2012). Falls efficacy among older adults enrolled in an evidence-based program to reduce fall-related risk: sustainability of individual benefits over time. *Family & Community Health, 35*(3): 256-263.

Snead, B., Pakstis, D., Evans, B., & Nelson, R. (2015). The use of creative writing interventions in substance abuse treatment. *Therapeutic Recreation Journal, 49*(3), 179-182.

Snyder, C.R. (2000). Hypothesis: There is hope. In C.R. Snyder (Ed.), *Handbook of hope: Theory, measures, and applications* (pp. 3-21). San Diego, CA: Academic Press.

Spence, S.J., & Schneider, M.T. (2009). The role of epilepsy and epileptiform EEGs in autism spectrum disorders. *Pediatric Research, 65*(6), 599.

Sprouse, J.K., Klitzing, S.W., & Parr, M. (2005). Youth at risk: Recreation and prevention. *Parks and Recreation, 40*(1), 16-21.

Starr, E.G. (1896). Settlements and the church's duty. *The Church Social Union, 28,* 1.

Statistics Canada. (2004). 2001 Census. Retrieved on January 20, 2005, from http://statcan.ca

Steinberg, L. (2002). *Adolescence* (6th ed.). Boston, MA: McGraw-Hill.

Stephan, Y., Sutin, A.R., & Terracciano, A. (2014). Physical activity and personality development across adulthood and old age: Evidence from two longitudinal studies. *Journal of Research in Personality, 49,* 1-7. doi:10.1016/j.jrp.2013.12.003

Steves, C.J., Mehta, M.M., Jackson, S.H., & Spector, T.D. (2016). Kicking back cognitive ageing: Leg power predicts cognitive ageing after ten years in older female twins. *Gerontology, 62,* 138-149. doi:10.1159/000441029

Stivers, C. (2000). Bureau men and settlement women: Constructing public administration in the progressive era. Lawrence, KS: University Press of Kansas.

St. Mary's Patient Library. (2016, Spring). *SMH Patients Library News.* [Patient Flyer]. Rochester, MN: Mayo Clinic.

Streifel, S. (1998). *How to teach through modeling and imitation* (2nd ed.). Austin TX: PRO-ED.

Stumbo, N.J. (2002). *Client assessment in therapeutic recreation services.* State College, PA: Venture.

Stumbo, N., Martin, L., & Ogborne, V. (2004). Collective voices, shared wisdom: On the need for a professional association to represent therapeutic recreation in Australia. *Annals of Leisure Research, 7*(2), 85-94.

Stumbo, N.J., & Peterson, C.A. (1998). The leisure ability model. *Therapeutic Recreation Journal, 32*(2), 82-96.

Stumbo, N.J., & Peterson, C.A. (2004). *Therapeutic recreation program design: Principles and procedures* (4th ed.). San Francisco, CA: Benjamin Cummings.

Stumbo, N.J., & Peterson, C.A. (2009). *Therapeutic recreation program design: Principles and procedures* (5th ed.). San Francisco, CA: Benjamin Cummings.

Sung, H.C., Lee, W.L., Li, T.L., & Watson, R. (2012). A group music intervention using percussion instruments with familiar music to reduce anxiety and agitation of institutionalized older adults with dementia. *International Journal of Geriatric Psychiatry, 27*(6), 621-627. doi:10.1002/gps.2761

Suzuki, H. (1995). *Therapeutic recreation: Recreation to reduce disability and maintain health.* Tokyo, Japan: Fumaido Publishing.

Swann-Guerrero, S., & Mackey, C. (2008). Wellness through physical activity. In T. Robertson & T. Long (Eds.), *Foundations of therapeutic recreation: Perspectives, philosophies, and practices for the 21st* century (pp. 199-214). Champaign, IL: Human Kinetics.

Sylvester, C. (1989). Therapeutic recreation and the practice of history. *Therapeutic Recreation Journal, 23*(4), 19-28.

Sylvester, C.D. (2015). Re-imagining and transforming therapeutic recreation: Reaching into Foucault's toolbox. *Leisure/Loisir, 39*(2), 167-192.

Sylvester, C., Voelkl, J.E., & Ellis, G. (2001). *Therapeutic recreation programming: Theory and practice.* State College, PA: Venture.

Takeuchi, Y. (2014, September). *Recreation therapy practice in the world: Global discussion— Japan.* American Therapeutic Recreation Association Annual Conference 2014, Oklahoma City, OK.

Tapus, A., Mataric, M.J., & Scasselati, B. (2007). Socially assistive robotics: Grand challenges of robotics. *IEEE Robotics & Automation Magazine, 14*(1), 35-42.

Tavassoli, T., Miller, L.J., Schoen, S.A., Jo Brout, J., Sullivan, J., & Baron-Cohen, S. (2018). Sensory reactivity, empathizing and systemizing in autism spectrum conditions and sensory processing disorder. *Developmental Cognitive Neuroscience, 29,* 72-77.

Taylor-Piliae, R.E., Newell, K.A., Cherin, R., Lee, M.J., King, A.C., & Haskell, W.L. (2010). Effects of Tai Chi and Western exercise on physical and cognitive functioning in healthy community-dwelling older adults. *Journal of aging and physical activity, 18*(3), 261-279.

Theurer, K., Mortenson, W.B., Stone, R., Suto, M., Timonene, V., & Rozanov, J. (2015). The need for a social revolution in residential care. *Journal of Aging Studies, 35,* 201-210. https://doi.org/10.1016/j.jaging.2015.08.011

Thibadeau, S.F. (1998). *How to use response cost.* Austin, TX: PRO-ED.

Thompson, P.D., Buchner, D., Piña, I.L., Balady, G.J., Williams, M.A., Marcus, B.H., . . . Wenger, N.K. (2003). Exercise and physical activity in the prevention and treatment of atherosclerotic cardiovascular disease: A statement from the Council on Clinical Cardiology (Subcommittee on Exercise, Rehabilitation, and Prevention) and the Council on Nutrition, Physical Activity, and Metabolism (Subcommittee on Physical Activity). *Circulation, 107*(24), 3109-3116. doi:10.1161/10.CIR.0000075572.40158.77

Tiger, L. (1979). *Optimism: The biology of hope.* New York, NY: Simon & Schuster.

Tousignant, M., Corriveau, H., Roy, P.M., Desrosiers, J., Dubuc, N., & Hébert, R. (2013). Efficacy of supervised tai chi exercises versus conventional physical therapy exercises in fall prevention for frail older adults: a randomized controlled trial. *Disability and rehabilitation, 35*(17), 1429-1435.

Trowbridge, R. (1988). *Therapy and recreation.* Melbourne, Australia: Centre for Continuing Education, Monash University.

Tsai, H.H., & Tsai, Y.F. (2011). Changes in depressive symptoms, social support, and loneliness over 1 year after a minimum 3-month videoconference program for older nursing home residents. *Journal of Medical Internet Research, 13*(4), e93.

Tsukamoto, M. (2013). Research on reconstruction of lives after retirement: Through participating in rice farming group for retirees. *International University of Health and Welfare Conference Paper, 18*(1), 34-45.

Twenge, J.M. (2000). The age of anxiety? Birth-cohort change in anxiety and neuroticism, 1952-1993. *Journal of Personality and Social Psychology, 79,* 1007-1021.

United Nations. (1948). The Universal Declaration of Human Rights. Retrieved from www.un.org/en/universal-declaration-human-rights/

United Nations. (2015). World population prospects: The 2015 revision. Retrieved from https://esa.un.org/unpd/wpp

United Nations Development Program. (2018). Human Development index. Retrieved from http://hdr.undp.org/en/content/human-development-index-hdi

U.S. Census Bureau. (2010). The older population: 2010. Retrieved from www.census.gov/prod/cen2010/briefs/c2010br-09.pdf

U.S. Census Bureau. (2018). Publications, briefs, reports from Census Bureau Experts. Retrieved from https://www.census.gov/library/publications.html

U.S. Department of Veterans Affairs. (2016). Case study: Veteran Affairs Medical Centers. Retrieved from http://eos.sirsidynix.com/wp-content/uploads/2011/12/Case-Study-VA-Medical-Centers.pdf

U.S. Public Health Service. (2002). *Closing the gap: A national blueprint for improving the health of individuals with mental retardation.* Retrieved September 15, 2005, from www.surgeongeneral.gov/topics/mentalretardation/retardation.pdf

Van der Ploeg, E.S., & O'Connor, D.W. (2010). Evaluation of personalised, one-to-one interaction using Montessori-type activities as a treatment of challenging behaviours in people with dementia: The study protocol of a crossover trial. *BMC Geriatrics, 10*(1), 3.

Van der Smissen, B. (2005). *Recreation and parks the profession: A comprehensive resource for students and professionals.* Champaign, IL: Human Kinetics.

Veal, A. (2016, June). *Leisure and human rights.* Key note presentation at the World Leisure Congress, Durban, South Africa.

Veblen, T. (1899). *The theory of the leisure class: An economic study of institutions.* New York, NY: Macmillan.

Velde, B.P., & Murphy, D. (1994). The therapeutic recreation (TR) profession in Canada. Where are we now and where are we going? In G.L. Hitzhusen, L. Thomas, & N. Frank (Eds.), *Global therapeutic recreation III: 3rd International Symposium on Therapeutic Recreation* (p. 108). Columbia, MO: University of Missouri at Columbia.

Vidoni, E.D., Johnson, D.K., Morris, J.K., Van Sciver, A., Greer, C.S., Billinger, S.A., . . . Burns, J.M. (2015). Dose-response of aerobic exercise on cognition: A community-based, pilot randomized controlled trial. doi:10.1371/journal.pone.0131647

Vincent, G.K., & Velkoff, V.A. (2010). The next four decades: The older population in the United States: 2010 to 2050. Retrieved from www.census.gov/prod/2010pubs/p25-1138.pdf

Vipond, R. (1991). *Liberty and community: Canadian federalism and the future of the constitution.* Albany, NY: State University of New York Press.

Visser, C.F. (2013). The origin of the solution-focused approach. *International Journal of Solution-Focused Practices, 1*(1), 10-17.

Wada, K., & Shibata, T. (2007). Living with seal robots: Its sociopsychological and physiological influences on the elderly at a care house. *IEEE Transactions on Robotics, 23*(5), 972-980.

Wardlaw, J.M., Murray, V., Berge, E., del Zoppo, G., Sandercock, P., Lindley, R.L., & Cohen, G. (2012). Recombinant tissue plasminogen activator for acute ischaemic stroke: An updated systematic review and meta-analysis. *Lancet, 379,* 2364-2372.

Washburne, M.F. (1904/1990). The labor museum. In M.L. McCree Bryan & A.F. Davis (Eds.), *100 years at Hull-House* (pp. 74-81). Bloomington, IN: Indiana University Press. (Reprinted from *Craftman,* September 1904, pp. 570-579).

Watanabe, H. (2006). Societal potential of adapted sports. *21st Century Social Design Research, 5,* 135-144.

Wehman, P. (2001). *Supported employment in business: Expanding the capacity of workers with disabilities.* St. Augustine, FL: Training Resources Network.

Weikart Center for Youth Program Quality. (2016a). Social and emotional learning challenge. Retrieved from www.cypq.org/SELChallenge

Weikart Center for Youth Program Quality. (2016b). Youth program quality assessment. Retrieved from http://cypq.org/assessment

Weil, E.F. (1913/1990). The Hull-House players. In M.L. McCree Bryan & A.F. Davis (Eds.), *100 years at Hull-House* (pp. 92-95). Bloomington, IN: Indiana University Press. (Reprinted from *Theatre Magazine,* September 1913, pp. xix-xxii).

Wenzel, K. (1998, May/June/July). President's message. *NTRS Report, 23*(3), 1-5.

West, P.C. (1984). Social stigma and community recreation participation by the physically and mentally handicapped. *Therapeutic Recreation Journal, 26*(1), 40-49.

Weuve, J., Kang, J.H., Manson, J.E., Breteler, M.M., Ware, J.H., & Grodstein, F. (2004). Physical activity, including walking, and cognitive function in older women. *JAMA, 292*(12), 1454-1461. doi:10.1001/jama.292.12.1454

Wilhite, B., Devine, M.A., & Goldenberg, L. (1999). Self-perceptions of youth with and without disabilities: Implications for leisure programs and services. *Therapeutic Recreation Journal, 33,* 15-28.

Wilhite, B., Keller, M.J., & Caldwell, L.L. (1999). Optimizing lifelong health and well-being: A health enhancing model of therapeutic recreation. *Therapeutic Recreation Journal, 33,* 98-108.

Williams, R. (2008). Places, models, and modalities of practice. In T. Long and T. Robertson (Eds.). *Foundations of therapeutic recreation: Perceptions, philosophies, and practices for the 1st century* (pp. 63-76).Champaign, IL: Human Kinetics.

Willis, S., Schai, K.W., & Martin, M. (2009). Cognitive plasticity. In V. Bengtson, D. Gans, N. Putney, & M. Silverstein (Eds.), *Handbook of theories of aging* (2nd ed.). New York, NY: Springer.

Winstein, C.J., Stein, J., Arena, R., Bates, B., Cherney, L.R., Cramer, S.C., . . . Zorowitz, R.D. (2016). Guidelines for adult stroke rehabilitation and recovery: A guideline for healthcare professionals from the American Heart Association/American Stroke Association. *Stroke, 47*(6), e98-e169.

Wise, J.B. (2015). Leisure. *Therapeutic Recreation Journal, 49*(2), 166-178.

Witman, J. (1992). *The Cooperation and Trust Scale.* Enumclaw, WA: Idyll Arbor.

Witt, P.A., & Caldwell, L. (2005). Principles of youth development. In P.A. Witt and L.L. Caldwell (Eds.), *Recreation and youth development.* State College, PA: Venture.

Witt, P.A., & Crompton, J.L. (1996). The at-risk youth recreation project. *Journal of Park and Recreation Administration, 14*(3), 1-9.

Witt, P.A., & Crompton, J.L. (2002a). *Best practices in youth development in public parks and recreation settings.* Ashburn, VA: National Recreation and Park Association.

Witt, P.A., & Crompton, J.L. (2002b). Programming for the future. *Parks and Recreation, 37*(12), 64-68.

Witt, P.A., & Ellis, G.D. (1989). *The leisure diagnostic battery: Users manual.* State College, PA: Venture.

Wolfensberger, W. (1977). The normalization principle, and some major implications to architectural environmental design. In M. Bedner (Ed.), *Barrier free environments* (p. 135). Stroudsburg, PA: Dowden, Hutchinson & Ross, Inc.

Woodham-Smith, C. (1951). *Florence Nightingale: 1820-1910.* New York, NY: McGraw-Hill.

Woods, R.A., & Kennedy, A.J. (1970). *The rise of urban America: Handbook of settlements.* New York, NY: Charities Publication.

World Health Organization (WHO). (1989). *History of the development of the ICD.* Geneva, Switzerland: Author.

World Health Organization (WHO). (2001). *International classification of functioning, disability and health.* Geneva, Switzerland: Author.

World Health Organization (WHO). (2002). *Towards a common language for functioning, disability and health: ICF—The international classification of functioning, disability and health.* Geneva, Switzerland: WHO.

Yoshioka, N. (2016). Can recreation exist in healthcare? Recreation therapy and its professionalization. *International Journal of Physical Therapy & Rehabilitation, 2,* 110. doi:http://dx.doi.org/10.15344/2455-7498/2016/110

Zabriskie, R., & McCormick, B. (2000). Accreditation and academic quality: A comparison with healthcare accreditation. *SCHOLE: A Journal of Leisure Studies and Recreation Education, 15,* 31-45.

Zander, R.S., & Zander, B. (2000). *The art of possibility: Transforming professional and personal life.* Boston, MA: Harvard Business School Press.

Zero to Three. (2016). *DC:0-5™: Diagnostic classification of mental health and developmental disorders of infancy and early childhood.* Washington, DC: Author.

Zijlstra, G.R., Van Haastregt, J.C., Ambergen, T., Van Rossum, E., Van Eijk, J.T.M., Tennstedt, S.L., & Kempen, G.I. (2009). Effects of a multicomponent cognitive behavioral group intervention on fear of falling and activity avoidance in community-dwelling older adults: Results of a randomized controlled trial. *Journal of the American Geriatrics Society, 57*(11), 2020-2028.

Index

Note: The italicized *f* and *t* following page numbers refer to figures and tables, respectively.

About the Editors

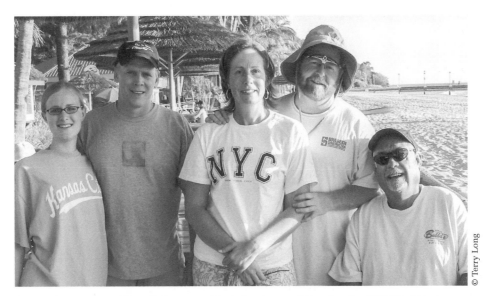

Editors Terry Long and Terry Robertson with their wives and friend at the 2005 World Leisure Symposium in Brisbane, Australia. Pictured from left to right, Anne and Terry Long, Shelly and Terry Robertson, and John Chambers.

© Terry Long

Terry Long, PhD, is a professor and the director of the School of Health Science and Wellness at Northwest Missouri State University, where he has worked since 2000. He is regarded nationally as one of the leading scholars in the field of therapeutic recreation, as evidenced by his teaching, research, applied experience, and service to the field.

Long has been on the editorial board of *Therapeutic Recreation Journal* for more than 10 years and served as editor from 2008 to 2011. He was an active member of the Northwest Missouri State faculty senate, serving his second term from 2012 to 2014, and was the faculty senate president for the 2014-2015 academic year. In addition to therapeutic recreation, Long's professional interests also include adventure-based therapy, inclusion, disability rights, and mental health. His interest in independent living has enabled him to be instrumental in fostering a partnership between Northwest Missouri State and Midland Empire Resources for Independent Living (MERIL).

Terry Robertson, PhD, is a professor and associate dean in the College of Health and Human Services at California State University at Long Beach.

Robertson was previously a clinical associate professor at the University of Utah; a professor and chair of the department of health, physical education, recreation, and dance at Northwest Missouri State University; and a research fellow at the University of Queensland. While at Northwest Missouri State, Robertson helped create a partnership with Midland Empire Resources for Independent Living (MERIL), for which he served on the board from 1994 to 2008, including six years as the chair. The Terry Robertson Community Partner Award was created in 2010 in honor of Robertson's service to MERIL.

In addition to his work on independent living, Robertson has had a considerable impact on the field of therapeutic recreation, working as an educator, practitioner, and consultant for more than 40 years. He is a past president of the National Therapeutic Recreation Society, the Missouri Therapeutic Recreation Society, and the Nevada Therapeutic Recreation Society. He also served on the Utah Therapeutic Recreation Licensure for six years and was the director of continuing education for the Midwest Symposium on Therapeutic Recreation for more than 20 years.

About the Contributors

Patricia Ardovino, PhD, CTRS, CPRP, is retired from her position as associate professor at the University of Wisconsin at La Crosse. She received her undergraduate and master's degrees in physical education and adapted physical education from Ohio State University and received her PhD from Indiana University. Before receiving her doctorate, Dr. Ardovino spent 22 years working with people with disabilities—as an instructor in an institution for people with intellectual impairments, the program director of a sheltered workshop, the coordinator of a respite program, and the director of a community-based therapeutic recreation center for the Memphis Park Commission. At the University of Wisconsin at La Crosse, she led four study tours of Italy that focused on leisure in the Roman Empire and accessibility for tourists with disabilities. Her teaching and research interests include therapeutic recreation in correctional settings, inclusive recreation, and the impact of the war in Iraq on recreation and therapeutic recreation.

Cari E. Autry, PhD, LRT/CTRS, is a faculty member in the recreational therapy program in East Carolina University's department of recreation and leisure studies. She received her doctorate degree in health and human performance, with a concentration in therapeutic recreation and a minor in special education, from the University of Florida. Dr. Autry has presented at state, national, and international conferences related to youth development, children and families who are homeless, therapeutic recreation modalities such as sailing and adventure therapy, virtual reality and simulation for people with disabilities, community development, social capital, and therapeutic recreation education. Dr. Autry has published in journals such as *Therapeutic Recreation Journal, World Leisure Journal, Leisure Sciences, International Leisure Review, Sociology of Sport Journal,* and *Leisure/Loisir.* She serves as the special interest group facilitator in leisure for children and youth for the World Leisure Organization. Dr. Autry serves as cochair of the American Therapeutic Recreation Association's research institute poster session. She has been an associate editor of *Therapeutic Recreation Journal* for the past 13 years. For leisure, she enjoys sailing, traveling, scuba diving, gardening, music, shelling, hiking, and fly-fishing.

Jessie L. Bennett, PhD, CTRS/L, is an assistant professor in the department of recreation management and policy at the University of New Hampshire. She received her bachelor's degree in therapeutic recreation from Green Mountain College, her master's degree in youth and family recreation from Brigham Young University, and her PhD in leisure behavior from Indiana University. After completing her baccalaureate studies, she worked as a recreational therapist (RT) for a residential rehabilitation center for children with developmental disabilities. During her graduate studies, she did recreational therapy for veterans with combat-related disabilities and their families. She has extensive clinical training as an RT, with most of her career working as an RT in adaptive sports programs for veterans with disabilities. Employing primarily mixed methodologies, her research is focused on examining the outcomes of RT programs for veterans with physical and psychological disabilities.

Jody Cormack, DPT, is the vice provost for academic programs and dean of graduate studies for California State University at Long Beach (CSULB). She received her bachelor's degree in physical therapy from CSULB. After working as a physical therapist in the rehabilitation setting, she returned to academia and earned master's degrees in biokinesiology and in education as well as a doctorate in physical therapy from the University of Southern California. She became a board-certified specialist in neurologic physical therapy and is certified as an advanced clinical instructor. Her clinical practice focused on facilitating functional and neurologic recovery for patients with neurologic disorders. In addition to her education degree, Dr. Cormack completed a fellowship offered by the American Physical Therapy Association (APTA) Educational Leadership Institute (ELI) that focused on leadership in higher education. She has served as a member of the boards of directors for several professional and community organizations.

Laura Covert-Miller, PhD, CTRS, is an associate professor in the health, human performance, and recreation department at Pittsburg State University in Pittsburg, Kansas, where she teaches therapeutic recreation and recreation courses. She received her doctorate degree in gerontology from the University of Nebraska at Omaha and has a master's degree in recreation (therapeutic recreation) and a bachelor's degree in recreation (therapeutic and corporate wellness) from Northwest Missouri State University. Dr. Covert-Miller has presented at state, regional, and international conferences related to healthy aging interventions in older adults. Prior to earning her doctorate degree, Dr. Covert-Miller was a personal trainer, group exercise instructor, and employee wellness coordinator with several organizations serving older adults. She is a member of the American Therapeutic Recreation Association and the International Council on Active Aging.

Melissa H. D'Eloia, PhD, CTRS, is an associate professor in the recreation program at Western Washington University. She received her doctorate and master's degrees in the department of parks, recreation, and tourism, with a concentration in therapeutic recreation and experiential education and a certificate in disability studies, from the University of Utah. Prior to earning her doctorate degree, Dr. D'Eloia worked as a recreation therapist with youth and adults in mental and behavior health settings as well as

therapeutic outdoor programs. Dr. D'Eloia has presented at state, national, and international conferences related to outcome measurement, therapeutic camp programs, and the application of solution-focused counseling techniques in recreational therapy practice. Her research has been published in *Therapeutic Recreation Journal*, *Journal of Leisure Research*, and *Journal of Youth Development*. Her leisure interests include skiing, dancing, gardening, camping, and traveling.

Mary Ann Devine, PhD, CTRS, is a professor of recreation, park, and tourism management at Kent State University. She received her doctoral degree in recreation and leisure studies from the University of Georgia. Her research interests are in the area of inclusion of individuals with disabilities in recreation, sport, and leisure services. Dr. Devine has conducted numerous studies examining aspects of the inclusion process such as social acceptance, social construction of disability, best practices, stigma, attitudinal barriers, and the application of the ADA in leisure setting. Recently, Dr. Devine has been examining the role of social justice related to inclusion as well as the role of leisure in helping individuals with intellectual disabilities transition from high school to college.

Rodney Dieser, PhD, CTRS, is a faculty member at the University of Northern Iowa. Dr. Dieser believes that classroom learning should be based on a professor who has one foot in research and the other in professional practice. As a researcher Dr. Dieser has published over 100 articles and five textbooks, and his writings have appeared in such journals as *Alberta Journal of Educational Research*, *Counselling Psychology Quarterly*, *International Journal of Applied Positive Psychology*, *Journal of Leisure Research*, and *Therapeutic Recreation Journal*. As a practitioner, Dr. Dieser works 10 to 12 hours a week as a certified therapeutic recreation specialist and a licensed mental health therapist at a community mental health agency in Waterloo, Iowa. His prior employment includes serving as an inclusion specialist for the Salt Lake City, Utah, school district, working with adults with developmental disabilities, and working as a licensed therapeutic recreation specialist in addiction rehabilitation and homeless outreach for Catholic Community Services of Salt Lake City. Rod completed his PhD in physical education and recreation at the University of Alberta in 2002 and a master's degree in mental health counseling at the University of Northern Iowa in 2014. Other degrees include a bachelor's degree in recreation and leisure and a master's degree in parks, recreation, and tourism from the University of Utah, as well as an associate's degree in therapeutic recreation from Lethbridge Community College.

Alice Foose, PhD, is an associate professor in the School of Health Science and Wellness at Northwest Missouri State University. She has worked in a range of park and recreation and social service programs, including clinical, community-based, and wilderness settings. With an extensive background in life span development, she has worked with children and adults with developmental disabilities in a variety of community settings, and she assisted with several research projects involving people with developmental disabilities while in graduate school at Indiana University in Bloomington. Her interests are the social context of recreation activities, volunteerism, and collaborative partnerships. She has presented both nationally and internationally and has been published in *World Leisure Journal*, *Mental Retardation*, and *Schole.* She holds degrees from Indiana University and the University of Kentucky.

Keith Fulthorp, EdD, has over 25 years of experience within the recreation field and is currently an associate professor at California State University at Long Beach in the department of recreation and leisure studies. Keith's research interests are in the areas of municipal recreation and parks in urban areas, leadership, team building, and solution-focused counseling. He obtained his doctorate degree from the University of Southern California in 2009 and continues to be closely tied to both the recreation and school counseling professions. Keith's municipal recreation research and education sessions have been presented at the California Park and Recreation Society (annually since 2004), the National Recreation and Park Association (annually since 2010), the American Therapeutic Recreation Association, the Midwest Therapeutic Recreation Symposium, and the Academy of Leisure Sciences Teaching Institute.

Jamie Hoffman, EdD, CTRS, is an associate professor and the recreational therapy program coordinator in the department of recreation, parks, and tourism administration at California State University at Sacramento. She received her doctorate degree in educational leadership from California State University at Long Beach and her bachelor's and master's degrees in recreational therapy at the University of Tennessee. Dr. Hoffman has presented at state, national, and international conferences related to recreational therapy modalities such as surfing, adaptive kayaking, swimming, and aquatic therapy. Her current research relates to international cultural perspectives of disability and how those influence recreation participation. Dr. Hoffman has been published in journals such as *Therapeutic Recreation Journal*, *Cogent Psychology*, and *Disability and Health Journal*. For leisure, she enjoys gardening, canning, traveling, scuba diving, deep sea and spear fishing, surfing, biking, and skiing.

Erick Kong, EdD, CTRS, RTC, is an assistant professor in the department of hospitality, recreation, and tourism at California State University at East Bay. He received his doctorate degree in educational leadership and management from Alliant International University. Dr. Kong has presented at international, national, state, and regional conferences. He has conducted numerous studies examining knowledge competencies, interventions, and quality assurance. Dr. Kong serves as chair of professional development and a member of the Standards of Practice Committee for the American Therapeutic Recreation Association. He is also part of the Item Writing Committee for the National Council for Therapeutic Recreation Certification. In addition, he serves on the Recreation Therapy Section board for California Park and Recreation Society and is part of the Licensure Task Force for recreation therapy licensure in the state of California. His leisure interests include rock climbing, hiking, sailing, biking, orienteering, geocaching, and kayaking.

Michal Anne Lord, PhD, CPRP, is the executive director of the Texas Recreation and Park Society (TRAPS). She is certified by the National Recreation and Park Association (NRPA) as a parks and recreation professional and is state certified. She taught for 13 years at Southwest Texas State University in the department of health, physical education, recreation, and dance and was the division coordinator of recreation administration, including the therapeutic recreation emphasis. She also has worked in community recreation for nearly 25 years. She has served on the NRPA board of trustees and as president of the National Therapeutic Recreation Society and the Therapeutic Recreation Branch of TRAPS. She currently serves on the board of directors of Special Olympics Texas and has chaired the National Advisory Council of Very Special Arts. Michal Anne has received the fellow award from TRAPS and the TR Professional of the Year Award from the TRAPS'

Therapeutic Recreation Branch, the fellow award from the NRPA Southwest Regional Council, and the NTRS Distinguished Service Award.

Susan Myllykangas, PhD, CTRS, is a professor in the parks and recreation program in the School of Health Science and Wellness at Northwest Missouri State University. She received her doctorate degree in leisure and human performance, with concentrations in gerontology and family studies, from Indiana University. Dr. Myllykangas has worked in the field of parks and recreation, specializing in therapeutic recreation, in both community and clinical settings, since 1983. She has presented at state, national, and international conferences related to therapeutic recreation issues and trends, parks and recreation management, and aging issues. Dr. Myllykangas serves as the undergraduate curriculum coordinator for both the parks and recreation and gerontology programs at her university. She is an associate editor for the journal *Schole* and has been invited as a reviewer for other professional journals and publishing companies such as Sagamore Venture, Taylor and Francis, and Sage Publications. Many community agencies have found her leadership contributions extremely beneficial, and she serves on many of their boards. For leisure, she enjoys photography, travel, cooking, reading, theatre, and Netflix binges.

Shinichi Nagata, PhD, CTRS, is an assistant professor in School of Health Science and Wellness at Northwest Missouri State University, teaching courses on therapeutic recreation, adapted physical activity, and research methods. Shinichi studies the role of leisure in coping with depression and the effects of socially assistive robots for older adults with depression. Shinichi received his bachelor's degree in disability studies at the University of Tsukuba in Japan. While he was in the program, Shinichi had an international internship at an inclusive sports facility in Canada. After completing his undergraduate degree, Shinichi worked for the Tokyo Sports Association for the Disabled (TSAD). He earned his master's degree in recreation, with an emphasis on therapeutic recreation, at Northwest Missouri State University. Shinichi completed his PhD in leisure behavior in the School of Public Health at Indiana University at Bloomington. Shinichi is an active member of a therapeutic recreation study group in Japan, sharing the current information about North American therapeutic recreation. Shinichi also serves for the International Therapeutic Recreation Coalition,

which was initiated by the National Council for Therapeutic Recreation Certification (NCTRC). For leisure, he enjoys playing badminton, walking on trails, and traveling the world with his family.

Shane Pegg, PhD, is a senior lecturer in the tourism discipline of the School of Business at University of Queensland in Australia. He has been involved in a wide array of research and consultancy projects related to tourism and event management. He has a particular interest in the coproduction of accessible tourism and leisure service experiences. Dr. Pegg received his bachelor's degree in recreation management from Griffith University, his master's degree and graduate certificate in gerontology from the University of Utah, and his MBA and PhD from Central Queensland University. A passionate advocate for therapeutic recreation in Australia, he has published a variety of refereed journal articles and book chapters and is a past recipient of the American Therapeutic Recreation Association's Outstanding Professional Award. In 2017, Shane's contribution to the field was internationally recognized with his election as a fellow of the Academy of Leisure Sciences.

Cameo Rogers, MS, CTRS, CDP, CDCM, is certified by the National Council for Therapeutic Recreation as a therapeutic recreation specialist and is certified as a dementia practitioner, dementia care manager, Alzheimer's disease and dementia care trainer, and dementia support group facilitator through the National Council of Dementia Practitioners. She has a bachelor's degree in recreation (therapeutic and corporate wellness) from Northwest Missouri State University and is currently completing her graduate degree in social gerontology from the University of Nebraska at Omaha. In her role as corporate life enrichment manager for Immanuel in Omaha, Nebraska, she leads, coaches, and consults with senior living communities. She passionately advocates for person-centered engagement and enhanced team member training on communication techniques for working with individuals with dementia. She was honored with the NCCDP Certified Dementia Practitioner of the Year award in 2018.

Sydney L. Sklar, PhD, CTRS, is a professor at the University of St. Francis and currently serves as chair of the recreation and sport management department. He earned a master's degree in recreation administration from Aurora University (1997) and a PhD in health and human performance at the University of Florida (2005). His professional experience includes practitioner work at Shands Vista Mental Health Center and Fox Valley Special Recreation Association. Syd's research includes outdoor adaptive sports, therapeutic recreation education, youth development, and adventure learning. His publications include chapters in therapeutic recreation textbooks and articles in journals such as *Therapeutic Recreation Journal* and *World Leisure Journal*. He currently chairs the Council on Accreditation of Parks, Recreation, Tourism, and Related Professions. His career includes service to state and national associations, and he has presented at local, state, regional, national, and international conferences. For leisure, Syd enjoys going on outdoor adventures with his family and playing guitar in a rock and roll band.

Heewon Yang, PhD, CTRS, FDRT, is a professor in the department of recreation and leisure studies at California State University at Long Beach. Heewon teaches both general recreation and therapeutic recreation courses. He is interested in developing intervention programs for people with mood and anxiety disorders, and brain fitness programs for older adults and people with brain injuries.

Ramon B. Zabriskie, PhD, TRS, CTRS, FDRT, is a professor at Brigham Young University in the Marriot School of Management, where he is currently the therapeutic recreation program coordinator. His primary line of research focuses on family leisure and family wellness and how different types of family leisure involvement and satisfaction relate to aspects of family functioning, communication, and satisfaction with family life. His work has been published in a variety of books and academic journals, including *Journal of Leisure Research*, *Leisure Sciences*, *Therapeutic Recreation Journal*, *Family Relations*, *Fathering*, *Adoption Quarterly*, and *Marriage & Family Review*. Dr. Zabriskie has been honored with numerous teaching and scholarly awards. He has served on the American Therapeutic Recreation Association board of directors, the Utah Recreation Therapy Association board of directors, and the Utah recreational therapy licensure board, and he is currently serving on the board of directors for the Academy of Leisure Sciences. He has been a guest editor or associate editor for several journals and is a fellow of the National Academy of Recreational Therapists. If you ask him, however, he is simply a husband, father, grandfather, and fly fisherman.